Voice Problems
of Children

Second Edition

D. KENNETH WILSON, Ph.D.

Consultant, Speech Pathology and Audiology
St. Petersburg, Florida

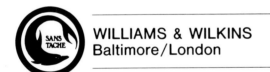

WILLIAMS & WILKINS
Baltimore/London

LYLLY JIM

Made in the United States of America

Reprinted 1979

Library of Congress Cataloging in Publication Data

Wilson, D. Kenneth
    Voice problems of children

    Bibliography: p.
    Includes index.
    1. Voice disorders in children. [DNLM: 1. Speech disorders—In infancy and
childhood. 2. Voice—In infancy and childhood. WV500 W747v]
RF511.C45W54 1978   618.9′28′55   78-2389
ISBN 0-683-09193-X

Composed and printed at the
Waverly Press, Inc.
Mt. Royal and Guilford Aves.
Baltimore, Md. 21202, U.S.A.,

Voice Problems of Children

Second Edition

To my wife
Frances Patton Wilson

Preface to the Second Edition.

The second edition of this book contains many new procedures based upon principles we have found successful in working with children and teenagers who have voice problems. We have modified and augmented our procedures as clinical reports and research findings have become known. We feel this edition represents the best of the modern concepts of vocal rehabilitation combined with and based upon principles and methods that have met the test of time. In addition we have reorganized and expanded almost all the material of the first edition. The first chapter contains a description of the classification of voice problems, their incidence, and the role of the speech pathologist in helping children with voice problems. The next three chapters contain descriptions of the causes of voice problems of children and teenagers: organic, organic changes due to vocal abuse and vocal misuse, functional causes, and contributing factors. Emphasis is placed on the role of vocal abuse and misuse in causing voice problems in many children. Examination procedures are presented in the next two chapters with emphasis on the tenet that therapy plans easily unfold as a detailed and accurate diagnosis proceeds. In the following five chapters we present procedures for various types of voice problems in children and teenagers. Basic to therapy planning is our 10 step voice therapy outline which we have refined from the first edition. Increased attention is placed on careful planning to eliminate vocal abuse and vocal misuse in children and teenagers with laryngeal pathology. Additional material is included in the chapter on improving oral-nasal resonance in children with velopharyngeal insufficiency. We have expanded the chapter on voice problems of hearing-impaired children as the role of the speech pathologist becomes more important in their education. The last chapter includes carryover of newly learned voice behavior, the role of the family, progress and dismissal criteria, and report writing.

My wife, Frances, has continued as my chief supporter. Her encouragement and professional assistance have made it possible for me to complete the second edition. My thanks go to colleagues and students who have given me suggestions for this edition.

D. KENNETH WILSON

Buffalo, New York
August 1978

Preface to the First Edition

This book focuses on the voice problems of children. While its primary purpose is for use in training speech clinicians, it is also designed to be used by practicing speech clinicians in various schools, colleges, university clinics, hospitals, and the community as well as by clinicians in private practice. The contents will also acquaint physicians and other allied health professionals with the voice problems of children.

Pertinent material from diverse periodicals and books in speech pathology, medicine, dentistry, psychology, and education is an integral part of the text. The causes of voice problems are reviewed and examination procedures are described. Remedial methods and techniques are presented for voice problems due to laryngeal dysfunction and defects of resonance, and also those associated with hearing loss. The examination and remedial procedures are structured to be used as a practical guide for the speech clinician with emphasis placed upon the team approach to the remediation of voice problems. It has been necessary, in many instances, to adapt adult procedures to children since much of the available information on voice problems concerns adults. These adaptations were made as judiciously as possible and are primarily based upon clinical experience with children with voice problems. The need for more research and controlled studies of voice problems of children is therefore apparent.

The anatomy and physiology of the speech and hearing mechanisms have not been included in this book since comprehensive presentations are readily available in texts of medicine, dentistry, speech pathology, audiology, and speech and hearing science.

The voice therapy art illustrations were designed for special use by the speech clinician and were drawn so that the clinician himself can easily make facsimiles for use in therapy.

Thanks are due to many persons. Special thanks go to my wife, who was my chief advisor, researcher, and consultant; without her this book would not have been written. Special thanks are also due to my cousin, Geraldine Balsam, Art Instructor, The Packer Institute, Brooklyn, New York, for her voice therapy illustrations, and to Melford D. Diedrick, Medical Illustrator, The State University of New York at Buffalo School of Medicine, for his illustrations of laryngeal pathology. Thanks are also given to Ruth L. Powell, Medical Librarian, Veterans Administration Center, Bay Pines, Florida, Noretha Harper, Medical Librarian, Bay Front Medical Center, St. Petersburg, Florida, and Anthony R. Tusa, Interlibrary Loan Librarian, State University of New York at Buffalo, formerly at the University of Florida, for their help in obtaining reference materials. Special recognition is given to my parents, Dales and Gladys Wilson, for their interest and encouragement during the writing of this book, and to my daughter, Shannon, who as an active teenager often wondered when "quiet hours for book writing" would end.

D. Kenneth Wilson

Buffalo, New York

Contents

ONE

Children's Voice Problems

Children with voice problems require a careful appraisal of the problem, a detailed diagnosis, and a comprehensive treatment plan. A voice disorder in a child presents a challenge to those concerned. Many times the causes are unknown or obscure, the diagnosis requires time, and the rehabilitation takes even more time, effort, and patience.

These procedures require the joint efforts of many specialists from several areas, including speech pathology, audiology, clinical psychology, social work, dentistry, laryngology, pediatrics, otology, allergy, radiology, plastic surgery, neurology, and psychiatry. A child with a voice problem may first be seen by any one of these specialists. For example, a child with severe hypernasality may be discovered in a survey by a school speech pathologist, or a child with a hoarse voice may be taken by his parents to the family physician or laryngologist. Children with voice problems are usually identified in the schools. Often they are first seen in community, hospital, or college and university speech clinics. Referral and consultation with other specialists are usually necessary.

Appraisal includes a detailed description of the voice problem in all its aspects: voice quality, loudness, pitch, and resonance. A complete case history is obtained. All the facts of the appraisal are gathered together and specific tests and examinations are selected to determine the cause or causes of the problem. The results of the tests and examinations are studied and the diagnosis made. The diagnosis is often difficult because the symptoms may be common to several different causes. For example, the causes of hypernasality include faulty learning, imitation, or a physical velopharyngeal insufficiency. It is necessary to differentiate these causes one from the other in order to find the basis of the hypernasality. A treatment plan is then devised and the prognosis, the prediction of the amount of anticipated progress, is formulated. The treatment plan may include voice therapy, medical, dental, and surgical procedures as well as psychological treatment.

The following example illustrates the basic approach to children with voice problems. When Chris was seen at 7 years of age he had been hoarse for over 3 months. A recent head and neck examination by a laryngologist revealed small newly formed bilateral vocal nodules at the junction of the anterior and middle thirds of the cords. Chris continually abused his voice by screaming and yelling. During the past 6 weeks the hoarseness had increased markedly to the point where Chris periodically lost his voice, and he often resorted to whispering to reduce the physical effort needed for talking. The teacher reported that Chris usually refused to recite in class and when he was required to speak he could not be heard because of excessive breathiness. When we saw him he was almost completely without voice, having a very weak laryngeal tone, and he was severely hoarse. Upon consultation with the laryngologist, voice therapy was recommended as the procedure of choice to see if reducing or eliminating vocal abuse and direct attention to improving the quality of the laryngeal tone would result in reduction or elimination of the vocal nodules. A vocal rehabilitation program was carefully structured and administered. An indirect laryngoscopy after 2 months of twice-weekly therapy revealed marked reduction in the size of the vocal nodules, and another indirect laryngoscopy 1 month later indicated that the vocal nodules were no longer present.

A NORMAL VOICE

In order to evaluate a person's voice it is necessary to know the essential elements of a

1

normal voice in contrast to the characteristics of a problem voice. A normal voice is essential for efficient speech communication. A good voice should have the following characteristics: (1) pleasing voice quality, (2) proper balance of oral and nasal resonance, (3) appropriate loudness, (4) a modal frequency level (habitual pitch level) suitable for age, size, and sex, and (5) appropriate voice inflections involving pitch and loudness. The rate of speaking should be such that it does not interfere with the five essential characteristics of a normal voice. This basic definition of a normal voice must be broad enough to allow a wide range of variation in any one or more of the essential positive characteristics.

Many interesting facts may be obtained from listening to a person's voice and speech (Laver, 1968): the size and physique, the sex and age, and the medical status. The latter includes laryngitis, pharyngitis, colds, and hormonal status. Also revealed are a person's general social behavior and background, including regionalisms and dialects and hypernasality associated with specific dialects.

A PROBLEM VOICE

To define a problem voice the five characteristics of a normal voice can be listed as negative characteristics, making the answer to the question "What is a problem voice?" fall quite easily into place.* A child has a voice problem if his voice shows one or more of the following characteristics: (1) disturbed voice quality caused by laryngeal dysfunction and characterized by hoarseness, harshness, or breathiness; (2) hypernasality and hyponasality caused by improper balance of oral and nasal resonance; (3) a voice too soft to be heard easily or so loud it is unpleasant; (4) a modal frequency level too high or too low for age, size, and sex; and (5) inappropriate inflections of pitch and loudness. Rate, if too fast or too slow, may interfere with adequate voice production. A problem voice may be distracting or unpleasant to the listener, and it may be severe enough to interfere with communication (ASHA, 1964; Peterson, 1946).

* Audiotapes of voice disorders collected by F. S. Brodnitz, M.D. (1974) are available from the Graduate Program in Communicative Disorders, University of Southern California, Los Angeles, CA 90007.

CAUSES OF VOICE PROBLEMS

The causes of voice problems in children can be divided into four categories: (1) organic, (2) organic changes resulting from vocal abuse and vocal misuse, (3) functional, and (4) factors contributing to the voice problem.

The causes of voice problems exist on a continuum with organic at one end and functional at the other (Moore, 1971a, pp. 535–536; Murphy, 1964, p. 2; Sokoloff and Rieber, 1966, pp. 321–322). Congenital or adventitiously acquired laryngeal, pharyngeal, oral, or nasal deviations lie at the organic end of the continuum. Voice problems due to emotional disturbances or poor voice standards in the environment lie at the functional end of the continuum. The continuum is a two way path because a pathology can result in a poorly functioning mechanism or a poorly functioning voice mechanism can result in organic changes or an organic condition (Moore, 1971a, pp. 535–536; Murphy, 1964, p. 2; Sokoloff and Rieber, 1966, pp. 321–322). It is difficult to make a clear distinction between organic and functional voice problems; while some form of organic disease or structural anomaly is the primary cause in an organic voice disorder, some functional elements may be present (Brodnitz, 1971a, p. 50). Sometimes the psychological reaction to an organic problem causes a voice problem " . . . far in excess of the organic impairment" (Brodnitz, 1971a, p. 50). Every vocal deficiency has a psychic effect, whether it is conscious or unconscious, acknowledged or secret (Tarneaud, 1958). A vocal dysfunction may continue long after the organic voice disorder becomes functional (Brodnitz, 1971a, p. 50; Sokoloff and Rieber, 1966, p. 322).

Structural or pathological changes occurring as the result of faulty use of the vocal mechanism lie in the middle of the continuum. Damsté (1973) termed these organic alterations of the vocal cords "secondary organic dysphonia." Brodnitz (1967a) stated patients who have developed an organic condition as a result of vocal abuse or misuse do not belong in the same category as patients with bona fide organic damage such as paralysis of a vocal cord. Our label for this cause is "organic changes resulting from vocal abuse and vocal misuse." Our fourth classification, factors contributing to the voice problem, includes such conditions as allergies and upper respiratory diseases which contribute to the other three causes and in some cases are the primary causes themselves. All four types of causes may be so intertwined that the specific cause or causes of a voice problem may be obscure.

CLASSIFICATION OF VOICE PROBLEMS

Voice problems are traditionally grouped into four categories: (1) voice quality problems, (2) resonance problems, (3) loudness problems, and (4) pitch problems. Deviations in rate in some instances are regarded as a fifth category of voice problems, although rate is often classified as a problem of articulation or rhythm.

Ineffective voice inflections are caused by a combination of poor loudness and pitch control. Van Riper and Irwin (1958, pp. 272–273) pointed out that while the four category classification is convenient, "Seldom does the abnormal variation exist along one dimension of voice alone." A hoarse voice may be low in pitch or a breathy voice may be weak in intensity. This interdependence of characteristics makes classification of voice problems difficult. Thus we will define specific characteristics individually and then see how they are intertwined. Our definitions are based on subjective descriptions and evaluations and on the results of acoustical analyses of defective voice.

Voice Quality Problems

The primary classification of voice deviations concerns quality of the voice. Quality disorders are disturbances in the laryngeal tone usually associated with sound generated at the level of the vocal cords. The disorders described as harshness, breathiness, hoarseness, and exclusive or excessive use of vocal fry are defects of tone generation.

Factors in Voice Quality

Before we specify the characteristics of voice quality problems it is necessary to consider the factors that make up voice quality. Voice quality is dependent upon four fundamental factors (Strother, 1942, pp. 209–210). (1) The basic structure of the vocal mechanism must be within the range of normal variation. Variations in structure of one or more parts of the vocal mechanism may ac-count for differences in voice quality. (2) The physiology of the muscles and surfaces of the larynx, pharynx, and nasal and oral cavities must also be within the range of normal variation. Punt (1974) stated the pharynx and larynx, especially the vocal cords, must have essential lubrication; the vocal cords must have an adequate amount of thin mucus supplied from glands in the laryngeal ventricles. Strother stated that if the muscles are tense or fatigued, if the surface tissues are abnormally dehydrated, if the surface tissues are covered with excess mucus, or if there is swelling or inflammation in any part of the vocal mechanism, the effects on voice quality will be deleterious. (3) Voice quality can be seriously affected by the individual's emotional status, either on a chronic or transient basis. (4) Voice quality is dependent upon good use of the vocal mechanism and may be affected by inadequate habits of voice production.

Marge (1964) studied speech and language of 143 children, 80 boys and 63 girls, nearly all of whom were in the sixth grade. Teachers and speech pathologists were requested to rate the children on 40 speech and language variables. As a result of a factor analysis voice quality was one of seven factors extracted. The variables which had high loadings for this one factor were quality of voice, articulation, appeal of voice, pronunciation, and flow of words. Thus basic to a pleasing voice is good articulation, correct pronunciation of words, and fluent speech.

Definitions of Voice Quality

Harshness. A harsh voice is unpleasant and rough (Hanley and Thurman, 1970, p. 209). Vocal fry may be present, considerable tension is localized in and about the larynx, and abrupt glottal attacks may be used frequently (Van Riper, 1972, p. 157). In an abrupt glottal attack the vocal cords come together tightly causing air to be impounded below the glottis. More pressure than normal must be applied to separate the cords resulting in the air being suddenly released with the voice sounding constricted and harsh (Fomon, Bell, Lubart, Schattner, and Syracuse, 1966). The harsh voice may be lower in pitch than is normal and also weak in intensity since many people find it difficult to obtain adequate loudness at low pitch levels

(Fairbanks, 1960, pp. 175–176). Bowler (1964) found a mean fundamental frequency of 95.4 Hz for harsh voices compared to 127.1 Hz for normal adult male voices.

Breathiness. A breathy voice is a combination of vocal cord sounds and the whisper-like noise components of turbulent air (Moore, 1971a, p. 537). The vocal cords do not fully approximate. This allows unvibrated air to escape between the cords adding a noise element to the voice (Fomon et al. 1966). The vocal cords vibrate but because closure is not firm there is continuous air flow causing a person to have limited vocal intensity and low pitch (Fairbanks, 1960, p. 179). A breathy voice may be mild or severe; in its mild form only a small amount of aspirate noise element is added, but in its most severe form all phonation is lost and there is only a whispered voice.

Werner-Kukuk and von Leden (1970) analyzed high speed motion pictures of the breathy glottal attack. They observed that the posterior portion of the vocal cords does not approximate, and even after stabilization of the vibratory pattern the arytenoid cartilages remain widely separated in the form of a permanent open triangle with the triangle base at the posterior commissure. The anterior section of the vocal cords opens briefly, while the middle portion has a fairly normal outline. At the beginning of a breathy initiation there is irregularity in the vibratory pattern, but soon all areas of the vocal cords show gentle abduction and adduction as the vibrations stabilize. In a breathy production Isshiki and von Leden (1964) found more than 150 cc of air are expelled before sound production begins.

Hoarseness. Hoarseness is quite common and occurs at some time in almost every person. It is at times overlooked and neglected by speech pathologists since it frequently accompanies and subsides with a common cold; thus there is a tendency to regard hoarseness as temporary and to feel the trouble will "clear up by tomorrow" (Damitz and Dill, 1940). However, hoarseness is the unique symptom of laryngeal involvement and may be a significant complaint in any medical and surgical condition (von Leden, 1958). Hoarseness lasting longer than 10 days to 3 weeks should never be ignored (Barr, 1938; DeWeese and Saunders, 1973, p. 106; Negus, 1939; von Leden, 1958).

Its cause should be determined and removed when possible and voice therapy given when indicated. The term hoarseness is frequently used for any type of deviation of the laryngeal tone. However, the speech pathologist should be able to distinguish a hoarse voice from a harsh or breathy voice.

Hoarseness in its simplest definition is a combination of harshness and breathiness with the harsh element predominating in some hoarse voices and the breathy element in others (Fairbanks, 1960, pp. 182–183). Jackson (1959, p. 576) described hoarseness as " ... a quality of voice that is rough, grating, harsh, more or less discordant, and lower in pitch than normal for the individual." The hoarse voice has been the topic of laboratory studies. Moore and Thompson (1965) analyzed ultra high speed motion pictures of the vocal cords and phonelegrams of hoarse vocal sounds produced by two subjects. They concluded hoarseness is characterized by random fundamental frequency variability. Isshiki, Yanagihara, and Morimoto (1966) found aperiodicity of the fundamental frequency present in hoarse voices, with noise components and frequency variations in a voice closely related to each other. An increase of noise components in a voice will intensify the frequency variation. Yanagihara (1967a, 1967b) studied five vowels produced by 10 adults who had varying degrees of hoarseness—slight, moderate, and severe. Through spectrographic analysis he classified hoarseness according to the amount of noise present. He found that the range and energy of noise components vary with the perceived degree of hoarseness and are more evident in the vowels /ɑ/, /ɛ/, and /i/ than in the vowels /u/ and /ɔ/. He classified voices into four main types based on the presence of noise components in the different formants of these vowels. The types ranged from a small amount of added noise to almost complete replacement of the laryngeal tone by noise. Shipp and Huntington (1965) rated and analyzed acute laryngitis in 15 adults with a mean age of 25.9 years, comparing the laryngitic stage to their normal voices after laryngitis had subsided. The fundamental pitch was the same under both conditions. The ratings indicated that breathiness was related to hoarseness but harshness was not. They cautioned these findings may apply only to hoarseness accompanying acute laryngitis. Thus research has shown that hoarseness is related to breathiness, that there is random fundamental frequency variation and aperiodicity of fundamental frequency in the hoarse voice, and that noise components added to the laryngeal tone increase according to the amount of perceived hoarseness.

Vocal Fry. According to Hollien, Moore, Wendahl, and Michel (1966), "Vocal fry results from a train of discrete laryngeal excitations, or pulses, of low frequency. . ." Vocal fry may be produced consciously by phonating quietly at the lowest possible pitch so the sound bubbles out of the larynx in discrete bursts (Zemlin, 1968, p. 197). Moore and von Leden (1958) proposed the name dicrotic dysphonia for the voice quality referred to as vocal fry; they established it as a physiological not a pathological entity. Vocal fry in itself when present in a minor degree in the normal voice does not constitute a voice deviation; only when vocal fry is used exclusively (Hollien et al. 1966) or excessively is it considered a voice deviation. We have seen children who have an excessive amount of the popping, cracking sound of vocal fry which is usually associated with quality deviations. Vocal fry typically has a fundamental frequency below the average range of frequencies for a normally pitched voice. It has been measured as ranging from 92 Hz (Murry, 1971) to as low as 2 Hz (Hollien and Michel, 1968). Timcke, von Leden, and Moore (1959) found simulated vocal fry had a frequency of 75 Hz compared to the frequency of 150 Hz before the change to a vocal fry.

A low rate of air flow (McGlone, 1967; McGlone and Shipp, 1971; Murry, 1971) and high subglottic air pressure (Murry, 1971) are associated with the production of vocal fry. But McGlone and Shipp (1971) found little difference for subglottic air pressure in vocal fry and modal registers. The speech pathologist should listen carefully to deviant laryngeal tones in order to differentiate vocal fry from various types of laryngeal dysfunction and to determine if a child is using vocal fry exclusively or excessively.

Resonance Problems

Hypernasality

Some nasal resonance is present in all speech. The /m/, /n/, and /ŋ/ are normally nasalized. When vowels are nasalized this type of resonance becomes objectionable and is then called hypernasality. Hypernasality may also be present on consonants, especially consonants requiring a buildup of breath pressure within the oral cavity, such as /s/, /k/, /ʃ/, /z/, and /g/. Sometimes these pressure consonants are nasally emitted with a characteristic snort. Assimilation hypernasality may be present when the vowels preceding or following /m/, /n/, and /ŋ/ are excessively nasalized because of their close proximity to the normally nasalized sounds. Fletcher (1972) stated hypernasality has been an elusive problem in rehabilitation because it may range all the way from a simple regional twang to a problem of such severity that the hypernasal resonance replaces all other features of speech. Further, Fletcher stated, hypernasality causes vowels to be blurred, some consonants to lose their crispness, and some consonants to be replaced by sounds which do not depend on a buildup of pressure in the mouth. These deleterious habits may result in unusual patterns of speaking resulting in serious disturbances in personality and behavior of the person.

A resonance problem may be the result of velopharyngeal dysfunction with or without an overt cleft palate. Hypernasality is not the best descriptive term for cleft palate type speech because often there is a combination of both hypernasality and hyponasality accompanied by an unusual cul-de-sac type of resonance. The speech of persons with imperfect velopharyngeal closure is characterized by excess nasal emission of sounds, hypernasality, and an inadequate oral breath stream with both voice quality and articulation often seriously defective (Ward and Wepman, 1964).

Hyponasality

Hyponasality is a lack of nasal resonance on the /m/, /n/, and /ŋ/ phonemes. The person sounds as if he has a cold, and in the extreme form of hyponasality /b/ is substituted for /m/, /d/ for /n/, and /g/ for /ŋ/, resulting in word confusions such as *be* for *me, dew* for *new,* and *rag* for *rang.* Sometimes hyponasality (Fairbanks, 1960, p. 170) and hypernasality are considered articulation defects since they are related to poor use of the articulators. However, hypernasality and hyponasality are usually classified as voice problems.

Loudness Problems

A child may habitually talk so loudly that all the neighbors know his business and his family's also! He can easily be heard above the din of the school lunchroom, the teacher constantly tells him to talk quietly, and he is the loudest singer in the class. In contrast, there is the quiet talker who can never be heard. Everyone asks her to talk louder and to repeat until she gives up talking except when necessary. When she reads aloud in class no one can hear her so the teacher may think she has a reading problem. Often she is regarded as an extremely shy child. Her only problem may be that she does not talk loud enough.

Results of various studies on loudness level vary according to the distance between the speaker and the sound measuring instrument. When measured with a sound level meter at about 40 in from the speaker's mouth without interfering background noise, loud talking is about 86 dB and soft talking about 46 dB (Fletcher, 1953, pp. 76–77). Draper, Ladefoged, and Whitteridge (1960) agreed with this 40 dB difference between quiet talking and what they called "parade ground shouting." Black (1961) found the range from soft to loud talking to be about 30 dB when measured 18 in from the speaker's mouth, that is, from about 70 dB for soft speech to 100 dB for loud speech. He found a normal or natural level of loudness to be about 80 dB measured 18 in from the speaker.

The most comfortable listening level may be used as a guide for proper loudness. Hochberg (1975) reported the most comfortable listening level for speech loudness at the level of the ear was 64.35 dB sound pressure level (SPL), and the comfortable level for speech intelligibility was 69.31 dB SPL.

Nichols, Dembowski, and Dewey (1971) compared 30 normally loud women (mean age, 20 years 1 month) with 30 women rated as "soft-spoken" (mean age, 19 years 11 months). The mean comfortable loudness level for the normally loud women measured 12 in from the mouth was 59.5 dBB and 50.5 dBB for the soft-spoken group.

Pitch Problems

A child has a deviation in pitch if his voice shows one or more of the following charac-teristics: (1) a modal frequency level that is either too high or too low, (2) a very narrow pitch range, (3) excessive pitch breaks, or (4) too-high or too-low pitch in specific situations. We are especially interested in a child's modal frequency level and whether it is appropriate for him. A too-low pitch in an 8-year-old girl making her sound like an adolescent boy is as incongruous as a too-high pitch in a 10-year-old boy which makes him sound like a kindergarten girl. We should also consider what the child, himself, thinks about his pitch level. One boy of 9 had what we considered a very high-pitched voice. However, the teacher and parents reported they thought his pitch level was all right but that he did not talk very much. Other children did not react to his high-pitched voice, and it did not seem to be a problem until we asked the boy himself what he thought about his voice. He replied, "I sound like a girl so I don't talk any more than I have to." Sadly he added, "You're a speech teacher, can't you make me talk more like a boy?"

The high voice pitch level of childhood continuing in a boy after the usual age of voice change should be considered a serious voice deviation. During the period of voice change a boy's voice drops approximately an octave and a girl's voice 3 or 4 semitones. A child of 12 who uses higher pitch levels in his conversational speech does not stand out as being particularly different. However, when the child is about 14 or 15, whether a boy or girl, the voice change should be well under way. The speech pathologist in a junior or senior high school should be especially cognizant of the period of voice change. If changes do not occur in a boy or do occur in a girl to lower her modal frequency level drastically, remedial measures should be considered. We recall one husky 17-year-old high school football player with a high-pitched voice. Examinations by the family physician, laryngologist, and psychologist revealed no organic or psychological basis for his high pitch. We were able to lower his pitch level approximately an octave during the initial therapy sessions and in about a month's time he was using the lower pitch level habitually in all situations.

INCIDENCE OF VOICE PROBLEMS IN CHILDREN

Many speech pathologists feel voice disorders in children are on the increase. Pressures of modern living and higher standards for school achievement are responsible for increased general tensions which result in vocal hyperactivity and a poor voice. Even so, some speech pathologists currently report that they have very few children with voice problems in their case loads. When asked to take a second look at children in their schools they find many more with voice problems. One school speech pathologist who is very aware of vocal disturbances reported for the past several years that the incidence of all types of voice problems in his schools has averaged between 5% and 6% of the school population with about half of them needing voice therapy on a regular basis and the remainder requiring attention from other specialists.

Results of Voice Surveys

Results of most voice surveys of children show approximately 6% to 9% with voice problems, which means between 60 and 90 children per 1000. However, one study by Silverman and Zimmer (1975), in a survey of 162 children in a private school in Wisconsin, kindergarten through eighth grade, found 38 (23.4%) children chronically hoarse with about half of them estimated to have vocal nodules. This was a school where high achievement was stressed and the authors felt this atmosphere may have contributed to the large number of children chronically hoarse. Twenty-six (68.4%) of the children with hoarse voices were in the primary grades, with the highest incidence of 46.0% in the third grade. For the fourth through eighth grades the incidence declined with no hoarseness observed among children in the eighth grade. In contrast to this study, Gillespie and Cooper (1973) found 1.2% of 5054 students in Alabama in grades 7 through 12 had voice problems.

Other surveys show approximately the number of children we expect to find with voice problems. Pont (1965) in California surveyed 639 children and found 9.1% of the kindergarten through eighth grade children with hoarse voices (8.8% in second grade and 9.4% in the other grades). Baynes (1966) in Michigan found 7.1% of 1012 first, third, and sixth grade children had chronically hoarse voices. James and Cooper (1966) in Ohio found 6.2% of 718 third grade children had voice problems with about half of them having combined articulation and voice problems.

Senturia and Wilson (1968) reported 6% of 32,500 school children ages 5 to 18 years in the St. Louis, Missouri, area had voice deviations. From these figures they estimated voice deviations occur in 3 million of the 50 million children in the United States in the age range 5 to 18 years. Assuming a more conservative estimate of 3% with communicatively handicapping voice deviations, Senturia and Wilson arrived at the figure of 1½ million children in the United States with voice problems. In a later article Wilson (1972) indicated about half (1.0% to 1.5%) of the total school population need voice therapy. He also stated the exact number of children surveyed was 32,542, with 1962 having some form of voice deviation. During the two years following the survey approximately 1000 of the children were seen for specific diagnostic procedures. Twenty-four per cent of the children when seen did not have voice problems, revealing the apparently transient nature of some voice disorders, although in most of them it was determined from interviewing the parents that the children had experienced some previous difficulty with voice. Seventy-six per cent had deviations in voice ranging in severity from barely perceivable to problems which severely handicapped communication.

Yairi, Currin, Bulian, and Yairi (1974) in Texas surveyed 1549 school age children first through sixth grade twice within a three month time span. The results showed a general incidence of hoarseness of approximately 13% but between 2.4% and 3.4% were judged as having a clinically significant problem. Pannbacker (1975) in Texas reported 8.6% of 93 first grade children had chronically hoarse voices. Manohar and Jayaram (1973) surveyed 1454 school children in Mysore City, India, finding 9% of the children aged 5 through 14 had voice problems, including quality, pitch, and intensity deviations. Schlanger and Gottsleben (1957) surveyed 516 residents of a school for the retarded. The mean chronological age was 28.9 years and the mean mental age was 7.8 years. Forty-seven per cent had voice problems with the outstanding problems being hoarse-huskiness, hypernasality, pitch, and rate.

It is interesting to compare the incidence of voice problems in children with the incidence of voice problems in adults. Laguaite (1972) screened 428 adults going through a series of tests in a multiphasic health screening unit. The patients ranged in age from 18 to 82 years with the average age of males 43.1 and females 45.7 years. Of those referred for laryngeal evaluation, 7.2% were males and 5% females, making an average of 6.5% of the population with abnormal voices.

Incidence in Case Loads of School Speech Pathologists

Voice problems should constitute about 5% of a school speech pathologist's case load. Surveys show the proportion of voice problems in the school speech pathologist's case load vary greatly from 1.6% to 15%. For example, Frick (1960) reported 50 school speech pathologists in Pennsylvania estimated their case loads should have about 5% voice problems, while in reality the percentage was 2.01%.

Voice problems represented 2.3% of the case load of over 1400 public school speech pathologists surveyed in a nationwide sampling (Bingham, Van Hattum, Faulk, and Taussig, 1961). Black (1964, p. 7) reported in Illinois public schools voice cases represented 4% of the speech pathologists' case load. Des Roches (1976) found in Montgomery County, Maryland, public schools for the school years 1968–1974 voice problems represented 1.6% to 2.3% of the case load; they also reported that from 3.8% to 5.7% of the case load were children with hearing losses. Neal (1976) reported on a 1973 survey of 64 secondary school speech pathologists in the United States. Their case load distribution included 3.0% hard of hearing, 2.6% voice problems, and 1.2% cleft palate.

The number of children with voice problems being seen by speech pathologists is larger in some reports. Shearer (1972) reported that before a special team diagnostic program was initiated in Illinois, speech pathologists' voice case loads consisted of approximately 2% to 5% of their total load, but by the end of the first year of special voice team clinics, active voice cases represented 5% to 15% of the public school speech pathologists' case loads. Further, in 1974 we surveyed 51 school speech pathologists attending our short courses in Ohio. The average case load included 6.7% children with voice problems. The three most numerous problems among these children were 23% vocal nodules, 18% hoarseness with no pathology, and 12% resonance problems (chiefly hypernasality).

THE ROLE OF THE SPEECH PATHOLOGIST

The speech pathologist must see that all efforts are made to insure proper attention for all children with voice problems. The basic goals for the speech pathologist in dealing with children with voice problems are as follows: (1) to aid in the prevention of voice problems, (2) to act as a member of a team of specialists contributing to appraisal and diagnosis, and (3) to offer a voice therapy program to modify or eliminate the voice problem.

Prevention of voice disorders in children is an important function of the speech pathologist. We have seen that about 3% of the school age population 5 to 18 years have communicatively handicapping voice problems (Senturia and Wilson, 1968). About one-half of these need voice therapy (Wilson, 1972). The other half do not need voice therapy because they have conditions requiring only medical, surgical, psychological, or psychiatric attention. However, those not needing voice therapy may involve the speech pathologist in some way. For example, in many instances it is the speech pathologist's responsibility to see that children with voice problems are called to the attention of the proper specialists.

The speech pathologist should be aware of even minor voice problems. Some voice problems signal the possibility of actual physical problems or pathology. For example, a child with mild hypernasality may have a mild velopharyngeal insufficiency, in which case an adenoidectomy might create a severe velopharyngeal insufficiency with a severe voice problem. A child who has chronic mild hoarseness or a child with periodic hoarseness after periods of vocal misuse or vocal abuse may not be considered to have a problem. However, if he continues to use his voice in an improper fashion the hoarseness may become worse and result in pathological changes in the vocal cords. Any unexplained prolonged hoarseness indicates a need for immediate medical attention.

Children needing voice therapy should have first priority in the therapy schedule. Zemmol (1977) presented a three priority system for scheduling children in schools. She regarded children with severely handicapping communicative disorders as first priority cases and included among them voice disorders, especially at the initial stages of vocal rehabilitation, speech problems related to moderate-to-severe loss of hearing, and hypernasality. In the second priority classification Zemmol placed moderate voice deviations and speech problems related to mild-to-moderate loss of hearing. Key questions the speech pathologist in the public school should ask, according to Bown (1971), in selecting a case load are: "(1) Does the child have an emotional reaction to his communication effort? (2) Does the child's speech and language interfere with communication? (3) Does the child's communication problem interfere with classroom achievement?" A "Yes" answer to all three questions makes therapy imperative.

The school speech pathologist should seek the cooperation of the classroom teacher in prevention of voice disorders. Many voice disorders of adults begin in childhood, especially in those children who go through much vocal strain including shouting, screaming, and singing in an unnatural range (Ellis, 1959). Kallen (1959) felt a planned school voice hygiene program should be instituted to protect the voice from misuse and strain from the day a child enters kindergarten until he is well past puberty. Classroom teachers should be urged to create an atmosphere in the classroom conducive to the development of a good voice (Pronovost and Kingman, 1959, p. 112). Froeschels (1940) stressed the importance of good vocal hygiene for children during reading instruction to prevent hyperfunction of the vocal apparatus.

Both the speech pathologist and classroom teacher should give special attention to a child who is hoarseness-prone. According to Boland (1953) this is a person who gets hoarse easily after sports activities, parties, colds, difficult work, or emotional crises. The vocal behavior in a hoarseness-prone person is characterized by excessive tension in the neck muscles with an inadequate mouth opening for speech; this gives the impression of talking in the back of the throat or down in the chest. A hoarseness-prone person may complain frequently of vocal fatigue and periodic hoarseness. The speech pathologist should identify hoarseness-prone children so that early consultation, appraisal, diagnosis, and treatment can be considered. White (1946) noted voice problems in preadolescents and young adolescents are often overlooked since they are simply regarded as part of the maturation process. He felt these voice problems should be investigated and when possible

eliminated. This avoids the development of an inadequate self image which together with the voice problem could later be handicapping both economically and socially. For example, an attractive high school girl who applies for a position as receptionist may be denied the position because of excessive hypernasality or a teenage boy may be ridiculed because of his high-pitched voice (Moore, 1967).

Martin (1975) advocated that a close relationship should exist between teachers and the school speech pathologist to avoid making teachers feel unsure about what constitutes a communication problem and when to seek help. The school speech pathologist should make it clear to the teacher that over-referral is better than under-referral.

Classroom teachers have difficulty identifying voice problems as such with accuracy. When a voice problem is combined with an articulation problem the accuracy of identification by teachers increases. Diehl and Stinnett (1959) compared teacher referrals and the results of a school speech testing program of second grade children. Teachers were able to identify voice disorders with only 36.9% accuracy, while children with both articulation and voice disorders were identified with 70% accuracy. James and Cooper (1966) found about 10% teacher referral accuracy with children who had voice disorders only. But when the voice disorder was combined with an articulation problem teacher accuracy was about 52%. Wertz and Mead (1975) found kindergarten, first, second, and third grade teachers rated an audio sample of a voice disorder as the least severe problem compared to stuttering, articulation, and cleft palate, making voice the most likely disorder to go undetected in the classroom. In contrast to this, Clauson and Kopatic (1975) found teachers identified the audiotape of a child with a voice problem 92% of the time when contrasted to other types of disorders. Teachers should be provided with information about normal and abnormal voice (Martin, 1974). How to improve teacher referral through in-service programs was reported by Deal, McClain, and Sudderth (1976). Teachers were given examples of various voice disorders by listening to the 1972 F. B. Wilson voice tapes.† Following this the teachers were

---

† Latest edition (1977) available from Teaching Resources, 50 Pond Park Road, Hingham, MA 02043.

instructed to listen to children in their class-rooms and refer those suspected of having a voice problem. The following check list of voice descriptions was given to the teachers. Children who had these problems were can-didates for referral to the school speech pa-thologist: (1) hoarse for 2 weeks or more, (2) laryngitis for 2 weeks or more, (3) modal frequency level too high or too low, (4) speak-ing through the nose, (5) talking too loud or too soft, (6) breathy voice, (7) strained voice, (8) numerous pitch breaks, and (9) monoto-nous voice. Seventy-seven children were re-ferred for laryngeal examinations as a result of this program. Thirty-four children had vocal nodules, seven had edematous cords, seven had allergies, four could not be exam-ined, and 25 had normal examination results. Sixteen boys had bilateral nodules and three had a unilateral nodule, while all 12 girls had bilateral nodules. The mean ages in the nod-ule group were 8 years 6 months for the boys and 8 years 7 months for the girls.

The speech pathologist and the classroom teacher may need to cooperate in advising the family about voice problems. Parents gen-erally are not concerned about voice devia-tions as long as they can understand their child's speech. They are primarily concerned about language development and clarity of articulation and pay little attention to the voice of their child unless it is quite defective. Either they dismiss the voice deviation as something the child will outgrow or they may not realize it is different. They may say, "His brother went through the same thing," or "Listen to the other children in the neighbor-hood." If they can understand the child's speech generally parents are not usually con-cerned about poor voice quality, deviations in pitch, or any other voice deviations.

Weiss (1974) stressed the importance of the role of the speech pathologist in handling children who are wearing a speech aid or dental prosthesis. The speech pathologist should be knowledgeable regarding the as-pects of wearing a prosthesis and the method of caring for it. Also the speech pathologist should have a working knowledge of the criteria used for selecting a speech aid, the methods of assessing the fit of a speech aid, and the reasons for referral for reassessment and adjustment. The speech pathologist should also be knowledgeable in the area of personal hearing aids, their operation and care.

Speech pathologists are essential members of the team in contributing to the appraisal and diagnosis of voice problems. They should be prepared to conduct voice screening sur-veys in schools or other settings. They must be ready to administer appropriate tests for the appraisal of voice problems and be able to contribute their findings to the diagnosis. They should be prepared to administer a thorough voice therapy regimen. They must have an understanding of (1) anatomy and physiology, specifically of the speech and hearing mechanisms, (2) the principles and basic methodology of learning, and (3) the fundamental and specific methodology for the rehabilitation of voice problems.

As a speech pathologist conducts voice therapy his role can be exemplified by an-swering Andrews' (1973) five questions. The first question is "What am I teaching the child?" Specific goals of therapy should be formulated and techniques and procedures selected that will result in observable changes in vocal behavior. This question also implies that where indicated the speech pathologist should be manipulating the environment so that as new behavior is learned it can be transferred to a child's everyday living. The second question, "Will I know whether or not my instruction has been successful?" implies the necessity for the speech pathologist to chart progress session by session so that he knows immediately the effectiveness of a spe-cific technique, and knows whether it should be included or discarded before the next ses-sion begins. The third question may be stated as, "Is this step in therapy neces-sary?" The speech pathologist should imme-diately determine whether a selected step is really necessary for the vocal rehabilitation program and proceed accordingly. Question four is, "What instructional procedures am I using to reach the goal?" Instructional pro-cedures must be carefully determined with methods and materials carefully planned to make sure each technique has a specific pur-pose or contribution to the ongoing therapy. Question five is, "Am I using reinforcement effectively?" A reinforcer should be truly re-warding and desirable to a child. Reinforcers may be tangible items such as tokens or they may be in the form of verbal praise as a reward. A reinforcer must be valued by the child and delivered immediately upon the production of the desired response. Reinfor-cers should be rewards for the desired behavior, not bribes toward the production of a desired behavior. Satisfactory answers to these five questions will assure the speech pathologist that the correct trail is being followed.

SUMMARY

About 1.5% of school age children 5 to 18 years of age need comprehensive voice rehabilitation programs. The coordinated efforts of the speech pathologist, parents, teachers, medical, dental, and health related professional personnel are necessary in these programs. Voice problems are identified, evaluated, and diagnosed, and then plans of therapy are formulated. A child's voice problem may be characterized by hoarseness, harshness, or vocal fry; improper balance of oral and nasal resonance; loudness differences; an inappropriate voice pitch level; or poor use of vocal inflections. Causes of these problems include organic, organic changes caused by vocal abuse and misuse, functional, and contributing factors. The role of the speech pathologist in helping children with voice problems includes conducting preventive programs for good voice use, acting as a member of a voice diagnostic team, and conducting voice therapy programs for children. The goal of all voice therapy is to help children learn to use their voices effectively so they speak with a pleasing voice quality, with properly balanced resonance, and with appropriate voice pitch level, loudness, and inflection.

TWO

Organic Causes
of Voice Problems

Some children have voice problems present on an organic basis. There are five primary sites of organic causes of voice disorders: the larynx, the velopharyngeal area, the oral cavity, the nose, and the ear. Voice problems due to laryngeal involvements include harshness, breathiness, and hoarseness, or inappropriate pitch; defects in the velopharyngeal area cause the voice to sound hypernasal, sometimes with a typical cleft palate type quality; defects of the palate and sometimes the tongue also cause hypernasality; and defects involving the nose usually result in hyponasal (denasal) voice quality. Hearing loss may affect loudness, pitch, resonance, laryngeal tone, and rate.

THE LARYNX

Organic causes of voice problems arising in the larynx and the immediate surrounding areas are as follows: (1) structural anomalies, (2) paralysis of any one or several of the nerves supplying the larynx, (3) growths in or around the larynx, and (4) trauma to the larynx.

Structural Anomalies

Structural anomalies may be present on a congenital or developmental basis. In some cases these anomalies can be treated by surgical operations. In selected cases voice therapy is indicated. Close attention should be paid to children with these types of problems as their voices develop to determine if voice therapy is needed. Let us look at specific structural anomalies.

Congenital laryngeal webs may be supraglottic, glottic, or subglottic; they generally involve the anterior portion of the glottis (Laupus and Pastore, 1967, p. 205) and consist of thin connective tissue. The ventricular bands also may be involved (Baker, 1954). Laryngeal webs may range from a small anterior commissure webbing to almost complete closure of the glottis (Holinger and Brown, 1967) (Figs. 1 and 2). A complete web is incompatible with life and requires immediate surgical attention (DeWeese and Saunders, 1973, p. 119). The symptoms of congenital laryngeal webs in the infant consist of hoarse, weak, or absent cry, and sometimes difficulty in breathing (Holinger, Johnston, and Schiller, 1954). The treatment of laryngeal web is in the hands of the physician and consists of excision or dilatation of the web (Laupus and Pastore, 1967, pp. 205–206). Kirchner (1974; 1975) reported on the effective use of microcauterization in treating laryngeal web. Using the operating microscope, tissue is destroyed by heat with cauterization temperatures ranging from 800 C to 1120 C. Hardingham and Walsh-Waring (1975) described the treatment of congenital laryngeal web where the web is divided under magnified vision, using a laryngoscope in coordination with an operating microscope. A Silastic keel is secured between the vocal cords at the anterior commissure by means of a loop of nylon passing through the thyrohyoid and cricothyroid muscles.

In some instances, after the web has been removed there may be vocal disturbances present sometimes manifested in a high-pitched and weak voice requiring voice therapy. The condition is not always diagnosed when the patient is an infant (Holinger et al. 1954). A small anterior web may not interfere with breathing and its only influence may occur at the age of expected voice change. In this instance the high pitch of childhood continues because of the shortened vibrating portions of the vocal cords (Moore, 1971b, p. 97). Teenage boys with high-pitched voices need a careful laryngeal examination to rule out the possibility of a web.

Underdevelopment of one vocal cord may be present on a congenital or developmental basis resulting in an aspirate voice (West and

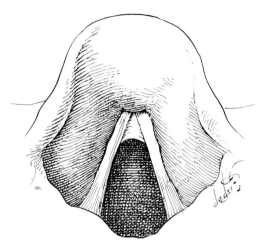

FIG. 1. Congenital web (small anterior). Illustration by Melford D. Diedrick.

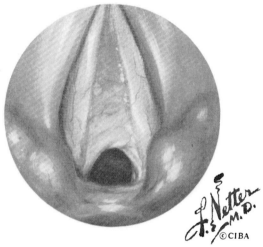

FIG. 2. Congenital web (incomplete) viewed through laryngoscope. Copyright *Clinical Symposia* by Frank H. Netter, M.D., published by CIBA Pharmaceutical Company.

Ansberry, 1968, pp. 220–221). The shape of the arytenoid and its attachment to the vocal cords may not be symmetrical (West and Ansberry, 1968, p. 221). In this condition also the child is likely to have a breathy voice quality because of inadequate approximation of the vocal cords (West and Ansberry, 1968, p. 221).

Some congenital laryngeal conditions are of interest to the speech pathologist if voice problems develop as the child grows. These include congenital supraglottic and subglottic

stenosis (Holinger and Brown, 1967). Congenital subglottic stenosis may be severe enough to require surgical or medical treatment or it may be mild enough to disappear as the child matures (Holinger and Brown, 1967). Huff and Magielski (1976) stated treatment of stenosis of the larynx in children should be conservative; dilatation and watchful waiting until the larynx has matured is recommended. In some instances surgical treatment may be necessary. Supraglottic stenosis may be repaired by excision of the stenotic area, inserting a stent and doing necessary skin grafting. In cases of cricoid stenosis a vertical incision is made in the thyroid, cricoid, and adjacent tracheal rings to provide for enlargement of the cricoid lumen. Inserting a stent and using skin grafts are necessary (Huff and Magielski, 1976).

Another congenital condition of interest to the speech pathologist is laryngomalacia (congenital laryngeal stridor). It is the most common of all congenital anomalies of the larynx (Holinger, Holinger, and Holinger, 1976). It is caused by a failure of the cartilages of the larynx, especially the epiglottis, to develop normally so that during inspiration, the epiglottis and the aryepiglottic folds collapse into the airway (Saunders, 1964) (Fig. 3). This results in a loud staccato repetitive crowing noise when the child inhales; the condition ordinarily disappears between the 12th and 18th month (Holinger and Brown, 1967).

Hyperkinetic dysphonia may be the result of a congenital structural anomaly and was described by Luchsinger (1965, pp. 303–306) as follows: "It is characterized by the excessive contraction of all muscles participating in phonation" including the laryngeal muscles, muscles of the respiratory apparatus, and the cervical suspension muscles of the larynx. The voice is harsh, strained, and sometimes muffled and sometimes overly loud. The child talks in this manner to overcome asymmetry or weakness of the laryngeal structure. The larynx shows the results of irritation in the form of hyperemia, swelling, and epithelial thickening of the vocal cord margins. Voice therapy is usually indicated.

Other congenital anomalies include absence of the epiglottis, deformities of the cricoid cartilage, and a laryngoesophageal cleft (Holinger and Brown, 1967). A few cases of congenital vascular anomalies of the larynx have been reported (Holinger and Brown, 1967).

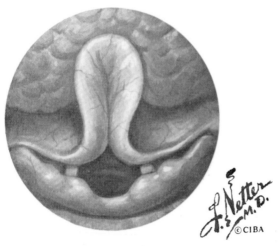

FIG. 3. Laryngomalacia (congenital laryngeal stridor). Copyright *Clinical Symposia* by Frank H. Netter, M.D., published by CIBA Pharmaceutical Company.

Vocal Cord Paralysis

Vocal cord paralysis, according to Holinger et al. (1976), is the second most common laryngeal anomaly, representing approximately 10% of all congenital anomalies of the larynx. The paralysis may be congenital or may appear as a result of acquired conditions such as trauma, growths, or inflammatory illness. It may affect one or both vocal cords (Holinger and Brown, 1967). Gacek (1976) reported on bilateral abductor cord paralysis in a father whose cords were in the midline position and two sons whose cords were almost in midline position (all had a significant stridor). Because of the difficulty in breathing, tracheostomy, according to Gacek, appears to provide the most effective treatment for this type of problem.

Typical vocal characteristics in laryngeal paralysis are hoarseness, a monotone, weak soft voice, and breathiness. The physiological condition is more serious if both vocal cords are affected with the cords fixed either in a paramedian position or in a fully adducted midline position. When the cords are in the paramedian position, the voice is excessively breathy; however, when they are fixed in the midline position the voice is good, although the person has much difficulty breathing and tracheostomy is indicated.

The actual incidence of vocal cord paralysis is unknown, but it should be noted that this type of problem is seen more frequently in children than previously recorded (Holinger and Brown, 1967). Holinger et al. (1976) reviewed 389 cases of partial or complete bilateral abductor vocal cord paralysis. One hundred forty-nine, nearly 38% of the patients, were infants and children 12 years of age or under. The paralysis was congenital in over half the children; in the remaining children the paralysis was an acquired condition.

When vocal cord paralysis appears in children the abductor muscles are the ones usually affected (Laupus and Pastore, 1967, p. 212). The paralysis may be either spastic or flaccid, but it is difficult to differentiate between them (DeWeese and Saunders, 1973, p. 100). Laryngeal paralysis is often accompanied by dyspnea or stridor (Cavanagh, 1955; DeWeese and Saunders, 1973, p. 103).

Cavanagh (1955) presented a comprehensive study of vocal paralysis in 37 children examined by direct laryngoscopy. The onset of symptoms occurred in 11 of them at birth and in the remainder up to 7 years of age. She could determine the cause of the vocal palsy in only eight of these children.

Congenital paralysis of one or both vocal cords in an infant is often associated with other abnormalities (Cavanagh, 1955; Holinger and Brown, 1967). Unilateral vocal cord paralysis in infants more frequently affects the left vocal cord (Holinger and Brown, 1967). The prognosis for voice function with right cord paralysis is good, for those with left cord paralysis only fair, since the latter is often associated with anomalies of the heart and great blood vessels (Holinger and Brown, 1967).

Laryngeal Growths

Papilloma in and around the larynx may cause hoarseness and sometimes aphonia. Laryngeal papillomatosis is a serious debilitating clinical problem both in children and adults (Holinger, Johnston, Conner, Conner, and Holper, 1962) and may involve air hunger and stridor (DeWeese and Saunders, 1973, p. 132). A papilloma is a wartlike growth thought to be caused by a virus (DeWeese and Saunders, 1973, p. 132) (Figs. 4 and 5). Cook, Cohn, Brunschwig, Goepfert, Butel, and Rawls (1973) reported on the treatment of nine children with laryngeal papilloma. Five of the nine children were delivered by mothers who had condyloma acuminatum

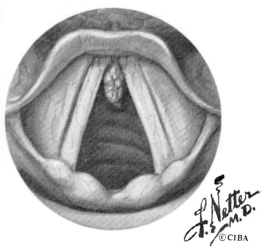

Fig. 4. Pedunculated papilloma at anterior commissure. Copyright *Clinical Symposia* by Frank H. Netter, M.D., published by CIBA Pharmaceutical Company.

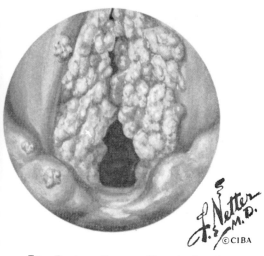

Fig. 5. Juvenile papillomatosis (laryngoscopic view). Copyright *Clinical Symposia* by Frank H. Netter, M.D., published by CIBA Pharmaceutical Company.

(wart of the genital organs) at the time of delivery. These five children required laryngeal surgery much earlier than the other four. An electron microscopic study of tissue specimens of these five children failed to find any actual virus particles. However, an electron microscopic study comparing the papilloma tissue with skin and genital warts showed ultrastructural details linking the three lesions. Lundquist, Frithiof, and Wersäll (1975)

described human laryngeal papilloma of the juvenile type as a benign epithelial tumor at the anterior part of the vocal cords, which has a tendency to spread along the epithelium, often involving also the aryepiglottic folds and regions as well as the ventricular folds.

Various methods of treating a child for papilloma are used, one of them being surgery; since they often recur, repeated surgery is common (DeWeese and Saunders, 1973, p. 132). Other procedures include microcautery (Kirchner, 1974; Kirchner and Duff, 1974), ultrasound (Fairman, 1972), carbon dioxide laser surgery (Strong and Jako, 1972; Strong, Jako, Polanyi, and Wallace, 1973; Andrews and Moss, 1974) and cryosurgery (Singleton and Adkins, 1972; Miller, 1973; Kärjä, Jokinen, and Palva, 1975). Great care must be exercised in removing papilloma or permanent hoarseness may result if vocal cords are damaged (DeWeese and Saunders, 1973, p. 132). Voice therapy usually is indicated when hoarseness persists after removal of the papilloma (Holinger, Johnston, and McMahon, 1952). Voice improvement is especially difficult in cases where surgery has resulted in a roughening of the free margins of the vocal cords.

Oleske and Kushnick (1971) reported on a child with papilloma of the larynx who was admitted to the hospital with acute respiratory distress when she was 2 years 1 month of age. Tracheotomy was performed immediately. Management consisted of repeated surgical removal of papilloma from the vocal cords and larynx. The papilloma continued to recur locally, but never beyond the laryngeal area. Direct laryngoscopy and tumor excision were performed 21 times in a 17-month period, averaging one procedure every 3.7 weeks. An autogenous vaccine was prepared from a sample of the papilloma and a total of 15 weekly injections were given. Two months later direct examination revealed that the papilloma had not recurred and that the vocal cords were intact. As a result the tracheotomy tube was removed and the patient was free of respiratory distress and was talking in a nearly normal voice. The girl was discharged after 716 days in the hospital.

The following is an example of a child who received voice therapy after successful treatment of laryngeal papillomatosis.

Tom was 7 years old when we first

knew him. His parents brought him to us for improvement of his voice after he had been hoarse all of his life. One day when he was 2 months old Tom had a series of choking episodes followed by severe respiratory distress. He was immediately admitted to a hospital where an emergency tracheotomy was performed. Later a laryngoscopic examination revealed papilloma on the ventricular bands and the vocal cords. These growths were removed and the pathology report indicated they were squamous papillomas. During the next 5 years Tom had 26 operations for removal of papilloma. After this the papilloma did not recur and the tracheotomy tube was removed. When we saw him he had been free from the papilloma for 2 years and the laryngologist reported the vocal cords were mobile, but the free margins were slightly roughened from the operations. Tom talked with excess tension in a strident pattern with audible breath escape as he phonated. He talked at a too-low modal frequency level with much effort, using a staccato-type initiation of words. The voice therapy goals were (1) tension-reducing measures, including relaxation and chewing exercises, (2) teaching easy initiation of tones to replace the staccato style, (3) raising the modal frequency level about 3 semitones (from B_3 to D_4, 245 to 295 Hz), and (4) improving the quality of the laryngeal tone. After voice therapy twice a week for 4 months Tom was speaking with very little effort and was initiating tones easily. His modal frequency level was higher with the quality of the laryngeal tone a bit breathy but within acceptable limits.

Congenital cysts may have their origin in the vocal cords, the ventricle, or the aryepiglottic folds (Baker, 1954). They may be discovered at birth or during childhood; successful treatment is by operation to remove the cyst (Baker, 1954). The voice is usually adequate after an operation; however, at times voice therapy may be indicated to overcome laryngeal insufficiency resulting from the operation.

A congenital laryngocele may be difficult to distinguish from a cyst (Holinger and Brown, 1967). It originates from the ventricle and is a sac filled either with air or fluid (Holinger and Brown, 1967). It may bulge out between the true and false vocal cords (Holinger and Brown, 1967). It may even be visible externally between the hyoid bone and the thyroid cartilage during coughing or straining (Laupus and Pastore, 1967, p. 210). The symptoms are hoarseness and dyspnea (Holinger, Johnston, and Schiller, 1954).

Malignant tumors as a cause of voice problems in children are rare (Laupus and Pastore, 1967, p. 208). There are reports of children who have undergone some form of therapy for cancer of the larynx, either partial removal of the larynx or total laryngectomy. However, these cases are so few that they are not of major concern to the speech pathologist.

Laryngeal Trauma

Hoarseness, breathiness, dysphonia, or aphonia in children may be associated with laryngeal trauma. Holinger and Schild (1972) reported on trauma to the larynx and immediate surrounding areas in three pediatric age groups and one young adult group. The first group of 42 children, 16 boys and 26 girls, were from birth to 1½ years of age. Fifteen of the infants had laryngeal findings associated with prolonged endotracheal intubation, and 22 of the infants suffered trauma due to aspirating foreign bodies such as safety pins, common pins, bits of glass, egg shells, and parts of plastic toys. In the second age group, 1½ years to 12 years, there were 57 children, 33 boys and 24 girls. Prolonged intubation was the cause of laryngeal injuries in 13 children, automobile accidents in 11, and foreign bodies in 19. In the third pediatric group, aged 13 to 18 years, there were 31, 17 boys and 14 girls. The pattern had changed as to causation, with 3 from prolonged intubation, 4 from aspiration of foreign bodies, and 21 from automobile accidents. In the group of young adults, 19 to 25 years of age, the causes included 1 from prolonged intubation, 1 from foreign objects, and 26 from automobile accidents. The figures are not complete for any of the groups since those classified under "other" were not included here. Injury may cause damage to either the joints or musculature of the larynx (Arnold, 1966) or may result in fracture of laryngeal cartilages (Holinger et al. 1952).

Intubation is a common cause of laryngeal trauma (Holinger et al. 1952). Intubation may be necessary to relieve respiratory problems in an infant who has difficulty breathing upon delivery (Holinger et al. 1952), or it may be done during an operation. Laryngotracheal complications which follow endotracheal intubation are inflammatory or allergic edema, ulceration of the laryngotracheal mucosa, laryngitis and tracheitis, glottic web, avulsion of a vocal cord (a forcible separation or detachment of the vocal cord), fracture of the cricoid cartilage, dislocation of an arytenoid cartilage, subglottic and glottic granulation tissue, and laryngotracheal stenosis (Smith, Hemenway, English, Black, and Swan, 1969). Jaffe (1972) reported approximately 3% of postoperative cases have hoarseness after an operation. Typically the hoarseness disappears after a few days; however, in some cases the hoarseness persists associated with severe pain on swallowing. Injury may arise during the act of intubation, from the endotracheal tube during the operation, or from the endotracheal tube during the postoperative course. Jaffe stated the specific treatment depends upon the type and the extent of the injury.

Johnsen (1973) described prolonged intubation as intubation lasting longer than 6 or 7 days. Johnsen described a group of 29 children with acute epiglottitis who were intubated for 2 or 3 days without lesions of the larynx or trachea that required treatment. In another group requiring intubation from 5 to 56 days, Johnsen stated the severity of the laryngotracheal damage was to some extent dependent upon the duration of the intubation, but this was not a rule without exception. Bowman, Shanks, and Manion (1972) reported on a child who had nasotracheal intubation from age 2 weeks to 40 months because of asphyxiating thoracic dystrophy. Laryngoscopies at 6 months revealed reddened vocal cords, at 10 months and 34 months normal structures, and at 46 months of age essentially normal function and structures, except there was a slight air loss between the arytenoids and a suggestion of asymmetry of vocal cord approximation. Goumaz (1973) presented information on 49 newborn infants who had been intubated because of respiratory distress. Intubation tubes remained in place from 20 hours to 41½ days. Thirteen infants had no objective lesions. The lesions in the other infants were ulcerations and various forms of glottic and subglottic changes. Hengerer, Strome, and Jaffe (1975) reported on injuries to the neonatal larynx from long-term endotracheal tube intubation. Acute findings were arytenoid and posterior commissure ulcerations and in some cases cartilage erosion.

In some cases of difficult breathing it may be necessary to perform a tracheotomy (Laupus and Pastore, 1967, p. 208). They stated this procedure does not necessarily result in permanent damage, but complications can occur, especially in infants and young children.

When a glottic web follows trauma the glottis is shortened resulting in a high-pitched voice. In general, pitch is raised in direct proportion to the shortening of the free vocal cord margins (Arnold, 1966). Huff and Magielski (1976) stated laryngeal webs that result from anterior laryngeal injuries respond well to thyrotomy and insertion of a McNaught keel. Under direct visualization the web is cut with a sharp knife to separate the two vocal cords. Then a tantalum keel is fashioned to keep the raw edges apart, and tabs are utilized to keep the keel from being displaced posteriorly. The strap muscles are closed over the tabs and the keel is left in place for 2 months.

Direct trauma to the neck may occur in an automobile accident (Holinger et al. 1952), often the result of hitting the dashboard or other obstructions within the car. Priest, Huff, and Banovetz (1967) stated laryngotracheal injuries of various kinds may occur in automobile accidents. They said, "At high speed an unseat-belted passenger is thrown forward with head erect, neck extended, and the larynx held firmly in position in front of the rigid vertebral column which serves as the anvil against which the larynx is hammered. Not only may the larynx be crushed and fragmented, but the cricoid may be torn off the cervical trachea or the larynx may be avulsed from the pharynx." Boles (1968) stated automobile and motorized bicycle accidents can cause crushing and fracturing injuries of the larynx; the symptoms are hoarseness, spitting of blood from the larynx or trachea, dyspnea, and subcutaneous emphysema of the neck. Harris (1972) stated in automobile accidents the type of injury usually falls into one of the following categories: (1) supraglottic tears and fractures, (2) transglottic injuries, (3) cricoid fractures, (4) avulsion of the trachea from the cricoid, and (5) lacerations or tears of the trachea. Children are less apt to have external laryngeal and tracheal trauma in automobile accidents than adults (Novick, 1967), but teenagers are more susceptible. Huff (1972) stated that with the increased use of snowmobiles there is an increase in the number of deaths and mutilating injuries including maxillofacial and laryngeal injuries.

Laryngeal trauma in children is more apt to be the the result of play activities such as falling against a fence (Novick, 1967) or falling against the handlebars of a bicycle. Chandler (1972) reported on an 11-year-old girl who suffered complete transection of the larynx and pharynx as a result of blunt trauma in the form of a ski rope injury when she was struck in the anterior neck by a rope towing a water skier behind a power boat, and after treatment her voice was a loud whisper. Ogura (1975) reported on a 14-year-old boy who struck his extended neck against a taut steel cable while riding a minibike on a golf course. There was complete laryngotracheal disruption and a paralyzed right cord. With treatment he eventually regained a useable voice. Cardoso and Gomes (1972) described an 8-year-old boy who had been shot in the larynx with an air gun. The pellet was imbedded in the left vocal cord and the pellet was easily removed following a midline thyrotomy operation. His voice was weak and slightly hoarse for about a month and then was normal. Damage to a child's larynx may also occur as a result of inhaling toxic (Holinger, Schild, and Maurizi, 1968) or caustic (Laupus and Pastore, 1967, p. 208) substances.

Voice therapy is recommended for voice problems resulting from various kinds of internal laryngeal trauma (Holinger et al. 1968) and may be indicated after recovery from external trauma.

THE VELOPHARYNGEAL AREA, ORAL CAVITY, AND NOSE

Resonance problems may be present in a child due to organic deviations in the velopharyngeal area, oral cavity, or nose. The presenting voice problem depends upon the physical site being misused. Velopharyngeal insufficiency may cause a voice problem characterized by combinations of hypernasality, hyponasality, and nasal emission (or snorting) of sounds. Sounds requiring a buildup of pressure within the mouth or pharynx are most frequently affected. Forty-three consonant sounds and blends are most fre-

quently misarticulated because of velopharyngeal insufficiency (Morris, Spriestersbach, and Darley, 1961) and are described in Chapter 6. The most common of the single consonants are /s/, /k/, /ʃ/, and /z/. Hypernasality is produced by relaxing the velum causing an opening into the nasopharyngeal port and using the nasal cavity as a cul-de-sac resonator. Induced hypernasality is present when the velum is raised but is very tense and even thin. Here the velum acts as a drum head to increase nasality. A sluggish velum may cause assimilation nasality on sounds adjacent to the normally nasal sounds /m/, /n/, and /ŋ/.* The causes of velopharyngeal insufficiency include: (1) cleft palate, (2) short hard and/or soft palate, (3) abnormal capacious pharynx, (4) velar paralysis, (5) submucous cleft palate, and (6) adenoidectomy. These causes can be present on congenital or developmental bases. Velopharyngeal insufficiency without an overt cleft palate ranges from 3.6% to 7.8% of the "cleft palate" population (Gylling and Soivio, 1965; Porterfield and Trabue, 1965; Rees, Wood-Smith, Swinyard, and Converse, 1967; Takagi, McGlone, and Millard, 1965).

Cleft Palate

About one child in 750 live births has a cleft palate. Cleft palates vary in extent of abnormality from a single cleft of the soft palate to bilateral clefts involving the soft and hard palate, the alveolar process, and the lip. After physical management many children need voice therapy to reduce hypernasality and nasal emission. Morris (1972, pp. 149–150) classified cleft palate as follows: Group I, those who have velopharyngeal competence with no nasal emission or hypernasality, where only the correction of articulation is the problem; Group II, marginal or borderline velopharyngeal incompetence, divided into two subgroups, (1) those who almost but do not quite achieve closure, and (2) those who sometimes but not always achieve closure; and Group III, the velopharyngeal incompetent person who has no ability to direct the airstream orally in speech in any context.

* An audiotape produced by B. J. Philips (1969) of children with cleft palate demonstrating their speech patterns including hypernasality and hoarseness is available from the University of Miami School of Medicine, P. O. Box 875, Biscayne Annex, Miami, FL 33152.

It should be noted that many children with cleft palate have voice problems in addition to hypernasality and nasal emission of air. The voice may sound hoarse and the laryngoscopic examinations often reveal the vocal cords to be hyperemic (reddened) and hyperplastic (thickened) (McDonald and Baker, 1951).

Brooks and Shelton (1963) found a greater percentage of cleft palate children with other voice problems than is usual for the general population. They found 10% of 76 cleft palate children between the ages of 6 years 5 months and 12 years had voice defects other than or in addition to hypernasality, including breathiness, hoarseness, and inappropriate pitch level. On the other hand, Takagi et al. (1965) reported only 0.6 of 1% of 1061 patients (including 83 with non-cleft palatal insufficiency) had voice disorders other than hypernasality.

Bzoch (1964) reported on 40 persons with cleft palate who received pharyngeal flap surgery. Before surgery, 14 of the subjects were judged to have breathy voice quality. Immediately following surgery this number dropped to eight and by the end of the study only two cases appeared to have breathy voices. In the initial preoperative speech evaluation 7 of the 40 cases had hoarse voices. Laryngeal examinations revealed no lesions of the vocal cords. Following surgery six cases presented hoarse voices, which remained characteristic in three of the seven cases at the time of final study. Breathiness in the voice is definitely reduced following such operative procedures, but hoarseness in the voice seems to persist in a certain number of such subjects. Therefore, it would seem that attention by the speech pathologist to hoarse quality in a cleft palate person is indicated.

McWilliams, Bluestone, and Musgrave (1969) reported on laryngoscopic examinations of 32 children with cleft palate (aged 4 years 10 months to 14 years 4 months) who had hoarse voices. Indirect laryngoscopy was done on 25 children with seven children requiring direct laryngoscopy. Twenty boys and three girls had vocal nodules. Four other children had atypical laryngeal conditions including a posterior glottic chink, bilateral vocal cord hypertrophy, slight anterior edema, and improper approximation of the vocal cords. Thus a total of 27 (84%) of the 32 children with hoarse voices were found to have vocal cord abnormalities.

Approximately 4.7 years after the initial evaluation, 27 of the original group of 32 children were reexamined and the results reported by McWilliams, Lavorato, and Bluestone (1973). One of the two who originally had normal cords now had vocal nodules, and the other hypertrophy. The one child who could not be viewed originally now showed vocal nodules. This made a total of 30 (94%) of the original group of 32 who eventually showed vocal cord abnormalities. On the reexamination 19 (70%) now had vocal cord abnormalities. Eight of the children who showed some atypical condition of the cords on both examinations had the same condition both times—in all cases vocal nodules. Of much interest are the changes that took place in seven children who originally were diagnosed as having vocal nodules: five changed from nodules to edema and two from nodules to hypertrophy. One other changed from posterior glottal chink to edema. Thus the condition of the vocal cords appeared to change for the better. The children who no longer showed any vocal cord pathology had an average age of 15 years 8 months, while those with retained or acquired abnormalities had an average age of 12 years 1 month, indicating that age may have been an important factor in remission. We feel an important finding of McWilliams et al. (1973) was that surgical removal of vocal cord nodules was an ineffective approach to management unless attention was paid to improving the velopharyngeal valving mechanism. Six children had surgical removal of vocal nodules during the period between studies. Two of these had physical management of velopharyngeal valving with no recurrence of the nodules but showed vocal cord edema. The other four did not have physical management of valving; three of them had recurrence of the nodules and the remaining one had a thickened right cord and severe hoarseness.

Lowry, Billings, and Leonard (1974) in a study of a cleft palate population found two with vocal cord abnormalities in a group of 74 patients (2.7%). One had thickened edematous and reddened vocal cords and the second patient appeared to have a very short vocal cord length in the anterior-posterior dimension. The average age at the first visit to the clinic was 7.1 years, the youngest being 3 weeks of age and the oldest 30 years 6 months of age. This study should not be contrasted with the studies of McWilliams et al. (1969) and McWilliams et al. (1973) because those studies dealt only with cleft palate children *with* hoarse voices.

Short Hard and/or Soft Palate

Various combinations of shortness of the hard and soft palate may occur. These are a short hard palate with a normal soft palate, a normal hard palate with a short soft palate, or a shortness of both the hard and soft palates (Kaplan, Jobe, and Chase, 1969). A bifid uvula may also be present. The incidence of bifid uvula was 1% in a school population of 10,836 kindergarten through high school children, as reported by Weatherley-White, Sakura, Brenner, Stewart, and Ott (1972). Studying the same population Stewart, Ott, and Lagace (1972) reported bifid uvula was found in isolation in 100 children, combined with a submucous cleft palate in eight, and combined with a cleft lip in two. Meskin, Gorlin, and Isaacson (1964) found the incidence of bifid uvula to be 1.34% in a population of 1864 dental patients of all ages, and 1.47% in 7837 entering students at a university. Taylor (1972) stated the bifid uvula is a definitive signal reflecting a disturbance in the embryological development of the palate and related structures. Taylor added that otologic sequelae and velopharyngeal incompetence may also occur in patients with a bifid uvula. Schendel and Gorlin (1974) reported individuals with Down's syndrome have a higher incidence of bifid uvula than the general population. In 389 patients, the incidence was 18 (4.63%).

Abnormal Capacious Pharynx

In some cases a child may have normal hard and soft palates but the pharyngeal area is abnormally deep making velopharyngeal closure impossible. Calnan (1971b) reported on 36 children, aged 5 to 7 years, and five adults who had nasal speech and apparently normal palatal pharyngeal mechanisms. However, clinical and cephalometric examinations revealed the pharynx to be larger than normal. Calnan described this condition as *congenital large pharynx*. The proportion of males to females was 3 to 1. Over 60% of Calnan's patients obtained normal speech after various types of pharyngoplasty.

Velar Paralysis

Structures may be normal in size and proportion, but a partial or complete paralysis may exist causing palate immobility, ineffective palate motion or inconsistent palate motion (Kaplan et al. 1969; Massengill, 1972, p. 20). For isolated palatal paresis Schweiger, Netsell, and Sommerfeld (1970) recommended a palatal lift prosthesis, which lifts the soft palate up and closes the velopharyngeal orifice completely anterior-posterior, leaving gutters on the sides for normal rest, breathing, and production of the nasals /m/, /n/, and /ŋ/. Kipfmueller and Lang (1972) described treating patients with velopharyngeal insufficiency where a normally sized soft palate did not elevate and where a palatal lift prosthesis was used successfully to improve speech. They also described a group of patients with velopharyngeal insufficiency where a palatal lift prosthesis with an added bulb resulted in improved speech. Kerman, Singer, and Davidoff (1973) reported on the successful use of a palatal lift prosthesis with two neurologically impaired young adults who had severe dysarthria resulting in palatal inactivity and hypernasality.

Submucous Cleft Palate

Submucous cleft palate is a congenital deformity involving an imperfect muscle union across the velum (Calnan, 1954). Arnold (1965, pp. 660–661) described the characteristics of submucous cleft palate. He noted the uvula may be normal, or it may be bifid. The hard palate may have a triangular defect at its posterior border and this bony defect is covered by healthy looking mucosa which is very thin, however, because it is not supported by intervening musculature. Upon phonation the mucosal covering becomes stretched and the bony defect can be seen. Sometimes transilluminating the palate with a nasopharyngoscope aids in the examination. The soft palate is usually too short and also weak so that it cannot elevate to produce nasopharyngeal closure. Beeden (1972) stated that a bifid uvula is present in almost all cases of submucous cleft palate, and a notch in the hard palate is present in every case. Calnan (1954) described submucous cleft palate as being characterized by a bifid uvula, a bony notch in the hard palate, and diastasis of the palatal muscles (muscle separation or clefting). Weatherley-White et al. (1972) found nine children with submucous cleft palate in their study of 10,836 school children, making an incidence of 1 in 1200. Stewart et al. (1972)

reported that of these nine children, eight had bifid uvula, one did not. In Down's syndrome, Schendel and Gorlin (1974) reported the incidence of submucous cleft palate was 3 in 389 patients.

Adenoidectomy

A problem resembling cleft palate speech may occur after removal of the adenoid. Prior to the operation the velopharyngeal area functions normally with the adenoid aiding in velopharyngeal closure. Goode and Ross (1972) advised the avoidance of an adenoidectomy when there are indications that hypernasal speech will result. They advised doing a lateral adenoidectomy leaving the midline bulk of adenoid tissue. Beeden (1972) advised that if a child has a bifid uvula and a palatal notch, adenoidectomy should be avoided. Lawson, Chierici, Castro, Harvold, Miller, and Owsley (1972) studied 40 children ranging in age from 4 to 17 years who were potential candidates for adenoidectomy. Evaluations had been requested because of suspected anomalous velopharyngeal area conditions based on the presence of certain deviant speech characteristics. All the children manifested some degree of hypernasality—seven minimal, 18 moderate, and 15 severe. Fluctuations in nasal emission occurred in some, and in others the hypernasality was noticeable only in continuous speech as contrasted to words in isolation. Cinefluorgraphic studies showed all but one of the 40 children had inconsistent velopharyngeal closure. Cephalometric measurements revealed one or more morphologic deviations in the palatal pharyngeal area in 27 of the 40 patients. These deviations included short or thin soft palate, thin pharyngeal wall, an unusual degree of concavity in the contour of the pharyngeal wall at the level of velopharyngeal closure, and excessive depth of the nasopharynx. Adenoidectomy was avoided except lateral adenoidectomies for cases where there was middle ear involvement.

Van Gelder (1974b) reported on 33 patients with hypernasality following tonsillectomy and adenoidectomy, the incidence being 1 in 3000 patients; there were also 4 cases of hypernasality following adenoidectomy alone, with an incidence of 1 in 10,000 patients. Van Gelder noted the following etiological factors in the 33 patients reported: congenital malformation or postoperative lesion of the soft palate, oblong configuration of the nasopharynx, lesion of nasopharyngeal wall, delayed or defective speech development, hearing disturbances, psychoneurotic behavior, and mental retardation. Roentgenographic examination showed 70% had an oblong nasopharyngeal configuration, 20% a lesion of the nasopharynx, and 60% a short soft palate or diminished velar motility. Calnan (1971a) reported on 19 patients, 16 children aged 6 through 14 years and three adults. Their speech history was identical in every case in that it had been normal before removal of the tonsils and adenoids and some even had a superior voice quality. After the operation speech became hypernasal and often unintelligible, including the three patients who had adenoidectomy alone. Calnan stated it is the adenoidectomy that is the chief cause of such speech problems, not the tonsillectomy. The main voice defects were audible nasal escape of speech and loss of voice projection. Radiological studies demonstrated a fully mobile soft palate, but with a gap between it and the posterior wall on /i/. The gap ranged from 2 to 10 mm with a mean gap of 5.1 mm. Buck (1954) found the gap on /i/ was 0.26 mm in a group of normal subjects. Calnan stated speech therapy for this group was without effect, but when the velopharyngeal gap was occluded by a cartilage implant behind the posterior wall of the pharynx speech returned to normal.

A child may have hyponasality immediately following removal of tonsils or adenoids because of postoperative edema. A waiting period of at least 3 weeks following the operation should be observed before attention to speech is given; by this time the edematous condition should be reduced and the hyponasality no longer present (Sloan, Brummett, Westover, Ricketts, and Ashley, 1964). After this, hypernasality may appear. Massengill (1972, p. 19) suggested that if hypernasality does not decrease 6 months to a year after removal of the adenoid, physical management and speech therapeutic procedures may be necessary. Goode and Ross (1972) stated that if speech does not return to normal in 2 to 6 months following adenoidectomy a careful evaluation should be made to assess the severity of the condition.

Hyponasality

Hyponasality is a lack of proper nasal resonance. Arnold (1965, p. 686) presented three cardinal diagnostic rules in assessing hypo-nasality: (*a*) the nasals /m/, /n/, and /ŋ/ always have a muffled sound, (*b*) nasal respiration, smell, and taste are disturbed in the organic forms, and (*c*) disorders of swallowing do not occur. Hyponasality is usually due to an obstruction in the nasal or nasopharyngeal passages (Fomon et al. 1966). Arnold (1965, p. 684) included among the causes deviated septum, bilateral turbinate hypertrophy, nasal polyps, enlarged adenoid tissue, allergic or inflammatory swelling of the mucosa, and traumatic injuries.

Choanal atresia may cause hyponasality. According to Cherry and Bordley (1966) choanal atresia is the condition in which the posterior openings to the nasal cavities are occluded by osseous (bony), osseous combined with membranous, or membranous material only. When choanal atresia is bilateral a surgical emergency exists especially with a newborn who does not know how to breathe through the mouth (Paisner, 1972). Cherry and Bordley (1966) advised that this condition may be diagnosed by passing soft rubber catheters through the nares during the newborn's pediatric examination. Of the 18 cases reported by Cherry and Bordley 84% were of osseous or osseous and membranous type, and 16% membranous only. Paisner (1972) stated it is important to determine whether a nasal obstruction is unilateral or bilateral. This can be done by closing off with a finger one nostril and then the other. A unilateral obstruction indicates either choanal atresia or a foreign body, while bilateral nasal obstruction usually indicates one of three things: hypertrophy of the adenoid, allergy, or deviated septum (Paisner, 1972).

Batza and Parker (1971) recommended that those with hyponasality should be investigated regarding eustachian tube patency. As we know, the eustachian tubes are normally closed, and they open only during a swallow, yawn, or a forcible blowing of the nose. In a few patients very small pressures, such as those created by phonation, open one or both eustachian tubes. The person then experiences what is known as autophony. This is a condition where the person's voice is amplified and sounds hollow in his own ears because his own voice is directed into the middle ear through the open eustachian tubes. Thus speech is reaching the middle ear from both sides of the eardrum. Likewise the sounds of

respiration are loudly heard and the patient often becomes a mouth breather. The patency of the eustachian tubes may vary in severity from a mild unilateral case to continuously open tubes bilaterally. Arnold (1965, p. 685) stated hyponasal speech may also be present on a functional basis, perhaps due to poor motor coordination, congenital dyspraxia, or faulty habits of verbal behavior. A hyponasal voice may persist long after the cause has been removed (Van Riper, 1972, p. 155).

In dealing with cases of hyponasality a thorough examination by the physician is essential. Surgical treatment is indicated when it is necessary to remove polyps or other obstructions causing the hyponasality. When swelling is present, congestion may be ameliorated by the use of medication (Arnold, 1965, p. 686).

NEUROLOGICAL, DEVELOPMENTAL, AND HEARING PROBLEMS

Myasthenia Gravis

Darley, Aronson, and Brown (1975, pp. 125–126) described speech changes in myasthenia gravis as follows: "As the patient continues speaking or reading aloud, fatigue of the speech musculature becomes evident in increase of hypernasality, deterioration of articulation, onset and increase of dysphonia, and reduction of loudness level. Finally his speech becomes an unintelligible, effortful blur. . . . After a period of rest the patient can resume speaking with more normal phonation, resonance, and articulation; but as he continues, the evidences of muscle fatigue again appear."† Voice changes can be the first and only symptoms of early neurologic disease (Aronson, 1971).

Wolski (1967) discussed an adolescent girl with myasthenia gravis. The chief complaint was nasal emission and hypernasal speech. This condition was described as a neuromuscular transmission problem with an apparent blockage of nerve impulses from motor nerve endings across the synapse to the motor end plate of skeletal muscles. Hypernasality followed a specific pattern. The girl was quite free from symptoms in the morning but as the day progressed her voice became more and more nasal. Treatment for this condition was medical with various drugs being used to control nerve impulses. Aronson (1971) pre-

† Quoted with permission.

sented a study of a 20-year-old girl with myasthenia gravis. Her chief complaint was a weak voice, and occasionally her articulation seemed imprecise. Her voice sometimes died out in the afternoon and was worse when she got home from work, but was fairly normal in the morning. She also had a slight breathy quality; after rapid and vigorous counting her voice became increasingly breathy with a deterioration of palatopharyngeal valving which resulted in audible hypernasality. Neiman, Mountjoy, and Allen (1975) reported on a 20-year-old girl with myasthenia gravis whose chief complaint was intermittent hoarseness of 4 years' duration, with each episode lasting from 1 to 2 weeks. Her voice was usually better in the morning and became more breathy with use. There was a minimal weakness of the palate and the vocal cords were flaccid and did not adduct completely. There was no hypernasality or articulation problem. Johnson and Ausband (1972) presented a discussion of twin infant girls with an unusual form of congenital myasthenia gravis. The main findings were a deformity of the posterior tracheal wall with occlusion of the tracheal lumen.

Primary treatment for myasthenia gravis is medical with various drugs being used to control nerve impulses. With adequate medical control, attention to speech and voice may not be necessary. Secondary treatment may involve the speech pathologist to help improve voice quality, resonance, and articulation. A palatal lift prosthesis may be helpful in reducing hypernasality and nasal emission when there is flaccid paralysis of the soft palate (Gonzales and Aronson, 1970). Here is another example of a child with myasthenia gravis.

Betty, age 10, was brought to our office by her mother. The chief complaint was hypernasality and some hoarseness which had become progressively more pronounced during the past 2 years. The mother reported, "When she gets up in the morning her voice sounds good, but when she comes from school, she's talking through her nose and she is hoarse. Her voice is better if I can get her to take a nap before supper. I usually can 'cause she's tired all the time." Betty was a quiet girl with a somewhat expressionless face and with mild ptosis of the eyelids.

We rated her as having severe hypernasality, mild breathiness, and a too-high modal frequency level (F_4, 350 Hz; Normal, C_4, 265 Hz). When asked to count rapidly she began to slow down when she reached 40, getting slower, more hypernasal and breathy until she quit at 70. Repeating vowels and nonsense syllables followed the same pattern. Betty was next seen by various medical specialists who arrived at the diagnosis of juvenile myasthenia gravis. Medication to control the problem was begun at once. Betty responded nicely with most symptoms (fatigue, facial expression) remarkably improved. When we saw her 2 months later she had moderate hypernasality and the hoarseness was gone but her pitch level was still high. Articulation tests, oral manometer ratios, and lateral head x-rays indicated Betty should respond well to behavioral management of her hypernasality. The voice therapy goals were directed toward (1) listening training for hypernasality and pitch, (2) developing adequate oral breath pressure and oral air flow to eliminate the hypernasality, and (3) lowering her modal frequency level 5 semitones (from F_4 to C_4, 350 to 265 Hz). She responded well to voice therapy twice a week for 3 months. She was then seen six times a year for 2 years because she needed supportive therapy over an extended period.

Multiple Sclerosis

Darley, Brown, and Goldstein (1972) reported on a series of 168 patients, 65 males and 103 females, with the diagnosis of multiple sclerosis. The patients ranged in age from 17 to 73 years with a median age of approximately 40, with four patients under 20 years of age. Impaired control of loudness, either too soft or too loud, unsteadiness in loudness, and harshness were noted in more than 70% of the patients. In about half of the patients articulation was defective. Poor control of variability for emphasis, poor pitch control, hypernasality, inappropriate modal frequency level, and breathiness were noted in 20% to 40% of the patients. Increased stress on usually unstressed words and syllables (scanning speech) was noted in 14% of the patients. Most speech deviations in multiple sclerosis become more prominent as additional motor systems become involved.

Scoliosis

Skelly, Donaldson, Scheer, and Guzzardo (1971) reported on hypernasality associated with spinal bracing in scoliosis. This is a lateral curvature of the spine and is a condition in which a series of vertebrae persistently deviate from the normal spinal axis. It is a deformity, not a disease. The deformity is generally noticed for the first time between 10 and 15 years of age, most often at 11 or 12 (Wiles and Sweetnam, 1965, in Skelly et al. 1971). Skelly et al. (1971) stated the Milwaukee brace is commonly used in treatment. Over a 4-year period they studied a total of 101 children with scoliosis between 6 and 15 years of age. Ninety-two cases of hypernasality were noted in this group compared to 69 hypernasality problems in 471 nonbrace patients. This represented a 14% incidence of hypernasality among nonbraced patients and 92% incidence among braced patients. Among the 92 brace cases hypernasality was rated in 61 as severe, 27 moderate, and four mild. In the four mild cases the modal frequency level was judged as too low with an additional description of harshness. In all cases judged as moderate to severe in hypernasality the modal frequency level was rated as too high.

Cerebral Palsy

Children with cerebral palsy may have a variety of voice problems depending on the type and severity of cerebral palsy. Mysak (1971, pp. 686–687) reviewed the literature on voice problems in persons with cerebral palsy. He presented the following voice characteristics as typical: An interruption of voicing, characterized by forced or intermittent voicing and phonation on inhalation (reverse phonation), may be present. The person may have difficulty coordinating the initiation of phonation with breath groups. Also, each phonation attempt may be short because of the difficulty in shifting from vegetative to phonatory breathing. The cerebral palsied child may have difficulty with pitch control and stability. The modal pitch often is low and the laryngeal tone characterized by breathiness. The spastic type usually has a hypertense voice and the athetoid type a hypotense voice. McDonald and Chance (1964, pp. 89–91) included among the laryngeal involvements an inability to initiate phonation because an adductor spasm holds the vocal cords tightly together. The opposite may also be present, that is an abductor spasm prevents the closing of the vocal cords for initiating phonation. McDonald and Chance listed typical breathing problems and associated speech symptoms: (1) only one or two syllables per exhalation, (2) an increase in tension occurs as longer vocalizations are attempted, (3) a noticeable escape of air before vocalization is initiated, (4) varied loudness of voice, and (5) interruptions of vocalizations. The voice problems of cerebral palsied children are so diverse each child's voice must be analyzed carefully so therapy can be efficiently planned.

Mental Retardation

The number of voice problems in retarded children is very high. As we reported in Chapter 1, Schlanger and Gottsleben (1957) reported 47% of those in a school for the retarded had voice problems. Descriptive terms given to the voice problems were hoarse-husky, aspirate, hypernasal, hyponasal, pitch, sing-song, monotone, and rate and volume disorders. Further, Saunders and Miller (1968) found that dysphonia and aphonia were present in a large series of retarded individuals in a hospital. Daly (1974) studied resonance in a group of 50 educable mentally retarded children aged 7 years to 19 years 1 month, whose IQ's ranged from 56 to 80. As measured by TONAR the incidence of hypernasality was found to be 38%, with 18% rated mild, 18% moderate, 0% severe, and 2% very severe. Daly (1977) later studied resonance in a group of 50 trainable mentally retarded children aged 7 years 8 months to 19 years 1 month, whose IQ's ranged from 31 to 55. As measured by TONAR II§ the incidence of hypernasality in this group was found to be 50%, with 36% rated mild, 6% moderate, 2% severe, and 6% very severe. Daly compared these groups to a normal intelligence group where the incidence of hypernasality was found to be 4%, all rated mild.

Speech pathologists should be particularly aware of voice and resonance disorders in children with Down's syndrome and should make an effort to identify and treat voice

§ TONAR II, Scientific-Atlanta, Inc., New Jersey Division, Randolph Park West, Route 10, Randolph Township, NJ 07801

disorders in these children (Montague and Hollien, 1973). Novak (1972) stated a subjective analysis of children with Down's syndrome revealed their voices to be harsh, rough, and characterized by vocal strain; in some children with Down's syndrome the voice has the same characteristics as ventricular phonation. Montague and Hollien (1973) had judges rate the voices of 10 boys and 10 girls with Down's syndrome and 20 normal children. The results indicated that the judges evaluated the Down's syndrome children as having more breathiness, roughness, and hypernasality then the normal children. Also the judges rated the girls with Down's syndrome as having significantly more breathiness and roughness in their voices than the boys with Down's syndrome. The hearing loss in the Down's syndrome group was approximately 35 dB for 500–1000–2000 Hz, which the authors stated may have presented a possible problem interfering with self monitoring of voice.

Montague (1976) found that children with Down's syndrome were perceived as being approximately 2.25 years younger than a normal group of the same chronological age. The judges listened to audiotapes of 18 words recorded by each of the children in both Down's syndrome (mean age, 10.42) and normal intelligence (mean age, 10.41) groups and asked to make judgments as to each child's age. The mean average rating for the normal children was 10.45 years and the children with Down's syndrome 8.17 years.

Studies of the modal frequency level of retarded children show varying results. Weinberg and Zlatin (1970) studied a group of 5- and 6-year-old children with Down's syndrome and compared them with children of normal intelligence. The results were as follows:

	Normal (Hz)		Down's Syndrome (Hz)
	No.		No.	
Boys 5 years	15	252.4	6	310.5
Girls 5 years	18	247.6	9	278.4
Boys 6 years	14	247.3	5	266.1
Girls 6 years	19	247.0	7	283.3
Group Mean		248.4		284.5
S.D. (semitones)		3.0		4.0

The group mean modal frequency level of the Down's syndrome children was significantly higher than that of the normal intelligence group.

On the other hand Montague, Brown, and Hollien (1974) studied 20 children with Down's syndrome, aged 7.8 to 13.5 years. The modal frequency level for the boys was 257 Hz with a standard deviation of 42.5 and for girls 228 Hz with a standard deviation of 20.3. They found no differences between the modal frequency levels of Down's syndrome children and intellectually average children of the same chronological ages. Hollien and Copeland (1965) studied the modal frequency level of nine 10-year-old girls with Down's syndrome. The mean was 244.8 Hz with a standard deviation of 1.31 tones. They stated the modal frequency level was slightly lower than that reported for normal girls but not enough to be considered abnormally low.

Novak (1972) studied 32 children 7 to 19 years of age with Down's syndrome and found the modal frequency level was 230 Hz for girls and 196 Hz for boys. The level in a group of mentally retarded children without Down's syndrome was 230 Hz for both boys and girls. Laryngeal examination of the children with Down's syndrome in this study found only light thickness of the mucosa of the vocal cords and no cases of thickened vocal cords; though in all of them the pharyngeal mucosa showed signs of atrophy and a tendency to drying. The otolaryngologic findings in 20 retarded individuals (aged 7 to 20 years) without Down's syndrome were normal except for one boy who had thickened vocal cords. Novak stated the voice deviations in the children with Down's syndrome could not be explained by the presence of endocrine disorders or pathologic findings on the vocal cords. Novak concluded that mental retardation is not the primary cause of voice disorders in children with Down's syndrome because if it were, retarded children without Down's syndrome would also have the harsh, rough, guttural voice usually associated with Down's syndrome. Further, Montague et al. (1974) stated that deviant voices clinically noted in persons with Down's syndrome are not related to modal frequency level but possibly are related to other vocal parameters yet to be determined.

Hearing Loss

Voice problems related to hearing loss vary considerably according to the type and degree of loss and the type of training program to which the child has been exposed. In many cases the voice problem is so intertwined with problems of articulation and language it is difficult to describe the voice problem in isolation. These speech and voice problems are related to the child's imperfect and often distorted reception of the speech and voice of others and to difficulty in monitoring his own speech.

Calvert and Silverman (1975, p. 183) observed that " ... deviations in voice and irregularities of rhythm are posing less of a problem than heretofore." They attributed this to increasing emphasis on maximum utilization of residual hearing at all stages of development. Ling (1975, p. 211) regarded problems related to voice as resulting from too much early emphasis on articulation skills when there has been insufficient attention paid to the control of breathing and early vocalization.

Improved teaching methods may have resulted in lessening voice problems, but they have not eliminated them. Typical voice problems of children with severe hearing losses are: breathiness, hypernasality, hyponasality, too high pitch (sometimes falsetto), monotony in pitch variation, loudness misuse—either too loud or too soft, too slow rate, monotony in rhythm and rate, hard glottal attack, and differences such as harshness and a hollow, nonresonant quality. Because of possible vocal abuse the speech pathologist should be alert to the possibility of vocal nodules in a child with a hearing loss (Arnold, 1965, p. 637). Habitual use of too-high voice pitch may cause vocal nodules (Ling, 1976, p. 213) particularly if his speech is characterized by breathiness.

Some of these same problems are encountered in children with moderate hearing losses, though they may take a different form and may be less severe. Silverman and Davis (1970, p. 427) indicated voice problems appear in children with hearing losses for speech of 56 dB (ISO, 1964) and greater. Fuller (1970, pp. 208–209) stated voice quality is affected in children with flat audiograms with threshold levels greater than 50 dB, or in children with losses 40 dB or greater in the low frequencies accompanied by greater loss in the high frequencies. Irwin (1965, p. 255) reported inadequate voice quality was noted in 22% of a group of 284 children referred to otological clinics.

Recent advances in medical and surgical treatment for conductive hearing losses and the increased use of hearing aids in all types of losses have reduced speech and voice problems of the hearing impaired. The speech pathologist should be aware that a person with a conductive loss may speak too softly since his own voice reaches him by bone conduction and seems loud while background noise may seem soft. On the other hand a person with a sensorineural loss may tend to speak too loudly in order to hear his own voice, regardless of the presence or absence of background noise.

SUMMARY

Voice problems may be present because of organic conditions. The larynx and adjacent areas may have structural anomalies, either congenital or developmental, including laryngeal webs and laryngomalacia. Vocal cord paralysis is a common congenital cause of voice problems. Laryngeal growths interfering with good voice production include papilloma, cyst, and laryngocele. Disturbed voice production may be the result of intubation, automobile accidents, aspiration of foreign objects, or play activities and sports where the larynx is crushed and fractured. Resonance problems arise from inadequate velopharyngeal valving due to structural deviations or accidents. Growths in the nose cause resonance deviations. Other voice problems are associated with neurological, developmental, and hearing problems. For example, children with cerebral palsy, retardation, or hearing loss often have problems of resonance, pitch, voice quality, and rate. Voice therapy is often indicated for organically based problems and is usually coordinated with physical management.

THREE

Organic Changes due to Vocal Abuse and Vocal Misuse

In the middle of the continum of causation we have voice problems caused by vocal abuse and vocal misuse. Mismanagement of the laryngeal mechanism can cause damage to the vocal cords themselves and also can disturb the muscular coordination necessary for a good voice. Damsté (1973) stated that when the glottis is not completely closed and a high rate of airflow is used, the suction effect (Bernoulli) and other traumatic practices can cause effusions and epithelial thickening to form along the borders of the vocal cords. Edema or nodules of the membranous parts of the cords, leukoplakia of the anterior half, and pachydermia of the posterior half of the glottis may occur. Damsté stated these are the consequences of detrimental voice habits, usually combined with smoking and drinking. Some vocal problems are directly caused by failure to inhibit the action of the extrinsic or swallowing muscles during the production of voice (Zerffi, 1939).

Either vocal abuse or vocal misuse may result in hyperfunction-hypofunction problems of voice. Brodnitz (1971a, p. 55) felt many voice disorders begin with excessive use of muscular force, which Froeschels (1943) termed hyperfunction. After prolonged hyperfunctional use, the muscles become exhausted until they are unable to produce the normal degree of tonus and a weakening sets in (Brodnitz, 1971a, p. 55) and there is reduced adductor laryngeal action (Aronson, Peterson, and Litin, 1964). Froeschels (1943) called this stage hypofunction. von Leden (1958) also stated persistent overexertion of the voice can cause weakness of the laryngeal muscles. Brodnitz (1971a, p. 55) pointed out hyperfunction usually involves the entire vocal mechanism although certain areas of the vocal mechanism may show more hyperfunction sites than others. Overexertion of the muscles of the larynx may cause irritation of the delicate tissues so they become swollen with blood (Harrington, 1950, p.

197). Brodnitz (1967b) stated the excessive vocal strain used by a person who sings or speaks over a cold can set up a pattern of hyperfunctional voice usage that persists after the infection has disappeared; the pattern of excessive muscular exertion and excess breath pressure then becomes a habit. When hypofunction sets in after prolonged hyperfunction, the voice sounds breathy and the cords show a bowing indicating weakness of the thyroarytenoid muscles (Brodnitz, 1971a, p. 57).

Hyperfunctioning vocal practices may result in various pathological conditions in the larynx which cause the voice to sound hoarse, harsh, or breathy, or a combination of these features. These pathologies include vocal nodules, polyps, polypoid changes, vocal fold thickening, hyperkeratosis, nonspecific laryngitis, hematomas, hyperemia of the vocal cords, and hyperplasia of the vocal cords. If there are incorrect vocal practices plus infection, such as in chronic laryngitis, there may be changes in the larynx causing chronic inflammation and thickening of the mucosa of the vocal cords (Moore, 1971a, p. 548).

Incorrect use of the voice is called vocal abuse and vocal misuse. We separate them as two different abnormal vocal practices for etiological, evaluative, and voice therapy purposes. Vocal abuse (Wilson, 1968) or poor vocal hygiene (Cooper and Nahum, 1967) includes traumatizing practices which may be quite detrimental. Vocal abuse is " . . . a combination of many injurious speech habits" (Holinger et al. 1968). Common types of vocal abuse include shouting, screaming, cheering, strained vocalizations, excessive talking, reverse phonation (vocalizing on inhalation), explosive vocalizations, abrupt glottal attack, throat clearing, coughing, and talking in the presence of high level noise. Cigarette smoking, intake of alcohol, and working in dusty places may also be considered vocally detrimental in some adolescents.

27

Vocal misuse refers specifically to improper use of pitch and loudness. Often there is an interplay between vocal abuse and vocal misuse with both present. Loud talking may accompany such vocal abuses as excessive talking and abrupt glottal attack. Vocal abuse and vocal misuse may be more pronounced in the living environment of some children. Loud talking families and large families are conducive to poor vocal habits. Many of the children Loré (1950) studied with laryngeal dysfunction lived in an environment conducive to abuse and misuse of their voices.

VOCAL ABUSE

There are two types of vocal abuse, sudden and violent straining of the voice or continuous use of vocally abusive practices (Kelly and Craik, 1952; Orton, 1951). Froeschels (1940) reported on a group of children under 16 years of age with various types of laryngeal dysfunction. There were 42 children with abrupt glottal attack, 15 children with too violent contraction of the pharyngeal constricting muscles, and 83 with both. Many undesirable vocal habits may originate in infancy and continue throughout childhood into adult life (Zerffi, 1939).

Shouting, Screaming, Cheering

When a person screams, shouts, or engages in cheering, excessive laryngeal tension is present which may result in irritation of the vocal cords. Shouting, screaming, and cheering are heard in children of all ages especially during play and during sports. A cheerleader may have voice problems, and many thousands of high school students are cheerleaders. Jensen (1964) found 12% of 377 female high school cheerleaders were judged to have hoarse voice quality. Shouting during sports activities is frequently heard in boys going through voice change (Peacher, 1952, p. 8). Habits of screaming and shouting during play may cause chronic hoarseness (Harrington, 1950, p. 198), disturbed muscular coordination necessary for phonation (Greene, 1972, p. 112), or vocal nodules (Luchsinger, 1965, p. 158). Vigorous shouting and cheering may cause vascular engorgement, injury to muscles or laryngeal joints, or hematoma (Moore, 1971a, p. 547). Children and adolescent boys are more likely to develop dysphonia than girls other than cheerleaders. This supports the general impression that boys tend to shout and cheer more strenuously than girls, prob-

ably due to the nature of their play and sports activities (Heaver, 1958).

Brodnitz (1971a, p. 57) pointed out "Sheer force is the main element in many voice disturbances. Children who use, and often misuse, their voices in youthful exuberance torture their vocal cords by shouting and yelling until screamers' nodules appear." The adolescent period is a time of muscular instability of the vocal mechanism when it should be free from all strain, yet it is the period when vocal exertion is likely to be very high; a youngster who returns from a ball game or other activity with huskiness, raspiness, and sometimes complete loss of phonation may be permanently damaging his voice (Uris, 1962).

Strained Vocalizations

Strained vocalizations include vocal imitation of cars, trucks, and airplanes during a child's play or when he is talking about noise sources. Usually extreme tension of the neck can be seen when strained vocalizations are made loudly. Strained vocalizations may produce hyperfunction in the vocal mechanism. This is evidenced by constriction of the muscles of the throat with the tongue sometimes thickened and pulled backward by contraction of its intrinsic muscles; in this instance the voice sounds restricted, strangulated, and harsh (Brodnitz, 1971a, p. 56).

Excessive Talking

A child who is vocally active doing much talking especially at a loud level and at an incorrect pitch is apt to have pathological changes in the larynx. West and Ansberry (1968, p. 216) maintained that if the voice is properly used no amount of vigorous vocalization can damage the edges of the vocal cords. Rubin (1964) stated with many singers " ... vocal strain can occur from excessive use of even the most ideally produced voice..." We maintain that prolonged vigorous talking by a child is a vocally abusive practice, sometimes resulting in vocal nodules (Wilson, 1961). Further, talking with normal loudness and pitch excessively from morning to night is also a vocal abuse (Orton, 1951; Perkins, 1957, p. 866; Wilson, 1961; 1962b).

Explosive Vocalizations and Abrupt Glottal Attack

Excessive use of explosive vocalizations and abrupt glottal attack result in irritation in the laryngeal area causing the voice to sound hoarse or harsh. Pathological changes, such as vocal nodules, may result from the overuse of this type of glottal attack. It may lead to hypofunctioning due to weakening of laryngeal muscles (Brodnitz, 1971a, p. 57). Koike and von Leden (1969) studied vocal initiation in adults with laryngeal pathology and concluded " . . . 1) the abruptness of the initiation increases in pathological phonations, and 2) laryngeal tumors are especially related to abrupt initiation." They found the mean rise time for the tumor group was about the same as the abrupt initiation exhibited by normal laryngeal subjects; their unilateral paralysis group's rise time was approximately the same as breathy initiation in normal subjects. Thus we can assume that abrupt initiation is characteristic of those with various types of tumor including laryngeal papilloma and vocal cord polyps. This was a study of the laryngeal performance of adults with voice pathology which we are applying to children. However, we have found that children with vocal nodules characteristically use an abrupt glottal attack.

Coughing and Throat Clearing

Many children with laryngeal dysfunction cough and clear their throats excessively. Senturia and Wilson (1968) found a history of recurrent coughing in half of 92 school-aged children with voice deviations. The percentage of children with a history of coughing was about the same for the group who had vocal cord lesions as for those who did not. Also vocal abuse may be associated with excessive laughing and crying. Analyses of high speed motion pictures of the larynx reveal vigorous changes in the larynx during even the mildest laughter or clearing of the throat (Timcke et al. 1959). von Leden and Isshiki (1965) studied laryngeal activities during coughing. An analysis of the high speed motion pictures indicated that a single cough impulse has three phases, " . . . an initial wide opening of the glottis, a protracted firm closure, and a complex vibratory (expiratory) phase." The vibratory or expiratory phase involves the vocal cords as well as the supraglottic structures and the mucosal lining of the posterior laryngeal wall. During a cough these structures undergo violent periodic undulations demonstrating the deleterious effect of a cough upon the delicate tissues of the larynx.

We have worked with children with vocal nodules who, with other vocal abuses, coughed excessively and vigorously. A cough may be a symptom of many different types of physical problems. A habitual hacking cough is symptomatic of allergic reactions to certain foods (Missal, 1961).

Punt (1974) stated lack of essential lubrication of the whole vocal mechanism by adequate mucus supply, especially from the glands in the laryngeal ventricles, may be self evident in listening to people who have to pause at intervals to clear their throats. Lack of adequate lubrication may be due to emotional factors, including stage fright, nose and sinus conditions, excessive smoking and drinking, the sicca (drying) syndrome, medications such as 'cold cures' which inhibit mucous and salivary secretion, and inadequate air conditioning.

An unusually long uvula sometimes causes a chronic cough, and it is sometimes amputated (DeWeese and Saunders, 1973, p. 35). We knew a 7-year-old boy who had a persistent cough which the laryngologist felt was one of the vocal abuses contributing to the vocal nodule formation. An examination revealed a very long uvula hanging down into the pharynx and touching the base of the tongue. The physician excised the tip of the uvula so it no longer caused a tickling irritation and the resulting cough. Schubert (1963) also described this problem in two patients who had persistent coughs; the simple excision of part of the uvula under local anesthesia rid these patients of their coughs.

Frequent throat clearing is probably one of the most common vocal abuses. This may be due to a variety of medical problems, including allergy to ingested foods (Missal, 1961). Any possible medical reasons for this should be checked, but often it is present on a habitual basis.

VOCAL MISUSE (PITCH, LOUDNESS)

The pitch and loudness of a child's voice need to be well controlled. Vocal misuse takes place when one or both of these aspects of voice are not used correctly. Usually we find children have modal pitch and loudness levels within the range of acceptability. However, in some children traumatizing misuse occurs through the intermittent but frequent and daily use of too-high and too-loud voices. Of course, these misuses can be present in some children on a continual basis. These misuses may take place during talking and singing. Habitual excessive loudness is detrimental to the vocal mechanism. Isshiki, Okamura, and Morimoto (1967) found distension of the trachea during loud phonation because of increased subglottal pressure. Thus we believe if excessive loud talking results in frequent distension of the trachea, muscle hyperfunctioning is created in this area. This can lead to chronic vocal abuse. The use of high intensity or high pitch levels is indicative of general incorrect use of voice (Perkins, 1971, p. 524). Vocal misuse may result in various types of laryngeal dysfunction characterized by harshness, breathiness, or hoarseness. The amount of talking in high level noise should be investigated when vocal abuse and vocal misuse are thought to be contributing to the cause of a voice disorder.

Talking in Noise

Normal speech communication, according to Miller (1974), can take place in noise levels of 66 dBA or lower at the usual distance from talker to listener of about 5 feet. At 5 to 12 feet between speaker and listener the background noise should be less than 50 to 60 dBA, and at public meetings or outdoor places where distances between the talker and listener are in the order of 12 to 30 feet the background noise should be kept below 40 to 55 dBA. Both vocal abuse and vocal misuse occur when a person talks in the presence of noise levels greater than these. Schiff (1973) stated speech to be understood must be at least 6 dB greater than the ambient noise level. He stated when one shouts in noise levels of 90 dB or greater for any length of time it is no wonder that sore throat, hoarseness, and vocal nodules commonly develop.

Vocal nodules are often found in workers who speak in high noise levels (Ferguson, 1955). The necessity for shouting to override excessive noise is enough to have a traumatic effect on the vocal cords if it continues over a period of time. However, the relationship of loudness and pitch is such that a person speaking in the presence of noise not only speaks loudly but also uses a higher pitch than he does habitually. Several studies have demonstrated an interrelationship between pitch and loudness.

What happens to loudness and pitch in a quiet environment? Brackett (1946) measured pitch levels of young adults under four loudness levels, soft conversational, conversa-

tional, interphone-aircraft, and shouting. The average pitch levels rose a total of 82.4 Hz (10 semitones) from 119.4 Hz to 201.8 Hz. The rises from one level to another were 16.6 Hz (4 semitones), 18.8 Hz (2 semitones), and 47.0 Hz (4 semitones). Black (1961), using 20 young adult males as subjects, had them say vowels and phrases. They were instructed to register 70, 80, 90, and 100 dB on a sound level meter; 70 dB was considered soft speech and 100 dB was considered loud speech. Rises in pitch with increased loudness were also measured in this study. The average total rise in pitch was 125 Hz (13 semitones) as the subjects went from 70 to 100 dB in loudness. The rise in pitch, however, was not equal among the different sound pressure levels studied. When the loudness increased from 70 to 80 dB there was a 13 Hz rise (2 semitones) in pitch, from 80 to 90 dB an additional 38 Hz rise (5 semitones), and from 90 to 100 dB an additional 74 Hz rise (6 semitones).

Ptacek and Sander (1963), in their study of 80 young adults, asked subjects to take a deep breath and phonate the vowel /ɑ/ as long as possible while monitoring intensity on a volume unit (VU) meter with a microphone 2 in from the mouth. Subjects were not asked to control the fundamental frequency of phonation. Soft phonation was held at 82 dB, moderate phonation 91 dB, and loud phonation 99dB. The Hertz rises were as follows. For the men the three median frequency levels were soft phonation 120 Hz, moderate phonation up 14 Hz (1 semitone) to 134 Hz, loud phonation up 21 Hz (3 semitones) to 155 Hz, a total rise of 35 Hz (4 semitones). For the women the three median frequency levels were soft phonation 225 Hz, moderate phonation up 12 Hz to 237 Hz, loud phonation up 11 Hz to 248 Hz, a total rise of only 23 Hz (2 semitones).

Pearsons, Bennett, and Fidell (1976) reported on speech levels in various environments. They stated the distance between the talker and listener is important primarily when conversation takes place in an outdoor environment where speech levels are reduced 6 dB for every doubling of distance between the talker and listener. This is not as true while talking indoors because the distance between talker and speaker is not as critical. They found that in background levels of ambient noise less than 48 dB people maintained an average voice level of 55 dB when the distance averaged one meter (39.37 in). In background levels above 48 dB and up to 70 dB, people began to raise their voice levels up to an average of 67 dB, at the rate of 0.6 dB per 1 dB increase in the ambient noise level, with the same distance of 1 meter between speaker and listener. Speech levels at various vocal efforts were measured in children in an anechoic chamber where the background level of noise was 16 dB. The means (and standard deviations) for five speech levels are as follows: Casual, 53.0 (5.0), Normal 58.0 (5.0), Raised 65.0 (7.0), Loud 74.0 (9.0), Shout 82.0 (9.0). Acoustical analyses of speech in the anechoic chamber indicated that vocal emphasis shifted from the low frequencies to the high frequencies as level of speaking went from normal to shout. Thus we can see that vocal intensity increases as the level of background noise increases, and as vocal effort increases the pitch of the voice is dramatically raised.

Harris and Weiss (1964) found in a group of adult male speakers there was an average increase in pitch of approximately 40% for loud speech and a decrease in pitch of approximately 12% for soft speech. Thus when we examine a child's use of pitch he should be observed when he is talking loudly, normally, and softly. When we decrease loudness we get a dividend in lowering the pitch level without paying much attention to the pitch itself.

We know high levels of noise are detrimental to the hearing mechanism and should be avoided. We are especially interested in the misuse and abuse of the voice when a person talks in a noisy environment. Talking in noise causes a person to talk louder as noise levels increase (Hanley and Steer, 1949). Mills (1975) stated noise levels of 60 to 65 dBA often require the speaker to increase the voice level and vocal effort, and that levels of 75 dBA often require the talker to shout. We will present some of the studies done on noise in the environment in order to illustrate the effect environmental noise may have on the loudness, pitch level, and vocal abuse in the voice. We are interested especially in those situations where children and adolescents are apt to be talking for prolonged periods of time in high level noise. These situations include riding in automobiles, using farm machinery, listening to rock music, and using motorized sports equipment. Shown below is the effect of noise on loudness and pitch of the voice in adult males.

Voice Loudness and Pitch Levels

Shouting Voice (100 dB)
(Pitch Rises 21–74 Hz)

↑

Very Loud Voice (90 dB)
(Pitch Rises 14–38 Hz)

↑

Raised Voice (80 dB)
(Pitch Rises 13–17 Hz)

↑

Normal Voice (70 dB)
(Normal Pitch Level)

The four loudness levels of voice shown are normal voice, raised voice, very loud voice, and shouting voice. The decibel levels for these speaking conditions are 70, 80, 90, and 100 dB (Black, 1961). The Hertz rises between each intensity level are 13 to 17 Hz, 14 to 38 Hz, and 21 to 74 Hz (Black 1961; Brackett, 1946; Ptacek and Sander, 1963). This information should be used conservatively because we have combined studies not originally designed to be combined. Also its use is limited because the data is on adult males. Let's take an example of how this information might be used as a rough guide in an actual situation. If a man with a normal voice and modal frequency level is talking at 70 dB and he raises his voice to 80 dB, then the voice frequency level goes up 13 to 17 Hz (2 to 4 semitones). If it is necessary to speak in a very loud voice, he increases the loudness to 90 dB and his voice pitch rises 14 to 38 Hz (1 to 5 semitones). If it is necessary for him to shout, his voice goes to 100 dB and the pitch rises another 21 to 74 Hz (3 to 6 semitones). This is a total rise in pitch ranging from ¼ octave to more than a full octave.

When riding in an automobile at high speeds it is necessary to talk in a very loud voice in order to be heard because of the level of noise created by the high speed movement of a car. The increase in loudness causes a rise in pitch, also an increased amount of vocal abuse. We have all had the experience of finding the volume of a car radio too loud when we slowed down from expressway speeds to 20 or 30 miles an hour on an exit ramp. Bolt, Beranek, and Newman, Inc. (1965) measured the noise in automobiles.

They found the amount of noise within automobiles went from 71 dB at 20 miles an hour to 78 dB at 40, and up to 82 dB at 60 miles an hour. This means a person would have to speak at a level of a shout at 100 dB to be heard one foot from the listener when a car is traveling 60 miles an hour (Beranek, 1947; Beranek and Rudmose, 1947; Rosenblith and Stevens, 1953).

If the child with a voice problem lives in a farm community, the possibility of his talking in the presence of machine noise should be explored. Many young farm children ride for hours with their father on a tractor and at an early age begin to operate the tractor themselves often with another child riding with them. Talking in such conditions may have deleterious effects on the voice. Jones and Oser (1968) found the noise level near the tractor operator's ear averaged 105 dB when the tractor was operated under full load. Ouzts (1969) reported the noise level of three different pieces of farm machinery measured approximately 1 in from the operator's ear on a plane parallel to the side of the head. Farm tractor noise was 96 dB sound pressure level (SPL), bean combine noise 102 dB SPL, and cotton picker noise 107 dB SPL. Also Lierle and Reger (1958) found noise levels in farm tractors measured 6 in from the ear ranged from approximately 85 dB SPL to 102 dB SPL (300 to 1200 Hz octave bands).Gupta (1977, p. 13, p. 42, p. 49) reported the noise level of farm tractors operating at full load measured with a microphone located near the right ear of the operator ranged from 78.5 dBA to as high as 101.5 dBA, and at the ear of a bystander 25 feet from the line of travel of the tractor the noise level was 100.15 dBA.

Talking while listening to rock groups, or to rock music in stereo earphones may be detrimental to the voice. The intensity of live rock music has been measured and found to range from 94 dB SPL to 150 dB SPL with an average of 120 dB SPL depending upon the distance from a group and the Hertz band being measured. Lebo, Oliphant, and Garrett (1967) measured the intensity of rock groups in the center of auditoriums as being from 109 to 122 dB LIN (the unweighted sound pressure levels between 20 and 20,000 Hz). Lebo and Oliphant (1968) measured rock group levels from the center of the performing hall as being from 100 to 116 dBA. Rupp and Koch (1969) measured sound pressure levels generated in a practice room of a rock

group and found the range to be 120 to 130 dBC. Lipscomb (1969) in an animal experiment used 122 dB as the peak level representing sound levels approximating those measured in dance halls. Flugrath (1969) found the level of rock music measured one foot from the midpoint of the stage and 6 feet above the dance floor ranged from 94.32 dB to 102.05 dB at the octave band level of 2000 Hz. Jerger and Jerger (1970) found rock group music ranged from 104 to 124 dB SPL in the octave bands 300–600 Hz and 600–1200 Hz with peaks as high as 130 dB. The modal signal level during a 4 hour period was estimated at 110 to 120 dB in the octave band 600–1200 Hz. These measures were taken at the center of the group with measurements on either side of the stage ranging from 108 to 116 dBC SPL. Flugrath, Irwin, Wolfe, Krone, and Parnell (1971) measured rock music at several different points in a basement dance hall without windows, 52 by 52 feet, with concrete block walls, asbestos tile floor, and acoustic tile ceiling. They found the levels ranged from 96 to 113 dBA and 104 to 117 dBC. Ulrich and Pinheiro (1974) reported on rock music measurements as ranging from 110 dB to 115 dB SPL with the loudest range in the spectral distribution from 75 Hz to 1200 Hz with a slight peak between 300 Hz and 600 Hz. At times during measurements the SPL peaked beyond the 150 dB maximum capacity of the sound level meter. Measurements were taken at different points around a large stage. Kuras and Findlay (1974) had a group of 25 rock music listeners, age range 18 to 25 with a mean age of 21 years, adjust the loudness level according to most comfortable loudness level while listening to recorded rock music through headphones. Two rock recordings were used: a standard recording selected by the experimenter and one brought in by each listener. The most comfortable loudness level adjusted by the subjects for the standard recording was 88.1 dBA, and the level was 92.7 dBA for their own recording. Wood and Lipscomb (1972) found the level of rock music measured in stereo earphones ranged from 75 dBA to 155 dBA.

Bess, Gale, Aarni, and Redfield (1974) reported the noise in snowmobiles reaching the ear of a driver without ear protection was 110 dB or slightly higher by octave band analysis for 500, 1000, and 2000 Hz. Also octave band analysis for 125 Hz to 8000 Hz indicated that the snowmobile noise was in excess of 100 dB. Bess and Poynor (1972) measured sound pressure levels in snowmobiles at the approximate height of the driver's head. For a 22 hp snowmobile at approximately midthrottle the SPL ranged from 86 to 113 dBA. Also the SPL for a 26 hp engine at full throttle ranged from 105 to 136 dBA. In another study Bess and Poynor (1974) found the typical racing snowmobile noise varied from 132 dBA to 136 dBA. Noise levels within the spectator area averaged 106 dBA and ranged from 103 to 108 dBA at a distance of 6 meters (about 20 feet) from the track. Exposure to noise during a snowmobile meet extended for 3 to 4 hours or more. We can thus see that not only the snowmobile driver himself but also spectators within a range of 6 meters experience high level noise, and talking in the presence of such noise either by the driver or spectators requires excessive vocal tension and abuse.

The farm machinery, rock band, and sports equipment levels indicate a child talking in these noise conditions would usually have to use a shouting voice.

THE ORGANIC CHANGES

Vocal Nodules

Vocal nodules are the most frequently occurring pathological change and are seen in over half the children with deviant voices (Shearer, 1972). Vocal nodules develop, according to Aronson (1973, p. 14), as a result of the friction of soft tissue against soft tissue with a building up of hyperkeratotic epithelium and the development of fibrosis underneath. A vocal nodule first appears as a tiny elevation on one vocal cord and then later on the other. The development of a vocal cord nodule usually involves three stages. First, a localized slight reddening appears on the free margin of the vocal cord with the submucosa showing dilation of the thin-walled blood vessels (Withers, 1961). This may be the sign of a very small hemorrhage (DeWeese and Saunders, 1973, p. 135) or a mucous gland beginning to close (Voorhees, 1934). Second, there then occurs a localized swelling or thickening on the edge of the vocal cord (Arnold, 1963; Levbarg, 1939) with or without reddening. Third, a definite nodule forms with the thickening being replaced by fibrotic tissue and the nodule appears white, the same color as the free margin of the vocal cord

(DeWeese and Saunders, 1973, p. 135) or sometimes grayish (Aronson, 1973, p. 14).

Grey (1973) provided a different developmental sequence for vocal nodules. He used a microlaryngostroboscope in his study. He stated vocal nodules and polyps which occur at the junction of the anterior and middle thirds of the cords are due to mucosal distortion on abduction and not the trauma of adduction. As the vocal cords abduct, a triangular fold of mucous membrane is raised. When the cords further abduct, this is the last point to separate and corresponds to the site of vocal nodules. As a result of this continued raising of mucous membrane a thickening of the mucous membrane occurs due to squamous hyperplasia. Hemorrhage may occur at this point as the mucous membrane is continually being lifted from its base with blood accumulating in the potential space formed. Eventually organization of a fibrous nodule or polyp takes place. The repeated raising of the mucous membrane may lead to the accumulation of edema fluid resulting in a low-grade inflammatory process (Grey, 1973).

Sometimes inflammation is present around the area of the nodule. Figure 6 shows newly formed vocal nodules. They are concentrated and well defined and accompanied by a minimum of inflammation. Figures 7 and 8 show more mature nodules which are more diffuse with more inflammation present. The nodule ranges in diameter from one to several millimeters (Withers, 1961) with 3 mm being considered a very large vocal nodule. Some laryngologists subjectively rate the vocal cords and the size of nodules on a 5 point scale: 1, clear cords; 2, tiny nodules; 3, small nodules; 4, moderate nodules; and 5, large nodules (Deal, McClain, and Sudderth, 1976). The mean nodule rating in the Deal et al. (1976) study was 3.74 for boys (mean age, 8 years 6 months) and for the girls 3.08 (mean age, 8 years 7 months). At no time is there usually any pain connected with this process from the very beginning to the formation of a mature fully formed vocal cord nodule (Aronson, 1973, p. 14; DeWeese and Saunders, 1973, p. 135).

Vocal nodules may be unilateral or bilateral and are typically located on the edge of the free margin of the vocal cord in the area where there is maximum vibration, that is at the junction of the anterior and middle thirds of the vocal cord (Aronson, 1973, p. 14; Brodnitz, 1971a, p. 73; von Leden, 1958; Withers,

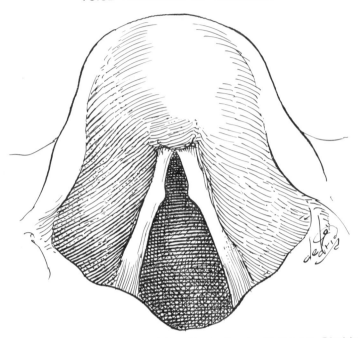

FIG. 6. Newly formed vocal nodules. Illustration by Melford D. Diedrick.

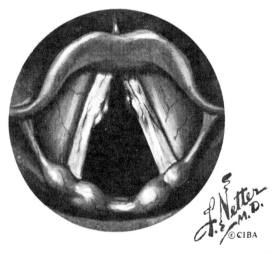

FIG. 7. Vocal nodules (inspiration). Copyright *Clinical Symposia* by Frank H. Netter, M.D., published by CIBA Pharmaceutical Company.

1961). When vocal nodules are described as appearing in the middle third of the cord, this description does not include the nonvibrating or cartilaginous posterior third of the cord (the vocal process) (Arnold, 1964; 1966). Actually the nodules are at the same location in both descriptions. Often two nodules are exactly opposite each other and contact during phonation (DeWeese and Saunders, 1973, p. 135). Size, composition, and location of the vocal nodules play an important part in the

degree of hoarseness present. Extremely small nodules produce no symptoms, while others produce hoarseness (DeWeese and Saunders, 1973, p. 135). Although a large mass generally produces more breathiness, a vocal nodule that is hard and not compressible can cause a faulty voice even though it is quite small (Moore, 1971a, p. 542).

Each child with vocal nodules has to be studied thoroughly in order to establish the cause or causes so the proper treatment pro-

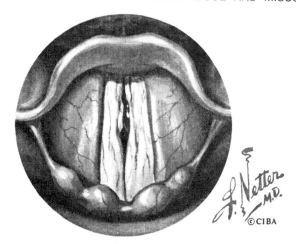

FIG. 8. Vocal nodules (phonation). Copyright *Clinical Symposia* by Frank .H. Netter, M.D., published by CIBA Pharmaceutical Company.

gram can be outlined. Thus following the discovery of vocal nodules the question, "Why has this child developed this problem?" must be answered. Anderson and Newby (1973, p. 270) stated it is difficult to explain why one child develops vocal nodules while another child can talk even more incessantly and yell even louder without developing vocal nodules. They stated it is not clear why one child's vocal organs just "can't take it." They further stated perhaps some allergy or structural weakness renders a particular child's larynx more susceptible to damage from strenuous use or from vocalization that would ordinarily be considered not unusual for his age. Other factors may be involved, including psychological, developmental, and hearing sensitivity.

The development of vocal nodules in children usually is the result of some sort of combination of (1) vocal abuse and vocal misuse, (2) chronic upper respiratory problems based on infections or allergies (Arnold, 1963; Withers, 1961), (3) the psychological living environment (home influence, size of family), (4) the physical living environment (air pollution), (5) the personality and general adjustment of the child (Arnold, 1963; Withers, 1961), and (6) endocrine imbalance especially thyroid (Arnold, 1963; Withers, 1961). Basic to all is a constitutional tendency toward development of vocal nodules (Arnold, 1963; Kelly and Craik, 1952; Luchsinger, 1965, p. 176).

Yelling, screaming, and arguing are common in children with vocal nodules and can signal chronically defective interpersonal re-

lationships (Aronson, 1973, p. 15). Wilson (1971) reported that vocal nodules can be physical symptoms of a child's emotional needs. In the St. Louis study it was shown that children with vocal nodules were about three times more talkative than their peers who did not have nodules; also, teachers indicated children with voice problems were among the more difficult to manage. Wilson concluded that vocal cord nodules are a symptom of generalized verbal aggression.

Vocal abuse and vocal misuse head the list of the basic reasons for the development of vocal nodules. Aronson (1973, pp. 14–15) stated vocal nodules are caused by vocal abuse, usually resulting from speaking, screaming, or singing at pitch levels that are excessively high. They occur in both boys and girls who shout, scream, or talk excessively. Vocal nodules are " . . . visible organic changes that are the consequence of a functional disorder" (Brodnitz and Froeschels, 1954). Specific misuse or abuse contributing to vocal nodules includes excessive laryngeal tension and the habitual use of too high pitch (Peacher, 1952, pp. 8–9). Aronson (1973, p. 14) stated vocal abuse related to nodules usually occurs at higher pitch levels because the area of trauma is in the anterior portion of the vocal cords. Others feel that using a too-low modal frequency level may explain the development of a nodule (Fisher and Logemann, 1970; Cooper, 1974). Other conditions can be the use of the voice at a pitch for which the larynx was not designed, as by cheerleaders and other speakers, prolonged vigorous use of the voice (Moore, 1971a, p.

547), or simply the use of the voice for too many hours a day (Withers, 1961). Habitually using a loud voice seems to be responsible for vocal nodules in many cases with a history of talking in noise, talking to people with hearing losses or yelling at high levels of intensity (Van Riper and Irwin, 1958, pp. 187–188). Long singing lessons (Van Riper and Irwin, 1958, pp. 187–188), the use of improper methods of singing (Orton, 1951), and singing during acute inflammation of the cords contribute to the formation of vocal nodules (Luchsinger, 1965, p. 178; Withers, 1961).

The following is a case report of a child with vocal nodules (adapted from Wilson (1961)).

Billy was 5½ years old when his parents first noticed occasional hoarseness. During the next 6 months the periods of hoarseness became more and more frequent until the child continuously talked with a hoarse voice. Billy's pediatrician referred him to a laryngologist. The laryngeal examination revealed bilateral nodules about the size of a pinhead at the junction of the anterior and middle thirds of the vocal cords. A referral was made by the laryngologist to the speech clinic. During the initial interview the parents stated that Billy was an active boy liking sports and outdoor activities where much yelling, loud talking, and other forms of vocal abuse were noticed.

Voice analysis revealed that the child's conversational voice was hoarse in a mild to moderate degree. Under some conditions the voice sounded high in pitch and at times the voice was dysphonic and even aphonic especially at the ends of breath groups. Isolated vowels were analyzed for hoarseness. A psychological evaluation showed the child to be above average in intelligence with no evidence of emotional problems. Treatment was started with Billy on the basis of two sessions a week. The parents were counseled periodically about helping the child at home with carryover activities. After 3 months a laryngeal examination revealed a significant reduction in the size of the nodules. Treatment was continued for another 3 months when again the laryngologist reported a continuing reduction in the size of the nodules. During the next 6 months the sessions were gradually reduced in number from twice a week to once a month. A recheck by the laryngologist 1 year after treatment had been started revealed the nodules had completely disappeared. The mother reported the child no longer had any undesirable vocal habits, his voice was free from hoarseness, and the pitch seemed generally lower. Periodic rechecks in the speech clinic during the following year indicated the child's voice was lower in pitch and completely free from hoarseness.

Polyps

Polyps of the vocal cord were described by Baker (1963) as follows. They are the most common of the benign tumors of the larynx. They are not true tumors because they arise as the result of abuse of the larynx either from continued abuse or a single traumatic episode. A sudden violent use of the larynx can cause a submucosal hemorrhage and an organization of the hemorrhage into the formation of a tumor composed of connective tissue and blood. Degenerations lead further to a clearing of the blood with a formation of tissue liquid and a translucent appearance. The polyp increases in size with continued use of the voice. A polyp is usually single and is attached to the junction of the anterior and middle thirds of the vocal cord. It may be on top of the cord or on the edge of the cord. Sometimes the polyp is subglottic (Fig. 9) arising from the under edge of the vocal cord. The polyp may be one of two types, pedunculated or sessile (Figs. 10 and 11). Hoarseness varies according to the size and location of the polyp. The patient clears his throat frequently. The presence of a polyp requires increased effort in phonating and as a result the patient becomes exhausted when he does much talking.

Polypoid laryngitis, which according to Baker (1963) is sometimes called chronic hypertrophic laryngitis and polyposis of the vocal cords, results from the continued misuse and abuse of the voice. He stated that this is a condition in which small vocal nodules undergo degeneration into small polypoid tumors which eventually involve the entire edge and the surface of both cords (Fig. 12). This condition is more common in adults than children.

Dysphonia Plicae Ventricularis

In some cases severe voice alteration is due to dysphonia plicae ventricularis which is the

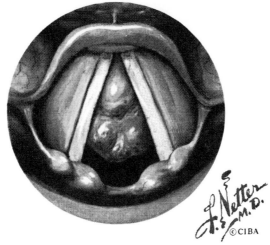

FIG. 9. Subglottic polyp. Copyright *Clinical Symposia* by Frank H. Netter, M.D., published by CIBA Pharmaceutical Company.

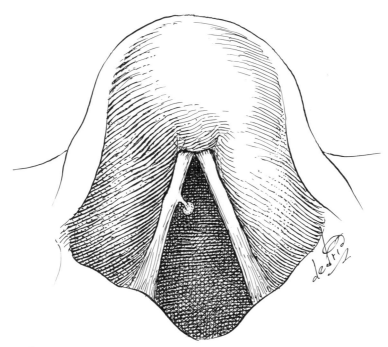

FIG. 10. Pedunculated polyp. Illustration by Melford D. Diedrick.

use of the false vocal cords instead of the true vocal cords for phonation. It is also called ventricular phonation and hyperkinesia of false cords (Fig. 13). As DeWeese and Saunders (1973, p. 116) stated this condition is a common cause of hoarseness frequently overlooked. The voice symptoms are quite distinct in this type of problem with the voice usually lower than normal in pitch with a restricted pitch range and with some characteristics of vocal fry present. Usually the laugh, the cry, and the cough are unaffected. Laryngeal examination reveals according to Fred (1962) that during quiet breathing the false cords appear normal although often thickened. When a person is asked to phonate, the false vocal cords close and are seen to vibrate. This problem may be due to vocal abuse, vocal misuse, or psychological stress; it may follow an operation; it may be present on a congen-

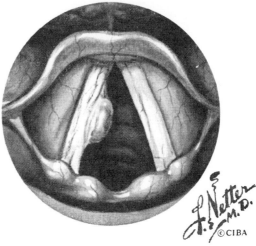

FIG. 11. Sessile polyp. Copyright *Clinical Symposia* by Frank H. Netter, M.D., published by CIBA Pharmaceutical Company.

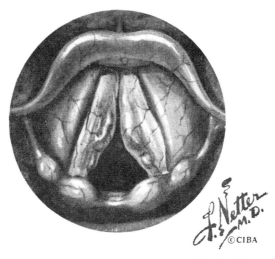

FIG. 12. Polypoid degeneration of true cords. Copyright *Clinical Symposia* by Frank H. Netter, M.D., published by CIBA Pharmaceutical Company.

ital basis with true vocal cords present or on a congenital basis in the absence of true vocal cords.

Vocal abuse and misuse can result in such severe pathology of the true vocal cords that a person is forced to use the false vocal cords for phonation. Talking in this manner may be temporary until the pathology of the true vocal cords is resolved or the person may continue to use ventricular phonation on a habitual basis. In psychogenic ventricular dysphonia the false cords are used for phonation even though the true vocal cords themselves are intact. This may occur according to Brodnitz (1971a, p. 82) after severe attacks of laryngitis or after removal of benign tu-

mors of the true vocal cords; thus the patient sometimes without being aware of it is afraid to use his vocal cords and substitutes ventricular phonation for true vocal cord phonation; this causes the person to tire easily and to complain about pains while speaking. Insecurity or neurosis may be the cause of this type of ventricular cord phonation (Freud, 1962).

Ventricular phonation may follow operations. Parisier and Henneford (1969) reported on an 11-year-old boy who had had three operations for the removal of juvenile laryngeal papillomas, one operation at 4 years of age and two at 5 years of age. After the last two operations the child developed persistent

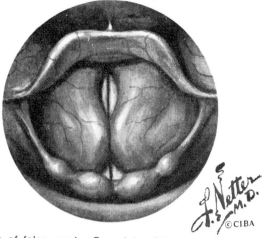

FIG. 13. Hyperkinesia of false cords. Copyright *Clinical Symposia* by Frank H. Netter, M.D., published by CIBA Pharmaceutical Company.

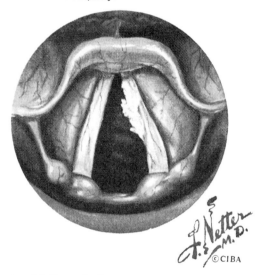

FIG. 14. Hyperkeratosis of left cord. Copyright *Clinical Symposia* by Frank H. Netter, M.D., published by CIBA Pharmaceutical Company.

hoarseness and mild dyspnea on extreme exertion. At 11 years of age a laryngeal web was discovered and removed. When his voice showed only minimal improvement during the next 6 months the laryngologist noted the child phonated with the false vocal cords and voice therapy was recommended for development of a more adequate voice. Obviously the elimination of false vocal cord phonation was the goal of voice therapy.

Hyperkeratosis

The beginning hyperkeratotic lesion in adults according to Cracovaner (1959) is a small red thickening on the edge of a vocal cord. It may be either on the anterior third or middle third of the vocal cord or both (Fig.

14). He felt hyperkeratotic lesions are due to chronic irritation including overindulgence in alcohol, excessive smoking, abuse of the voice, and inhalation of dust and fumes. Laryngeal examinations of elementary school children in the Baynes and Wendling (1965) study revealed hyperkeratotic plaques on the edges of the vocal cords in 57 of 242 children with harsh or breathy voices. Hyperkeratotic lesions in children are no doubt due to abuse of the voice, inhalation of dust and fumes, or chronic infection of the sinuses or pharynx. Baynes and Wendling (1965) described a hyperkeratotic plaque as a somewhat irregular white thickening of the mucosa, on the edge of the middle third of the vocal cord with the cord showing evidence of inflammation. Ro-

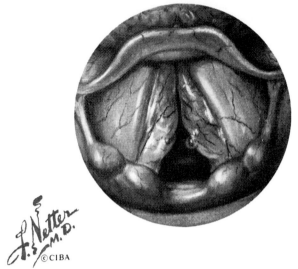

FIG. 15. Edematous vocal cords in chronic laryngitis. Copyright *Clinical Symposia* by Frank H. Netter, M.D., published by CIBA Pharmaceutical Company.

sedale and Nowara (1960) described hyperkeratosis as a " . . . typical pearly raised thickening of the mucosa with apparently normal movement of the vocal cords."

Nonspecific Laryngitis

In nonspecific or chronic laryngitis there is thickening and reddening of the vocal cords due to vocal abuse (Fig. 15). The diagnosis of nonspecific laryngitis can be made if vocal abuse can be demonstrated and all possible sources of infection or irritation excluded (Brodnitz, 1971a, p. 72). Hoarseness is a primary symptom. There may be no indicated medical treatment with voice therapy proving beneficial when vocal abuse and vocal misuse are the factors maintaining the nonspecific laryngitis (Van Thal, 1961).

SUMMARY

Organic changes in the larynx take place because of vocal abuse and vocal misuse. The development of pathology may occur or the fine muscle coordination required in a good voice may be disturbed. Vocal abuse can be a sudden violent use of the phonatory system, such as cheering at a ball game, or more continuous use such as excessive talking. Other vocal abuses are shouting, screaming, strained vocalizations, reverse phonation, explosive vocalizations, abrupt glottal attack, throat clearing, and coughing. Vocal misuse occurs when a child talks at a high level of vocal intensity or at a pitch level not appropriate for the laryngeal structures. Both vocal abuse and vocal misuse take place when talking in the presence of high level continuous noise. In many noisy situations a person must raise his vocal intensity to 90 or 100 dB, and at the same time the pitch level rises from one-fourth to more than a full octave. Noisy situations include talking while riding in automobiles, around farm machinery, listening to rock music, and using motorized sports equipment. The organic changes include vocal nodules, polyps, dysphonia plicae ventricularis, hyperkeratosis, and nonspecific laryngitis.

FOUR

Functional Causes and Contributing Factors

FUNCTIONAL CAUSES

In a functional voice disorder there is nothing wrong with the vocal mechanism. Even though a child has a healthy larynx, oral structures, and a healthy body, the use of voice quality (laryngeal dysfunction), resonance, loudness, or pitch is inadequate. Damsté (1973) used the term *habitual dysphonia* for laryngeal dysfunction. He stated that characteristically this type of problem occurs in a person whose voice has never been very good, with the problem having a gradual remote onset over a long period of time. The symptoms are constant and there is a history of voice strain—usually during mutation—or frequent occurrences of laryngitis, upper respiratory infections, and bronchitis. The voice problem may be present on a psychological basis or may be the result of imitation. Many children with voice abnormalities have no visible dysfunction or pathology upon laryngoscopy. This problem, according to Moore, White, and von Leden (1962), may be due to unusual or abnormal vibratory patterns of the vocal cords in the absence of actual pathology. A functional voice disorder may be characterized by normal laryngoscopic examination results with or without abnormal stroboscopic examination results; the dysphonia is more severe than any lesions or inflammations appear to warrant; and the problem may be of nervous origin but may in turn be conducive to the formation of organic lesions (Perello, 1962). A functional voice disorder is reversible and disappears when the vocal organs are used correctly (Perello, 1962).

Functional causes of voice problems of children can be divided into four categories: (1) disturbed mutation, (2) psychological, (3) imitation, and (4) faulty learning. All functional voice problems may have some organic factors included in the cause. For example, disturbed mutation may have a bona fide organic cause, but we are discussing it here because the problem is usually functional or psychogenic.

Prepubertal and Pubertal Changes in the Voice

During puberty there is normally a change in the modal frequency level of the voice due to growth changes in the larynx. This process is called mutation. A boy's pitch lowers about an octave and a girl's 3 to 4 semitones. In most males, according to Aronson (1973, p. 59), complete mutation of voice takes place within 3 to 6 months. During this time the neck lengthens and the larynx descends as well as grows in size. Zemlin (1968, p. 212) reported that at 15 years of age the vocal cords are about 9.5 mm in length for both sexes. During mutation the male vocal cords grow about 10 mm and become thicker. The female vocal cords grow about 4 mm. According to Kaplan (1960, p. 144) adult male vocal cords range from 17 to 23 mm and the female vocal cords from 12.5 to 17 mm. Most children, both boys and girls, go through voice change without any residual voice problems. However, in some instances there is disturbed mutation. Luchsinger (1965, p. 193) classified disturbed mutation in boys according to three clinical forms: (1) delayed mutation—the vocal changes do not take place until several years later than usual; (2) prolonged mutation—a persistence of the clinical signs of voice change over several years instead of just a few months; (3) incomplete mutation—the voice does not fully develop into the normal voice of an adult. In all three forms the voice is characterized by high pitch, chronic hoarseness, and many voice breaks. Continued use of the high pitch level of childhood is called mutational falsetto, or simply falsetto voice. The mechanical reason for mutational falsetto voice is the overcontraction of the cricothyroid muscles, and there is a pronounced elevation of the entire larynx during phonation (Arnold, 1966).

Aronson (1973, p. 60) described the physiological mechanism of falsetto: (1) Through action of the thyrohyoid and suprahyoid musculature the larynx is elevated high in the neck. (2) Through action of the stylohyoid muscles, the larynx is tilted downward resulting in maintaining the vocal cords in a state of laxity. (3) Even though the vocal cords are in a flabby state, the contraction of the cricothyroid muscles causes the vocal cords to be stretched thin. (4) The vocal cords are now reduced in mass and offer low resistance to infraglottal air pressure. (5) Only the medial edges of the vocal cords vibrate because on phonation infraglottal air pressure is at a minimum. Respiration during speaking generally is shallow.

Since the normal change in a girl's voice is a lowering of only 3 or 4 semitones her voice may not be considered deviant if it does not change although she may be considered to have a rather high-pitched and childish voice. However, if the pitch of her voice lowers significantly a pitch problem develops called perverse mutation. A mutational bass voice may occur in a preadolescent boy who has forced his voice down even lower than normal through imitating adults with very low pitches (Weiss, 1950). A boy over 14 or 15 years of age with a high-pitched voice is usually classified as being effeminate. It is possible to confuse the use of effeminate pitch inflections after the voice has changed with the problem of persistent falsetto. Therefore, before attempting to lower pitch the speech pathologist should make sure the older male teenager really has a too-high modal frequency level not just effeminate sounding pitch inflections. According to Coleman (1976) the degree of maleness and femaleness in the voice is a function of the laryngeal fundamental frequency and has little to do with vocal tract resonance characteristics.

Many voice problems arise during the period of voice change. Harrington (1950, pp. 192–193) stated, "Many of the voice disorders of the adult have their origin in the period of adolescence and are outgrowths of the voice problems related to this rather crucial period." Brodnitz (1971a, p. 61) noted many deviations of voice can be traced back to voice change during puberty.

Causes of Disturbed Mutation

Mutational disturbances of the voice are based on functional or organic causes or a combination of both. Functional causes of disturbed mutation include psychological involvements (Arnold, 1966; Timcke et al. 1959), sexual conflict related to a protest against social or sexual maturity (Van Riper, 1972, p. 150), and infantile or juvenile personality (Arnold, 1966; Luchsinger, 1965, p. 196; Van Riper, 1972, p. 145). A high-pitched voice may be used as a defense against pitch breaks or as a method of preventing a hoarse voice (Van Riper, 1972, p. 150). The physical examination usually shows normal sexual development in mutational falsetto voices (Arnold, 1966; Luchsinger, 1965, p. 195). Organic bases include laryngeal asymmetries (Weiss, 1950), small vocal cords (Fomon et al. 1966), congenital or acquired anterior laryngeal web which shortens the cords (Arnold, 1966), incomplete mutation in girls complaining of irregular menstruation (Luchsinger, 1965, p. 194), and endocrine disturbances (Fomon et al. 1966; Luchsinger, 1965, p. 188; Weiss, 1950). However, ordinary laryngoscopy usually reveals no major abnormalities in cases of suspected endocrine pathology (Luchsinger, 1965, p. 188).

Laryngeal Findings

In functional mutational disturbances the laryngological examinations are negative as far as size, structure, and function of the larynx are concerned. Hyperemia or congestion of the vocal cords may be present (Arnold, 1964; 1966; Luchsinger, 1965, p. 196), but these signs are the result not the cause of the habitual use of the falsetto voice (Luchsinger, 1965, p. 196). Allen and Peterson (1942) presented a case report of an 18-year-old male with a falsetto voice who had considerable inflammation of the entire laryngeal area. After pitch had been lowered to a normal level this inflammation was greatly relieved. They felt that in this case the inflammation had been caused by his use of a falsetto voice. In mutational disturbances the glottis assumes a typical oval shape upon phonation and in some instances the posterior half of the glottis may close incompletely (Arnold, 1966).

A good illustration of the necessity of a careful examination by a laryngologist in all cases of mutation problems in males was reported by Montgomery and Smith (1976). They reported on a 21-year-old male who had a persistently high-pitched voice after puberty. A careful examination revealed nonfusion of the thyroid laminae. The thyroid laminae were closed and a defective anterior glottis was repaired resulting in a normal airway with normal vocal cord length and the voice of a male adult.

We are including the following example because we have been asked about Teflon injection in instances where the vocal cords have not assumed the mass necessary for a lower pitched voice. Zwitman and Calcaterra (1975) described a 30-year-old man with severe hoarseness seen after Teflon injections in both vocal cords had been performed in order to lower an abnormally high pitch which had been present since puberty. Pitch analysis, using voice spectrography on audio samples of voice before and after Teflon injection revealed no significant drop in modal frequency level of the voice. The fundamental frequency of three vowels pre-Teflon speech averaged 175 Hz and the fundamental frequency of the patient's post-Teflon speech phonating a vowel was identified as 175 Hz. The hoarseness was presumed to have resulted for three reasons, (1) glycerin absorption, (2) inflammation of the vocal cords, and (3) asynchronous vibration of the cords. Removal of the Teflon is not possible so surgical treatment was not indicated. The authors concluded that Teflon injection to increase vocal cord mass is not refined sufficiently to consider its use in lowering vocal pitch. The authors advised that for this type of problem vocal cord injection should not be attempted until its usefulness has been proven.

Singing during Mutation

In general both boys and girls should be discouraged from choral singing during mutation (Brodnitz, 1971a, p. 64; Luchsinger, 1965, p. 159; Weiss, 1950). This is particularly true for boys who show voice breaks (Brodnitz, 1971a, p. 64). Brodnitz (1971a, p. 65) stated as a rule the singing voice requires a year or two longer to develop than the speaking voice. He advised that formal singing training should not be started in boys before the age of 17 or 18 and in girls not before 16 years of age. Overexertion of the intrinsic muscles of the larynx while singing may cause permanent impairment of the vocal coordination necessary in phonation (Greene, 1964, p. 91). The untrained singer may develop laryngeal symptoms which may be temporary or permanent if he persists in singing in outdoor classes, at summer camp, in the church choir, and in other situations for which he is not trained (Baker, 1962). Rubin (1964) mentioned the following as conditions likely to result from abusive singing: acute laryngitis because of infection or trauma to the vocal cords, chronic vocal corditis, vocal nodules, circumscribed or diffuse submucosal hemorrhage, and hypofunction or myasthenia resulting from deterioration in the tonus of the laryngeal muscles.

We have worked with several adolescents who had misused their voices during singing and developed hypofunction manifesting itself in a bowing of the vocal cords during phonation. More frequently we have seen teenagers who were in training to become professional singers and had been referred with the problem of vocal nodules. Others are rock singers with little or no singing training who violate all the rules of proper singing techniques.

Here is an example of a young rock singer we saw recently.

Rick, a 15-year-old rock singer with his own group, is a good example of a musically talented youth gone vocally astray. He was a self taught singer who formed a group and was immediately popular in the area of the state where he lived. About 6 weeks before we saw him he began to have trouble hitting higher notes, and some pitch breaks began to show up first during singing and then during speaking. A few days later he began to have periods of hoarseness lasting a day or two, usually following an evening of especially vigorous and loud singing. Three weeks before he came in he developed severe hoarseness, causing him to seek advise from his personal physician who sent him to a laryngologist. The diagnosis was bilateral vocal nodules at the junction of the anterior and middle thirds of the cords, with some enlargement of both ventricular bands. It was the laryngologist's impression that Rick had developed vocal nodules with chronic hoarseness because of vocal strain during singing and attempting to reach notes difficult for him. Medical or surgical treatment was not advised. Rick was referred to us by the laryngologist. Our problem was twofold: (1) to provide a voice therapy program of correct voice use with elimination of the nodules the goal, and (2) to direct him eventually to a qualified singing teacher. We asked Rick to take a leave from his group. We first placed him on a 10 day restricted talking program limited to scattered 1 minute doses for a maximum of 30 times in a 24 hour period. Each day he charted the 30 talking times according to place and time of day and reported to us daily by telephone. After the 10 days the hoarseness was almost gone and Rick rejoined his group but now as a guitarist with no singing a rule. We then saw him once a week for 2 months to eliminate other vocal misuses and abuses, including abrupt glottal attack, and to do direct voice therapy to improve his voice. A laryngeal examination now revealed the nodules were almost gone; then 6 weeks later a reexamination showed the nodules no longer present. After consultation with the laryngologist we sent Rick to a music teacher who was experienced in teaching singing to youths with Rick's history. The last time we saw him he brought us an audiotape of his "new singing style"—still rock, but following the rules of good vocal hygiene.

Psychological

Many functional voice disorders, especially those of deviations in flexibility, quality, pitch, and loudness, may be explained as a result of psychological disturbance or maladjustment (Curtis, 1967, p. 208). We have discussed functional mutation problems. Psychological factors which may cause a functional voice disorder in children include personality differences, character defects, emotional disturbances, and disturbed parent-child relationships. These factors are overlapping and intertwining and are not always easily separated. At times we see children with voice problems quite directly related to only one of the factors, but in many children a disturbance is seen in more than one factor. Murphy (1964, p. 32) discussed disturbed parent-child relationships as a cause of voice problems. He stated, "Many of the apprehensions or anxieties connected with vocal dysfunctions are traceable to disturbed earlier child-adult relationships, at least in part." He felt positive identification between parent and child is necessary to establish efficient

communication between them and if this identification malfunctions and the parent has an undesirable voice quality, he becomes a negative model, with the child developing " ... anxiety-reducing behavior, some of which may take the form of psychogenic voice symptoms."

Psychological factors may result in a variety of vocal symptoms. Some of these are hoarseness, harshness, breathiness, hypernasality, loudness problems, aphonia, and hypertense voice problems. For example, over aggressiveness may be one of the personality differences resulting in a habitually too loud voice (Pronovost and Kingman, 1959, p. 112). Hoarseness can be closely related to emotional disturbances or psychic trauma (von Leden, 1958). A child who is unmanageable and hyperactive may have a rough hoarse voice reflecting a character defect, congenital or acquired. When a child is emotionally disturbed, either neurotic or psychotic, almost any type of voice problem may be present.

In some children voice problems due to vocal abuse and misuse, such as vocal nodules, may be due to expression of psychological problems, hostility, and aggression. Also other children may be more repressed and thus show more inner tension in the laryngeal areas specifically (Mosby, 1970; 1972). Therefore, for some children the speech pathologist should be alert to psychological factors in voice problems. Excessive laryngeal tension may be caused by emotional conflicts (Peacher, 1952, p. 9). Any type of personality conflict may be revealed in a hyperfunctional voice problem.

Various psychological factors or upsets may be a factor in vocal abuse and vocal misuse. The result may be the formation of vocal nodules. Heaver (1958) obtained psychiatric evaluations of 50 patients ranging in age from 3½ to 73 years. The vocal cords of each of these patients were reddened, swollen, and thickened or had nodules or polyps with hyperkinetic action of the vocal cords. He concluded disordered emotional states tend to engender vocal abuse which could result in nodules or edematous fibromata. Callahan (1958) also said many people who exhibit abuse of the vocal cords have emotional strain and insecurity in their immediate background. He presented a report of an investigation of 20 adults with varying degrees of abuse of the vocal cords who had not been able to develop a normal voice after operation for benign tumor. The results of psychological projective tests revealed unstable emotional reactions including inadequacy, anxiety, and hostility. Callahan concluded continued vocal abuse is caused by emotional disturbances characterized by unconscious conflicts and frustrations.

However, one study demonstrated that children and adolescents with voice problems do not have personality differences as measured by the Minnesota Multiphasic Personality Inventory, nor difficulty in interpersonal relationships as measured by social status ratings by peers. Muma, Laeder, and Webb (1968) studied the personality and social status of 78 junior and senior high school students who had been rated "extremely clinical" in voice quality deviations, including chronic breathiness, harshness, hoarseness, and hypernasality. The social status was determined by ratings from peers regarding desirability of personal association in common school activities. It was found that those with obviously different voice qualities did not differ appreciably in peer evaluations or in personality characteristics in comparison with those who have normal voice quality.

Hysterical Aphonia and Dysphonia

Aphonia is a complete loss of voice which is usually present on a psychosomatic basis (Lewy, 1963; McCaskey, 1946; von Leden, 1958) and is commonly referred to as hysterical aphonia. Dysphonia is a partial loss of phonatory ability and may range from a mild condition to one approaching complete loss of voice. These types are also termed functional, psychogenic, or conversion aphonia or dysphonia (Aronson, 1973, p. 24). Damsté (1973) described these problems as having the following typical characteristics: sudden onset, with the dysphonia being of short duration; prior to onset the voice has been normal and generally the dysphonic symptoms are inconsistent in their presence; there is a history of emotional stress or mental conflict.

Brodnitz (1969) stated hysterical aphonia usually has a sudden onset with some patients losing their voice from one day to the next, or at some specific moment of the day. The lack of voice may be the presenting symptom of a major emotional disturbance with aphonia representing an avenue of escape

from a difficult dilemma (McCaskey, 1946). Aronson (1973, p. 21) stated it is due to mental stress, it is inseparable from the psychodynamics of the patient's reaction to the stress, and it is precipitated by definable emotional conflict.

Hysterical aphonia in children before the age of adolescence is very rare, but dysphonia in the absence of vocal strain is relatively common in children and may be considered a hysterical symptom (Greene, 1972, p. 192). Barton (1960) described the syndrome of hysterical dysphonia. The condition may vary from a mild dysphonia to complete loss of voice. He described a distinct clinical type called *whispering dysphonia* which is most commonly found in women and may appear any time between puberty and menopause. The patient speaks in a halting whisper without hoarseness and at times the phonation is normal. Most of Barton's case descriptions are of adult patients although he refers to one girl 16 years of age. During the laryngeal examination, according to Barton, the vocal folds move properly, they approximate accurately, and are free from any tumors or inflammations.

Some children have bowed vocal cords as the result of a hysterical condition. In some patients with deviant voice patterns including complete aphonia a mirror examination of the vocal cords shows a bowing and imperfect approximation in phonatory effort typical of hypofunctioning resulting from hyperfunctioning; this appears even though the midline approximation usually occurs in coughing or laughing (Lewy, 1963). Brodnitz (1969) stated the vocal cords appear normal in outline; however, if complete aphonia has been present for a lengthy time the unused cords may look unnaturally white. With a slight cough good adduction of the cords may be seen. Lesions are rare in aphonia caused by environmental stress (Aronson, 1973, p. 21). Aronson (1973, p. 24) and Van Riper (1972, p. 139) stated laryngoscopic examinations often show good adduction of the vocal cords to the midline on vocalizing and coughing, indicating neuromuscular normalcy. However, the larynx is elevated and positioned rigidly (Aronson, 1973, p. 24).

We have worked with some teenagers where the onset of the aphonia or dysphonia has been sudden, while with others the onset has been gradual and intermittent. The voice may return to normal as suddenly as it went into a whisper. In several teenagers we have seen, the voice suddenly went into a whisper for several days or weeks followed by a sudden complete and permanent recovery. In one teenage girl we saw, her dysphonia occurred intermittently and usually corresponded with some problem crisis in her life. Her dysphonia varied, so that at times her voice would be only slightly breathy. Placed in a crisis situation, within a few minutes she would get more and more dysphonic until she was completely aphonic. Her communication deteriorated to pantomimic speaking accompanied by a rush of air instead of phonation. Soon, however, she would resort to pad and pen as a substitute for any attempt to talk. In Chapter 9 we will present the voice therapy program which was conducted in cooperation with her physician, the school psychologist, and the guidance counselor.

Incipient Spastic Dysphonia

A few children have the beginnings of spastic dysphonia. As Cooper (1971a, p. 609) stated, a bright outcome can be noted for incipient spastic dysphonia. The cause is somewhat obscure but it is usually classified as a psychogenic disorder with probably some organic features with a neurological basis (Aronson, Brown, Litin, and Pearson, 1968a; 1968b; Aronson, 1973, Ch. 4). A 16-year-old boy we saw recently had a hoarse tremulous voice and had been diagnosed by a laryngologist as having beginning spastic dysphonia. Upon phonation, vocal cord spasm was seen localized at the junction of the middle and posterior thirds of both cords. We will discuss our therapy with him in Chapter 9.

Imitation

Murphy (1964, pp. 31–32) contended, "Throughout the vocal learning process, the voice acquired by the child depends upon how he imitates or identifies with important adults in his environment." He further stated the amount of pleasure a child gets from his early vocal play will influence how well he can master normal vocalization. He pointed out for normal growth preverbal language including babbling and vocal play must receive approval and success early in the child's life.

It is possible for a child to have a voice problem as a result of imitation of others with voice problems in his environment (Pronovost and Kingman, 1959, p. 112). Klinger (1962), for example, wrote about a child who imitated a cousin's cleft palate speech. Van Riper (1972, p. 151) stated stereotyped inflections may be due to foreign language influence. Eisenson and Ogilvie (1977, p. 312) included imitation of poor models as one of the reasons for voice disturbances in children. They remind us that a child learns both his language and the manner in which it is produced auditorially. Thus the mother, as she teaches her child the name of something new, is also teaching the child the manner in which the naming is done. A shouting mother results in a shouting child. As a child grows and becomes acquainted with other children and adults, he may select certain children and adults as his voice models. Usually such imitation is unconscious, but occasionally a child will consciously imitate another child or an adult in order to identify with them. Imitation of this type may begin quite early in life and continue through and beyond adolescence. Eisenson and Ogilvie stated classroom teachers have a great responsibility for the voices of children in their room; a well-liked teacher is imitated, a disliked teacher mimicked in voice as well as other aspects of behavior.

Faulty Learning

An overly loud voice is not necessarily a sign of overaggressiveness but sometimes a result of poor speech habits (Fabricant, 1962). The patient may have no organic lesion to account for the inefficient vocal cord vibration causing breathy voice (Fabricant, 1962). Murphy (1964, p. 33) cited as an example of faulty learning the child who has parents with hearing losses and who may be required to raise loudness and pitch levels and thus develop a pitch or quality disorder.

Eisenson and Ogilvie (1977, pp. 312–315) described faulty habits of vocalization. These include unsuitable modal frequency level, resonance problems, and poor breath control. Eisenson and Ogilvie stated some children may succumb to the pressures to vocalize in a manner which is physically difficult for them. These include an inappropriate modal frequency level and a voice quality which the child uses because he thinks it is more fashionable to talk in certain ways. For example, the use of abnormally high- or abnormally low-pitched voices may be consciously developed by a child.

CONTRIBUTING FACTORS

A variety of conditions may contribute to voice problems present on a functional basis, an organic basis, or on the basis of organic conditions resulting from vocal misuse and abuse. These contributing conditions include glandular conditions, allergies, upper respiratory conditions (chronic pharyngitis, sinusitis, deviated nasal septum), and premenstrual and menstrual problems. These contributing causes are intertwined with the three basic causes of voice problems, in fact it may be difficult to find the exact relationship of causes. For example, an allergic tendency is a common symptom in childhood vocal nodules (Greene, 1972, p. 124). The following case history illustrates this.

Ken, a 10-year-old boy, had been periodically hoarse for 5 years when we saw him in the clinic. The indirect laryngeal examination revealed essentially normal laryngeal structures except for nonspecific laryngitis with the vocal cords red and swollen. Further exploration revealed two reasons for the laryngitis: allergy to airborne pollens (present most of the year where he lived) and excessive shouting and loud talking when playing. Antihistamines were prescribed to relieve the edematous condition of the vocal cords. Voice therapy was administered by a speech pathologist for the purposes of reducing vocal abuse during play, eliminating the intermittent use of abnormally high pitch, and teaching the boy to use correct loudness in all situations. Within a period of 6 months the combination of medical and voice therapy resulted in a voice much improved in quality with the periodic hoarseness eliminated (Wilson, 1968).

Glandular Conditions

Metabolic disorders due to a dysfunction of the endocrine glands should be carefully investigated because the endocrine condition may affect laryngeal structures. An enlargement of the larynx may be seen in certain malfunctions of the anterior pituitary gland (Burke, 1968). Also hoarseness or huskiness may be present in myxedema and thyroid and parathyroid tumors (Burke, 1968). A chronically high-pitched voice in a male is usually functional but may be caused by the larynx failing to develop to a normal size because of glandular difficulties, for example hypogonadism (Moore, 1971a, p. 539).

Hyperthyroidism may be reflected in the voice when a person has a limited vocal range and a husky voice (Brodnitz, 1971b). Vocal quality may be influenced by changes in metabolic and hormonal balances (Brodnitz, 1962) with a low metabolic rate resulting in a retention of body fluids in the surface tissues in the laryngeal and tracheal areas (Brodnitz, 1954). Congenital hypothyroidism may result in different cry characteristics in infants. Michelsson and Sirvio (1976) analyzed 40 different cries from 4 infants of 10 days to 4 months of age with hypothyroidism. They were measured by sound spectrographic methods and compared with the crying of 75 healthy infants of corresponding ages. Both the minimum and maximum of the modal frequency level and the maximum pitch of shift were significantly lower in the infants with hypothyroidism and shifts occurred less often. The hypothyrotic infants attained a maximum pitch of 470 Hz with a minimum pitch of 280 Hz compared to 610 Hz and 390 Hz for the normal infants.

In borderline degrees of hypothyroidism a person may have mild dysphonia. This has been seen in singers who complain of limitation of the upper vocal range and of vocal fatigue; the vocal cords are normal or slightly gray (Brodnitz, 1971b). Bicknell (1973) reported the chief complaint in mild hypothyroidism is voice change, usually a weak voice which tends to be more noticeable in the evening. Other symptoms include strain in talking, difficulty in singing, and a lowering of the modal frequency level. There may be a dry irritating cough and a hoarse voice. According to Bicknell, the clinical appearance of the vocal cords varies, with some cords appearing quite normal while others may show bilateral edematous thickening and others may be distinctly polypoidal. Bicknell stated the treatment of choice is thyroxin and it usually takes at least 6 weeks before noticeable improvement in the voice is apparent; treatment must be continued indefinitely. Brodnitz (1971b) stated vocal symptoms of extreme thyroid deficiency include the rough, hoarse voice of the cretin and the person with myxedema.

Allergy

The speech pathologist should be acquainted with various types of allergy and allergic management as they apply to children. Many children with voice problems have allergies that may have contributed to the voice problem and in some cases are the primary cause. Allergic sensitivity to both airborne and ingested substances may contribute to voice problems through swelling of the mucosa of the nose, mouth, throat, larynx, trachea, and lung structures. Brodnitz (1954) estimated that at least 3% of the population in the United States has some form of respiratory allergy which may influence laryngeal function. Senturia and Wilson (1968) found a family history of allergy present in about 25% of the children with laryngeal dysfunction.

The etiological factors in allergy, according to Williams (1972) include perennial inhalants, such as house dust, molds, feathers, animal dander, and volatile oils or emanations from plants. In addition seasonal problems may be due to various pollens of the plant kingdom. Williams stated food antigens may also produce mild to severe edema of the laryngeal structures. He added that foods as well as inhalants may show a specificity of reaction, that is, one particular food may produce edema of the epiglottis only while another may produce edema of the uvula. Edema in any portion of the larynx, which appears as a pale glistening of the structures involved, is highly suggestive of allergic etiology.

According to Clemis (1976), food allergy in infancy most commonly affects the skin and the gastrointestinal tract. After the 1st year of life these symptoms may disappear for many months, only to reappear in the later preschool years as upper airway allergy with middle ear effusion. A past history of asthma, hives, unexplained skin rash, allergic dermatitis, hay fever, food intolerance, drug sensitivities, and contact allergy help to identify the allergic patient. Clemis stated that family allergy history need not extend beyond the immediate family: when both parents have a history of allergy there is a two in three chance of allergy in their child, two in

five chances with one allergic parent, and one in five when neither parent has allergies. According to Clemis (1976), Rapp and Fahey (1973), and Sanders (1967) physical symptoms of the allergic person may be Dennie's sign, that is, an extra line fold under each eye (Morgan, 1948); a transverse nasal crease and broad nasal root; allergic shiners—dark circles under the lower eyelid or dark circles under the eyes. Another common symptom is the allergic salute, that is, the rubbing of the end of the nose with the finger, hand, and forearm.

The tissue that is affected by an allergy is called the shock organ (Sanders, 1967). The mucuous membrane linings of the mouth, throat, and larynx are likely to be the primary shock organs of ingested substances (Missal, 1961). In some cases the contact may be relatively brief but when it is repeated frequently, drinking milk for example, allergic reactions may result (Missal, 1961). The lingering coating effect on the mucosa of some dairy products, especially high fat milk and ice cream, results in increased time for allergic reaction to take place. Milk and ice cream of low fat content are preferable as they have little coating effect. Because food remains in the body for hours antigens can be absorbed from the intestinal tract reaching the mucosa through the circulatory system thus causing a delayed allergic reaction (Missal, 1961).

Respiratory allergy may result from airborne irritants such as pollens (Wilson, 1968), dust (Frank, 1940; Moore, 1971b, p. 99), powdered substances of various kinds (Moore, 1971b, p. 99), and chemical substances (Frank, 1940). Ingested allergens include foods and liquids. According to Sanders (1967) the shock organ may be the respiratory tract or a part of it, such as the nasal mucosa, or the reaction may be localized in a very small area of the body. He added the most common symptom of food allergy is fatigue; it occurs in the morning even though the person has had a normal amount of rest, and usually there is less fatigue in the middle of the day. He stated headaches are common in the allergic patient and when due to food they often start 2 to 4 hours following the ingestion of the allergen.

In some areas of the nose, mouth, and throat there may be hyperemia, a reddening due to increased blood concentration. Reactions to allergic symptoms may include such vocal abuses as chronic coughing and throat clearing which in turn aggravate the swelling and inflammation and may result in organic changes. As Bawden (1968, p. 29) reported, if the throat clearing action is frequent and violent, vocal cord edema causes the voice to become hoarse and husky. Allergic reactions may be a factor in the formation of vocal nodules (Williams, 1972). A dry cough is often caused by an allergy due to food, with the cough varying in intensity, time, and onset. Some people cough soon after eating a particular food, others 4 or more hours later. The cough may also take the form of a deep or hacking cough, and there may be a sensation of tickling and a desire to clear the throat (Sanders, 1967).

Williams (1972) stated in allergic laryngitis, varying degrees of edema may involve the entire larynx or just specific portions of it. In its most severe form the entire larynx is involved, including the epiglottis, arytenoids, and vocal cords; this may require immediate restoration of the airway through intubation or tracheotomy. Williams added that less severe allergic reactions produce mild to severe hoarseness and are usually the result of edema of contact surfaces of the vocal cords.

The swelling and reddening of the mucosa of the nose may result in hyponasality (Arnold, 1965, p. 684). In some instances the turbinates are pale, translucent, or boggy bluish (Clemis, 1976).

A book by Rapp (1972) provides useful information in question and answer form for parents about the problems of allergies in children. Consultation with an allergist is indicated when allergy is suspected.

Upper Respiratory Conditions

Infections of the upper respiratory tract are a source of laryngeal difficulties (Cracovaner, 1959; von Leden, 1958). In the presence of impaired nasal respiration and the resulting mouth breathing, the mucous covering of the cords becomes dry leaving the cords unprotected (Kelly and Craik, 1952). Purulent postnasal discharge bathing the vocal cords has often been observed in patients with vocal nodules (Kelly and Craik, 1952). Sinusitis is often an accompanying problem in cases of chronic laryngitis (Murphy, 1967). Kelly and Craik (1952) found marked nasal obstruction or sepsis in 23% of their cases with vocal

nodules. Senturia and Wilson (1968) noted in their studies of voice-deviant children about one-half of the children had increased amounts of mucus, pus, or mucopus in each nasal fossa.

Premenstrual and Menstrual Problems

Hoarseness may be associated with premenstrual tension. Edematous conditions occurring a few days preceding the menstrual period may cause an increase in the bulk of the vocal cords and result in lowered pitch and vocal instability with voice breaks (Frable, 1962). Van Gelder (1974a) described *laryngopathia menstrualis* a condition mainly seen in singers who complain of voice changes just before and during menstruation. At this time the voice varies from dull and colorless to raucous and hoarse. Laryngeal examination reveals in some cases hyperemia, edema, or hemorrhage of the vocal cords. In other cases tension of the vocal cords is reduced, which results in a husky voice and if singing is forced small hematomas of the vocal cords may result. Therefore, if hoarseness is noted in surveying older girls, a recheck should be made at some other time and inquiry made about the periodicity of the hoarseness and its relation to the menstrual cycle. This hoarseness or vocal instability occurring for a few days each month should not be of great concern to the speech pathologist. However, if voice differences do appear in association with menstruation, girls should be cautioned to avoid singing and overuse of the voice on certain days.

SUMMARY

Many children exhibit normal vocal mechanisms but have voice problems present on a functional basis. These problems include disturbed mutation, psychological factors, imitation, and faulty learning. At puberty a boy's pitch level lowers about an octave and a girl's 3 or 4 semitones. Delayed, prolonged, or incomplete mutation may occur. Psychological problems may be reflected in various types of voice problems such as hoarseness, breathiness, harshness, or hypernasality. In some children the psychological problems are reflected in partial or total loss of voice. A child may model his voice after a favorite person, film star, or television personality, resulting in a voice quite inappropriate in pitch, quality, loudness, and resonance. Other children have different voices simply because they have learned incorrect speaking methods. Often other problems contribute to or even cause voice problems. A child's endocrine system may be imbalanced causing pitch and voice quality problems. A child with allergies may have resonance and voice quality problems because of swelling and vascular engorgement of the delicate structures involved in voice production. Frequent colds, sinus problems, and other upper respiratory problems may cause a child's voice to be deviant either intermittently or chronically. Older girls may have voice problems related to premenstrual or menstrual days. Recognizing the functional and contributing factors related to a child's voice problem makes it possible to plan a treatment program to overcome the voice problem.

FIVE

Examinations: I

Voice Team, Head and Neck, Case History

Children with voice problems require special examinations. The findings form the basis upon which voice therapy is planned. Many specialists may be involved. The most effective procedure for examining children with voice disorders is in the framework of a team situation.

THE VOICE TEAM

Examinations of children with voice problems include those made by various specialists in a team situation. A team approach assures comprehensive care of children with voice problems from the time the problems are first discovered through examination, consultation, treatment, and follow-up. Before a voice therapy program begins it is necessary to coordinate the relevant examinations conducted by the team. For example, a child with a chronically hoarse voice will require a head and neck examination. He may also need a general physical examination, an audiological evaluation, and examinations and tests for allergy. The child may need psychiatric or psychological attention, the parents may need counseling, and the child may need voice therapy.

We advocate a team approach to the diagnosis and treatment of children with voice problems to coordinate these services in an efficient and effective manner. Every major center of population should have a voice team similar to a cleft palate team, a hearing team (Kodman, 1964; Roeser, Campbell, and Brown, 1976; Wilson, 1962a; Yater 1972), a communication disorders team (Bown, 1972; 1973), and a learning center team (Parker, 1972).

Support for the team approach to diagnosis and treatment of voice disorders comes from many sources. Moore (1967) emphasized the need of a child with a voice problem for an overall approach. O'Neill and McGee (1962) felt a team approach should be used. Brodnitz (1971a, p. 83) emphasized the necessity for close cooperation between the speech pathologist and the laryngologist. He stated (Brodnitz, 1971a, p. 85) vocal rehabilitation requires a total approach and emphasis should be placed on the medical, functional, and psychological factors present in a person with a vocal disturbance. The voice team approach has been used successfully in schools. Wilson (1972) stated the ideal situation for treating voice disorders in children in schools should include cooperative efforts between parents, pediatrician, otolaryngologist, and speech pathologist.

Baynes (1965) and Freeman (1961; 1969) described the team approach in the public schools of Oakland County, Michigan. One aspect of this service is especially for children who have chronic voice disorders. Four or five times a year the consulting laryngologist examines children for abnormalities of the vocal cords. Local speech pathologists attend these examinations to review findings and to formulate recommendations with the examining physician. Their team includes the otolaryngologist, the teachers, parents, principals, psychologists, school social workers, and school nurses.

The details of a working voice team at Northern Illinois University were described by Shearer (1972). The team met four times a year and consisted of a speech pathologist, laryngologist, and school psychologist, with the University providing audiological services. The referring speech pathologist accompanied each child through the examination procedure. Each clinic lasted a full day and at each meeting 10 new referrals were seen, in addition to the children who were returned for a check on clinical progress. At the end of the day staffing was held by all members for all children seen that day and recommendations made in the various areas of rehabilitation. The conclusions of the team

51

together with recommendations for therapy and referrals were given to the appropriate speech pathologist and written reports were prepared. As time allowed, demonstration voice therapy was conducted.

Organization of Voice Team

A team approach to children with voice problems may be organized in different ways. It may function successfully with as few as two continuing members, a laryngologist and a speech pathologist, with arrangements for referral or consultation with other specialists as circumstances dictate. We feel, however, the ideal voice team is one in which specific members of the team meet regularly scheduling half-day sessions as frequently as the number of children with serious voice deviations warrants. The specialties represented at any one team meeting depend on the problems of the children being seen. This type of team approach is advocated with the realization that a more loosely knit organization may be adequate in some communities.

A team coordinator schedules and plans the sessions. Typically the coordinator is either a laryngologist or a speech pathologist. The team coordinator establishes a roster of all specialists who might be called upon to examine, diagnose, and treat children with voice problems and to conduct follow-up examinations as necessary. In addition to the speech pathologist and laryngologist, other specialists who may serve as members or consultants to the team include a pediatrician, neurologist, psychiatrist, psychologist, audiologist, social worker, and school personnel. Children are referred to the team by any of its members or by other specialists. The team approach includes four stages: initial evaluation, team staffing, progress evaluations, and follow-up. At a single meeting the team members may see children in any stage.

Stage I: Initial Evaluation

A list of children with voice problems is accumulated by the coordinator. The coordinator and one other team member, the laryngologist and the speech pathologist, meet on a regular basis. At these meetings they select the tests and examinations indicated for each child. The coordinator informs the parents of the recommended tests and examinations and it is the parents' responsibility to see that the child is examined by the specialists of their choice. For example, the

following may be recommended: a head and neck examination, a voice examination, a general physical examination, and psychological evaluations. Any immediate treatment indicated is given as the child is seen by each specialist. For example, a child may need medication to relieve allergic conditions affecting the nose and throat.

Stage II: Team Staffing

After the examinations have been completed the coordinator accumulates all the reports. The team members actively concerned with the group of children under consideration then meet for a staffing. The children are presented at this time, with some team members demonstrating the results of their detailed examinations. As the members of the team look over his shoulder the laryngologist can show them the child's vocal nodules. The speech pathologist may wish to conduct a brief session with the child to demonstrate the child's vocal capabilities and disabilities. Each member of the team presents his report. The team then agrees on the severity of the voice problem by rating it on a 5 point scale based upon one suggested by Muma et al. (1968) with 1—not clinical, 2—barely clinical, 3—obviously clinical, 4—severely clinical, and 5—extremely clinical. The team decides on the overall treatment for the child. The parents are informed of the planned course of action, and when indicated and appropriate the child is told of the treatment plan.

Stage III: Progress Evaluations

All children are scheduled at regular intervals in the course of their treatment for team evaluation and impressions of their progress. These evaluations include rechecking pathologies and evaluating effectiveness of certain therapies. Some children are seen by the team when a team member runs into specific problems requiring discussion and decisions by the team. Questions may arise about certain aspects of the treatment and other team members may make suggestions for a change in treatment. Decisions about dismissal from active treatment are also made by the team.

Stage IV: Follow-up

Following formal or regular aspects of treatment the child is seen periodically by the team. Usually children are rechecked every 3 to 6 months. The number of rechecks depends upon the problem and the child. This follow-up assures carryover of new voice habits and freedom from physical or psychological complaints. The voice team is the most desirable approach to the rehabilitation of children with voice problems. The comprehensive team approach can be adapted to the needs of a specific community.

The following is a case illustration of the four team stages (adapted from Wilson, 1968).

Jeff, an extremely active and loud-talking 6-year-old boy, was first seen by a school speech pathologist during a kindergarten speech and voice survey. His voice was hoarse, especially after periods of excessive loud talking and shouting during games. The school speech pathologist consulted with the coordinator of the local voice team who was a speech pathologist in the city speech and hearing center. They met with a laryngologist and the following recommendations were made: general physical examination, head and neck examination, neurological examination, and voice tests (Stage I).

Results of these examinations were presented at a team staffing (Stage II) as follows. A laryngeal examination revealed small nodules on the free margin of each vocal cord at the junction of the anterior and middle thirds. The laryngologist felt these vocal nodules were due to improper use of the voice and were too small for removal. The general physical and neurological examinations were negative. The voice tests revealed the child had a moderate to severe hoarseness, a too high modal frequency level, an exessively loud voice, and many vocal abuses including shouting, screaming, strained vocalizations when imitating jet planes and racing cars, and explosive release of vocalizations. The physicians prescribed a mild tranquilizer to help the child relax. The social worker agreed to see the parents for counseling in an effort to help the child reduce his excessive activity. The psychologist reported the child was essentially emotionally stable and of normal intelligence. Voice therapy was recommended and the speech pathologist saw the child for 16 voice therapy sessions of 45 min each

over a period of 3 months. Vocal abuse and loud talking were given attention and his modal pitch level was lowered. During this period the child was seen by the team after 10 voice therapy sessions for a progress evaluation (Stage III) at the request of the speech pathologist and laryngologist. The purpose was to demonstrate improvement in the boy's voice and show that the nodules were definitely reduced in size. He was also seen after the 16 sessions for another progress evaluation at which time he was dismissed from active voice therapy. The period of intensive voice therapy was followed by a series of check-ups to insure continuation of improved speaking habits (Stage IV). A laryngeal examination 6 months after the initiation of voice therapy revealed the vocal nodules were reduced in size. Another laryngeal examination a year later showed they were no longer present.

HEAD AND NECK EXAMINATION

The head and neck examination includes a careful evaluation of the neck, ears, nose, oral cavity, nasopharynx, and larynx. Special attention is given to those areas related to the chief complaint connected with the voice problem.

Neck

According to Saunders (1964, p. 80) palpation of the neck is part of the complete examination of the larynx and is described as follows. A cyst of the thyroglossal duct may be felt by the physician in the space between the thyroid cartilage and the hyoid bone. The space between the thyroid and cricoid cartilages is palpated to check for lymph nodes; the space is shortened as the patient prolongs /i/ at a high pitch showing normal function of the cricothyroid muscle and its nerve supply, the superior laryngeal nerve. The neck is palpated for swelling and enlargement of lymph nodes which may reveal glandular disease. The sternocleidomastoid muscles are checked for lymph nodes. The shape of the thyroid cartilage is noted (DeWeese and Saunders, 1973, p. 22).

Ears

The ears are carefully examined using the following procedures described by Collins

(1964, pp. 83–86). The physician first examines the external ear noting inflammatory spots, fissures, or ulcers. The back of the ear is examined especially for eczema. The ear canal is next examined, the physician pulls the ear upward, outward, and backward and inserts an aural speculum. The ear canal is inspected. Inflammations, discharges, and amount of wax are noted. The tympanic membrane is carefully inspected. It should be slightly concave and pearly grey with a lustrous surface. Normally the handle of the malleus can be seen near the center of the membrane. The short process of the malleus can be seen in the upper third of the membrane. In a retracted membrane the handle of the malleus appears foreshortened and the short process prominent (Collins, 1964, p. 322). Any perforations of the membrane are noted (Collins, 1964, p. 88). Fluid in the middle ear can be seen if the membrane is fairly transparent (Collins, 1964, p. 89).

Nose

Collins (1964, pp. 76–79) described the physician's examination of the nose. A nasal speculum is inserted into a nostril and the naris spread for better viewing. The septum is examined. It should be smooth and pink, located centrally in the nose, and not deviated to one side. The turbinates are examined for swelling. Nasal polyps and mucopus are noted. If the mucous membrane of the nose is purplish and boggy, especially with excess mucoid secretion, an allergic condition is suspected.

Oral Cavity

DeWeese and Saunders (1973, pp. 13–15) described the physician's examination of the mouth. The tongue is inspected and palpated. It should be red and not coated. The frenum is checked for length and is normal if the patient can protrude the tongue between the teeth. The floor of the mouth is examined and palpated for growths. The salivary glands are examined for normalcy. The teeth are checked for cavities and abscesses and gingivae for freedom from bleeding. The palatine or faucial tonsils should not project beyond the tonsillar pillars. The posterior pharyngeal wall is examined by depressing the tongue with a tongue depressor. Examination of this area includes noting the amount of mesial movement in the lateral pharyngeal walls

during phonation (Spriestersbach, 1958). The size of the nasopharyngeal isthmus is noted (Calnan, 1954).

The hard and soft palates are carefully examined. They should show a distinct difference in color, the soft palate pink and the hard palate whiter; the uvula can be bifid (DeWeese and Saunders, 1973, pp. 14–15). The relationship in length of the hard and soft palates is evaluated. Arnold (1965, p. 662) pointed out the soft palate is normally about half as long as the hard palate; however, in cases of congenital velar insufficiency it may be only a third or a fourth as long. The hard palate may be disproportionately shortened in varying degrees in the presence of a normal soft palate (Kaplan et al. 1969). In some cases, both the hard and soft palates may be short. The soft palate is carefully inspected for movement. This includes checking the symmetry of movement during the elevation of the soft palate and noting whether there is general or localized movement during phonation (Spriestersbach, 1958). The physician palpates the palate to detect absence of muscle union in the soft palate and a notch in the hard palate which may indicate a submucous cleft of the palate (Calnan, 1954). Calnan (1954) noted that intraoral examination of a submucous cleft palate reveals a short palate and a large nasopharyngeal isthmus. The uvula is often bifid or gives the impression it is bifid because it may look more broad and squat than usual with a "gutter" running down it. There is also a definite "gutter" along the midline of the velum with the median raphe absent. Further the velum fails to occlude the nasopharyngeal isthmus, but its mobility and degree of elevation are not markedly impaired although the velum may not elevate during swallowing as it does in a person with a normal palate. Calnan (1954) stated a submucous cleft palate should not be confused with other types of palatal insufficiencies such as congenital short palate. He pointed out the median raphe of the velum is usually well marked in the congenital short palate indicating a sound muscle union, although hypernasality is usually present since the nasopharyngeal isthmus appears to be large and the velum may elevate inadequately and asymmetrically.

Intranasal transillumination aids in the diagnosis of submucous cleft palate. During this procedure the midline defect of muscle union is seen as a bright area which extends anteriorly to a notch in the hard palate (Calnan, 1954). Massengill (1966) described a special technique for doing this. A light source is placed in a nostril and a photoelectric cell is placed under the palate. Light is registered on the photoelectric cell if a submucous cleft is present.

Calnan (1954) listed another type of velopharyngeal insufficiency described as cerebral agenesis which results in hypernasality and poor speech. In these cases the palate moves poorly or not at all. There is no history of neural disease or evidence of other paralysis although Calnan noted there is sometimes a weakness of the muscles of the lips and tongue. If this condition is suspected, the examiner can have the patient sustain vowels such as /ɑ/ while the examiner notes whether the velum continues to be in an upward position throughout the sustained phonation; a muscle weakness may be indicated if the velum relaxes during sustained phonation (Bloomer and Wolski, 1968).

Nasopharynx

DeWeese and Saunders (1973, pp. 16–18) described the examination of the nasopharynx. A postnasal mirror is inserted into the pharynx almost touching the posterior pharyngeal wall. The examiner views the posterior opening of the nose and the posterior end of the vomer located centrally in the opening. The turbinates are viewed. Drainage from the maxillary sinus may be seen. The adenoid (pharyngeal tonsil) grows from the roof and posterior wall of the nasopharynx. Increased size of the adenoid may occlude the eustachian tubes and obstruct nasal breathing.

Subtelny and Koepp-Baker (1956) stated the peak of lymphatic growth of the adenoid is somewhere between 9 or 10 years of age and 14 or 15 years of age. The adenoid can first be seen in x-rays at about 6 months to 1 year becoming quite well defined at 2 years. By adulthood adenoid atrophy is usually complete. This normal atrophy is gradual and slow and when all structures otherwise are normal the palate and the pharyngeal wall can make increasingly compensatory movements in order to maintain adequate velopharyngeal closure (Subtelny and Koepp-Baker, 1956). In Chapter 3 we noted that after adenoidectomy during childhood there is usually hypernasal speech present from a few weeks up to one year. However, in some cases hypernasality persists if a patient is left with a capacious nasopharynx or when a submucous cleft palate is unmasked.

Larynx

Indirect Laryngoscopy

Indirect or mirror laryngoscopy requires a laryngeal mirror, a head mirror with a good light source, 2 × 2 in gauze, and to warm the laryngeal mirror, an alcohol lamp, hot water, or forced hot air from a small hair dryer (Loré, 1973, p. 710). A metal container warmed by an incandescent bulb can also be used. The patient is asked to sit in an erect position with the base of the spine snugly against the back of an examining chair (Loré, 1973, p. 710). The knees should be held together and the chin slightly forward (DeWeese and Saunders, 1973, p. 18). The patient is asked to relax his shoulders, neck, and arms and to breath regularly and moderately deeply to minimize gag reflex and throat spasm (Loré, 1973, p. 710). A laryngeal mirror, No. 3 to No. 6 depending on oropharyngeal width, is warmed and its temperature tested on the back of the physician's hand. The patient protrudes his tongue; the examiner using a piece of gauze gently grasps the tongue between the thumb and middle finger; the index finger is used to retract the upper lip (Loré, 1973, p. 710). As the laryngeal mirror is inserted into the pharynx the uvula and soft palate are pressed upward (DeWeese and Saunders, 1973, p. 19). Emphasis is placed on having the patient breathe quietly through the mouth, if necessary panting like a dog will help prevent gagging (DeWeese and Saunders, 1973, p. 19). Another method that has come into use within the past few years employs fiberoptic light bundles to supply illumination to the distal end of a laryngoscope. Gould (1973) described his laryngoscope using the fiberoptic principle which provides satisfactory magnification over its entire field of view. The light is "cold" with no shielding required for the instrument. Improved viewing is attained allowing the physician to get a completely unobstructed view of the epiglottis and the laryngeal surfaces, and the anterior commissure. The patient appears to be more relaxed and cooperative since traction on the tongue is no longer necessary once the laryngoscope has been inserted.

Domenec (1973) described a bit different way of doing laryngoscopy with the "Storz" cold light nasopharyngoscope. After the nasal passages are sprayed with a local anesthetic the nasopharyngoscope is inserted through the nasal passage. The view of the larynx is especially good because there is no outside pressure and activity can be noted under more normal situations instead of having the tongue extended or having a laryngoscope inserted into the mouth. Also swallowing movements and motions of the posterior tongue can be noted. Domenec stated this method can be used on patients as young as 4½ years of age.

The physician examines the larynx during breathing and during phonation of a prolonged high-pitched /i/ (DeWeese and Saunders, 1973, p. 19). Loré (1973, p. 711) suggested the following check list in examining the larynx: (1) vocal cords (free edges and superior surfaces) and their motion, (2) arytenoid cartilages and their motion, (3) ventricles and ventricular bands, (4) anterior and posterior commissures, (5) subglottic space (wall of trachea), (6) aryepiglottic folds, (7) lingual and laryngeal surfaces and free edges of epiglottis, and (8) the glossoepiglottic folds. Structural deviations, motion problems, and pathology are carefully noted and described.

Figure 16 shows the high points of the laryngeal examination. For more detailed explanation of the head and neck examination the reader is referred to Loré (1973), DeWeese and Saunders (1973), and Collins (1964).*

Direct Laryngoscopy

Young children who cannot be examined by undirect laryngoscopy because of lack of cooperation or an extreme gag reflex can be examined directly under general anesthesia; most infants must be examined this way. A laryngoscope is used for this examination. A laryngoscope is a hollow metal tube with a distal light source illuminating the area beyond the end of the tube; different sizes and shapes are available to accommodate the size of the orifice (DeWeese and Saunders, 1973, p. 152).

The patient lies on the examining table with his head beyond the end of the table; an assistant supports the head, moving it for examination procedures while another assistant handles suction apparatus (DeWeese and Saunders, 1973, p. 155). DeWeese and Saunders (1973, p. 157) described the procedure as follows: "To make a direct examination of the larynx, the endoscopist stands above the head of the supine patient. A laryngoscope is introduced into the patient's mouth over the tongue. . .the patient's neck is slowly extended, and the laryngoscope is passed carefully over the posterior face of the epiglottis. . .to expose the vocal cords."

RADIOLOGICAL AND ULTRASONIC EXAMINATIONS

Radiological examinations are used for two main purposes in the evaluation of voice problems. One is the use of x-rays for diagnosing laryngeal lesions, the other for assessing velopharyngeal competency. Johnson and Feist (1971) discussed laryngography as the procedure of choice for diagnosing benign laryngeal lesions. Contrast laryngography with cinefluorography has also proved to be a useful procedure in evaluating infant swallowing abnormalities and vocalization difficulties. Laryngomalacia and laryngostenosis are two specific areas where these studies have been helpful in diagnosis and treatment planning. Johnson and Feist (1971) described the procedure as follows: A topical anesthesia is sprayed into the oropharynx and larynx and a contrast medium is then introduced to coat the pharynx and larynx. Both a routine series of roentgenograms and cinefluorography may be taken and are obtained in posterior-anterior and lateral projection. Random vocalization of infants can be recorded by roentgenography and cinefluorographic studies. Older children are usually cooperative during the examination once the anesthetic is introduced and the cough reflex is abolished. Roentgenograms of these children are made in quiet respiration, during the phonation of /a/ and /i/, during a modified Valsalva maneuver performed by requesting the patient to hold his nose and blow air out through pursed lips slowly and steadily as if whistling, and while producing /i/ using reverse phonation. Johnson and Feist (1971) stated laryngography allows for examination of areas that are difficult to observe by either indirect or direct laryngoscopic examination.

Xeroradiography is described by Holinger, Lutterbeck, and Bulger (1972). It is a tech-

* A life size head-neck model can be used to acquaint the student with indirect laryngoscopy and to view slides of normal and pathological larynges. The Lancer Laryngoscopic Manikin is available from Sherwood Medical Industries, 1831 Olive St., St. Louis, MO 63103.

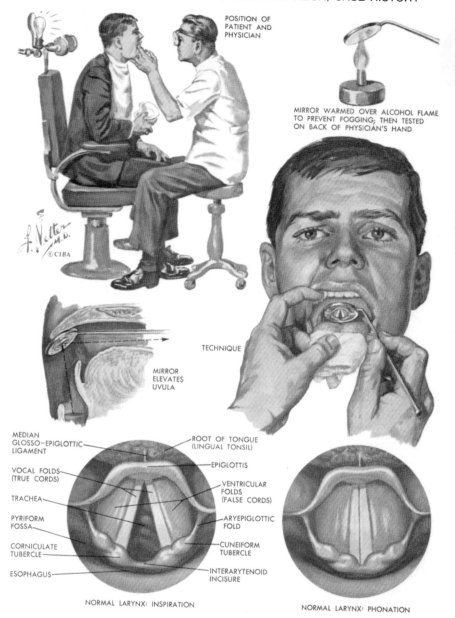

POSITION OF PATIENT AND PHYSICIAN

MIRROR WARMED OVER ALCOHOL FLAME TO PREVENT FOGGING; THEN TESTED ON BACK OF PHYSICIAN'S HAND

TECHNIQUE

MIRROR ELEVATES UVULA

MEDIAN GLOSSO-EPIGLOTTIC LIGAMENT

VOCAL FOLDS (TRUE CORDS)

TRACHEA

PYRIFORM FOSSA

CORNICULATE TUBERCLE

ESOPHAGUS

ROOT OF TONGUE (LINGUAL TONSIL)

EPIGLOTTIS

VENTRICULAR FOLDS (FALSE CORDS)

ARYEPIGLOTTIC FOLD

CUNEIFORM TUBERCLE

INTERARYTENOID INCISURE

NORMAL LARYNX: INSPIRATION

NORMAL LARYNX: PHONATION

Fig. 16. Examination of the larynx. (Copyright *Clinical Symposia* by Frank H. Netter, M.D., published by CIBA Pharmaceutical Company. Reproduced by permission.)

nique for examining the soft tissue of the neck which results in very excellent images with all densities of tissues recorded in detail and with good contrast. The margins of soft tissue and calcifications are accentuated and easily visualized. A xeroradiograph is made on an aluminum plate rather than on a photographic film. The plate is positioned under the patient and exposed to an x-ray beam passing through the patient. Woesner, Braun, and Sanders (1974) considered xeroradiog-

raphy a convenient technique requiring minimal patient cooperation. The procedure requires no topical anesthesia or contrast material. They stated it is especially useful in diagnosing neoplasms of the laryngopharyngeal area.

Hamlet (1973) described the ultrasonic method of assessing vocal cord vibration. A continuous-wave ultrasound is beamed laterally into the larynx by one transducer positioned on the neck and received by a second transducer on the other side of the neck. The transducers have to be placed so the transmission pathway is through the closed vocal cords. Then when the vocal cords open the ultrasound is reflected back from the glottal rim. Thus a series of ultrasonic pulses reflect the open quotient of the laryngeal vibratory pattern.

Children with velopharyngeal insufficiency usually require some type of x-ray examination to determine the extent of the defect. Lateral head plates may be taken with the palate at rest and while the child sustains various sounds such as /u/, /ɑ/, /i/, and /s/. Cinefluorography, x-ray motion pictures at 24 frames per sec, may be used for a more detailed analysis of velopharyngeal function during these sounds as well as during blowing and swallowing (Isshiki, Honjow, and Morimoto, 1969).

Lubker and Morris (1968) compared cinefluorographic film measurements with single-exposure still lateral x-ray film measurements. They found that if only one single-exposure film is to be used for estimating velopharyngeal opening, a still film taken during sustained /s/ seems to be the best choice. Massengill and Brooks (1973) suggested the /i/ sound is the best sound to employ during cinefluorographic study to determine if a patient can obtain velopharyngeal closure. Another techique is to use an ultrasonic beam aimed at the lateral pharyngeal wall until an echo is obtained. Kelsey, Ewanowski, Crummy, and Bless (1972) described this procedre by which it is possible to measure motion of the lateral pharyngeal wall of 1 mm or greater during speech. Ultrasonics are usually used in coordination with cinefluorographic studies. Still another techinque for asessing velopharyngeal closure is by endoscopy using a laryngeal telescope 6 mm in diameter (Zwitman, Sonderman, and Ward, 1974; Zwitman, Gyepes, and Ward, 1976).

X-ray film measurements are made of the distance between the soft palate and posterior pharyngeal wall. Generally an opening under 2 mm, measured in a lateral view, has no adverse effect on articulation or resonance. However, larger openings are acceptable for vowels preceding and following nasal sounds. Some speakers with velopharyngeal insufficiency with openings larger than 2 mm have acceptable speech and resonance. The reverse may also be true, some speakers with open-

ings under 2 mm may have noticeable articulation or hypernasality problems. For example, Shelton, Arndt, Knox, Elbert, Chisum, and Youngstrom (1969) reported that a group of children with borderline palatal pharyngeal closure with judged perceived hypernasality had a mean closure of 1.54 mm with a standard deviation of 0.72. Thus when receiving reports of measurements of lateral x-ray films the speech pathologist should recognize the limitations of this type of measurement.

Further guidelines for interpreting lateral x-ray reports may be helpful. Buck (1954), studying a group of normal subjects, measured lateral head plates to determine the smallest velopharyngeal opening during phonation. The results were /æ/ 0.36 mm, /i/ 0.26 mm, /ɑ/ 0.15 mm, and /u/ 0.12 mm. Moll (1962) studied 10 adults with normal speech by cinefluorography. Measurements of velum-pharynx distance on vowels were usually zero except for vowels preceding and following /n/. The mean velum-pharynx distance on vowels preceding /n/ averaged 4.45 mm while the distance following /n/ averaged 2.15 mm.

Hagerty and Hoffmeister (1954) measured velopharyngeal closure of cleft palate patients using lateral x-ray head plates. Three views were taken, with the palate at rest and during the production of /ɑ/ and /s/. The measurements were related to degree of articulation problem.

Articulation Problem	Palate at Rest	/ɑ/ Sound	/s/ Sound
None	7.6 mm	2.0 mm	0.25 mm
Minor	8.6 mm	3.3 mm	2.25 mm
Moderate	9.9 mm	4.8 mm	3.50 mm
Severe	12.7 mm	10.9 mm	11.40 mm

They also presented measurements on the relationship between minimal velopharyngeal distance and nasality. They stated it is possible to predict nasality from x-rays with about 75% accuracy.

Amount of Nasality	Velopharyngeal Opening
None	0–1 mm
Minor	2–3 mm
Moderate and Severe	4 mm or more

Subtelny, Koepp-Baker, and Subtelny (1961) found hypernasal speech was associated with moderate velopharyngeal openings from 3.5 to 7.0 mm. Van Demark (1974b) found a velopharyngeal gap greater than 2 mm on 92 % of 108 children with cleft palate who had been judged as having velopharyngeal incompetency.

CORRELATING THE VOICE EXAMINATION WITH THE PHYSICAL EXAMINATION

The analysis of a child's voice should be correlated with the physical examination. Positive physical findings such as vocal nodules of a specific size and location or an inactive soft palate guide the speech pathologist in his choice of examinations, in determining goals of voice therapy, and in selecting therapy measures. We can hypothesize how physiological insufficiencies and pathologies can affect the voice (West and Ansberry, 1968, p. 366). The reverse is true, that is, it is possible to hypothesize the physiological insufficiency or pathology according to the presenting vocal symptoms.

Arnold (1966) presented some guidelines used by laryngologists. (1) The voice disorder is related to the state of the vocal cord margins. He stated, "Any irregularity of the vibrating vocal cord margin causes incomplete glottal closure." This incomplete closure results in breathiness or air escape. Arnold stressed the more marked the alterations in the edges of the vocal cords the greater the voice deviation will be usually manifesting itself in a roughness of tone. (2) The site of the lesion should be considered. The anterior-posterior position of a lesion on a vocal cord generally determines the severity of the voice problem. Lesions in the anterior commissure cause the most severe voice disorders while variations in the posterior section of the cords result in less severe vocal disturbances. (3) If there is paralytic atrophy or traumatic deficiency there will be breathiness, a waste of air, a loss of vocal intensity, and shortened phonation time.

According to Moore (1971a, p. 555) when a speech pathologist listens to vocal production the physiological condition can be hypothesized as follows. Some weighting of the cords might be suspected as with edema or growths if the pitch is regularly very low combined with a rough hoarseness. A growth on a vocal cord, such as a nodule, or inadequate arytenoid approximation is suggested if the voice becomes increasingly breathy at higher pitches. One might suspect edema, growths, or inflammatory conditions producing excess mucus if the voice is hoarse at low pitches and becomes clear at high pitches. A high pitch may be due to an anterior laryngeal web or failure of laryngeal development. Baynes (1965) found children with a predominately harsh voice quality had a hyperkeratotic condition while those with a breathy voice quality had a well defined pathology such as vocal nodules. Hypernasality in a child may cause the speech pathologist to suspect velopharyngeal inadequacy or anterior growths in the nose. Hypernasality also may be the result of imitation or part of the learned pattern of speaking because of the particular region where he lives. When hyponasality is present one may suspect a partial or complete obstruction in the nasopharynx or posterior nasal passages.

The laryngologist's report must be available as the speech pathologist prepares and conducts the voice examination. Special attention should be given to all physical deviations noted by the laryngologist and they should be correlated with the results of the voice examination.

Many physicians and speech pathologists have forms to be completed for exchange of information. Figure 17 is an outline to be used in structuring a report form (Dweck, 1975, pp. 55–56; Fox and Blechman, 1975, pp. 66–67; Knight, 1973). Contents of the report form depend upon the job setting and information desired. Some physicians prefer to write a short letter about the pertinent findings of the head and neck examination. In either case a phone call to the physician should be made to acknowledge receipt of the information and, if desired, to ask specific questions. In some situations the referrral and examination results are done only by telephone. The voice team is the ideal situation for information exchange.

THE CASE HISTORY

It is necessary to obtain a special case history of the child's voice and voice problem from infancy to the present. The physician and speech pathologist cooperate in obtaining this information. The voice case history is designed to explore the etiology of the voice disorder as well as the factors contributing to the problem. This is in addition to a general case history which includes the general background of the child's growth and development including speech and language. Out-

Patient_____Date_____Physician — _____

Speech pathologist's description of voice problem:

RESULTS OF PHYSICIAN'S EXAMINATION

Ears: (Right   Left): External   Auditory canal   Tympanic membrane

Nose: Septum   Turbinates   Color   Polyps   Other obstructions   Sinus infection   Nasal allergy

Neck: Adenopathy (glandular disease, swelling and enlargement of lymph nodes)   Location

Oral Cavity: Teeth   Gingivae   Tongue   Pillars   Hard palate   Soft palate   Uvula   Symmetry of muscle contraction

Pharynx: Tonsils   Adenoid   Growths   Other abnormalities   Symmetry of muscle contraction

Larynx:

Description. General size: normal, larger than normal, smaller than normal. Color of surrounding tissue. Epiglottis: size, shape. False vocal cords. Appearance of vocal cords: color, thickened, edematous, inflamed, injected, malformed, scars.

Function of vocal cords. Tension: flaccid, normal, excessive. Symmetry of closure. Bowing of one or both cords. Manner of vocal cord closure: normal, hard, incomplete. Position of vocal cords at rest.

Presence of vocal pathology. Nodules, polyps, cysts, ulcers, other. Size of pathology. Appearance of pathology: hard, soft, other. Illustrate pathology on a diagram.

Other:

Does the patient have allergies, hypothyroidism, anemia, or any other chronic condition which might contribute to the abnormal voice quality? Has the patient's abuse and misuse of voice contributed to abnormal structure or function? Do the physical findings explain the abnormal voice quality? Is it possible that a continuation of present voice use may contribute to future or increased disorders of the mechanism?

Recommendations:

Are any of the following recommended: Silence, duration. Limited use of voice, duration. Training by a speech pathologist to help patient establish easy, efficient use of the vocal mechanism? If yes, note any restrictions, such as length of a voice session, outside practice, negative practice. Other recommendations: Medical, surgical, psychological-psychiatric.

Fig. 17. Outline for head and neck examination.

lines for a general case history can be found in standard texts (Dickson and Jann, 1974; Johnson, Darley, and Spriestersbach, 1963; Milisen, 1971; Nation and Aram, 1977). The suggested outline for a history of the voice problem follows.

Voice Case History Interview

Nature of Disorder

What is the parent's or patient's description of the voice disorder? How much of a problem is the disorder? Under what circumstances is it most troublesome?

Causes and Onset

What does the parent or patient regard as the cause? When was the disorder first noticed? By whom? Under what circumstances? Was its appearance sudden or gradual? Did it follow an illness?

Severity

Does the severity of the disorder vary? Describe the changes. Has it been better or worse recently? Does it vary according to the season? time of day? geographic location? weather? fatigue? mood (e.g., happiness, discouragement)?

Family History

Does any other family member have a voice, speech, or hearing problem? Does the child sound like any other family member when he talks? Does he sound like a friend or his teacher? Has the child ever lived in any other part of the country? Have his parents lived elsewhere?

Voice Use

When the child was an infant did he cry and scream more than other babies? Did he have any abnormality in respiration such as noisy breathing? Has he been a noisy or talkative child? Does he yell, shout, or scream excessively when he plays? How much talking does he do when riding in a car at high speeds? How much singing does he do? Does he sing solos or in a chorus or choir? Does he participate in dramatics or cheerleading? Does he spend much time talking in noisy places? Is his voice ever confused with that of anyone else on the phone?

Medical

When was his last medical examination? What was the physician's name? What were the findings? What medications does he take regularly? List all operations and give the hospital and date for each. Was his voice different after an operation? Has he had any serious illnesses? At what ages? Has he been in any accidents? Does he have allergies? hay fever? asthma? Does he have many colds? Has he ever had any eye trouble? Has he ever had any general breathing problems?

Has he ever had a metabolism test? If so what were the results? Was he given medication? What is his usual body temperature? Are his skin and hair dry? Does he perspire more or less than others? Do you know what his pulse rate is? Is he often fatigued without apparent cause? Has he ever been anemic? do you know what his blood count is?

Ears

Has he been examined by an otologist? Who? Where? When? What were the findings? Has he ever had ear trouble? Injury to the ears? Operation on the ears? Has he had medical treatment for an otologic problem? Does he have patulous eustachian tubes? What are the results of any hearing tests?

Nose and Nasopharynx

Has there been injury to the nose? Has he had sinus infections? Has he ever had a deviated septum? A broken nose? Has he ever had trouble breathing through his nose, one side or both? Is he a mouth breather? Has he had difficulty with the sense of smell? are /m/, /n/, and /ŋ/ adequately nasalized? Do they have a muffled sound? Has he ever had an adenoidectomy? Has his voice been different since then? Removal of nasal polyp?

Oral Cavity

Has there been injury to the mouth? Has he ever had a tonsillectomy? Has his voice been different since then? If he has had an operation on the palate why was it performed? Describe the surgery. Did it change his voice? Does he have a bifid uvula? Does he have difficulty producing speech sounds requiring oral breath pressure? Are some speech sounds emitted through the nose? What are they? Is there audible nasal emission of air as he talks? Has he ever had difficulty with the sense of taste? When he talks does he have facial grimaces or pinching of the nostrils? Has he ever had difficulty swallowing? Choking? Have liquids or food ever gone into his nose when swallowing? Can he blow up a balloon? Can he whistle? Can he drink from a fountain? With a straw?

Larynx and Hypopharynx

Has he ever been examined by a laryngologist? Who? When? Where? What were the findings? Has there been any injury to the neck? Has he ever had laryngitis? Lost his voice? Does he cough a great deal? Clear his throat often? Has there been any medical treatment for a laryngeal problem? Has there been an operation on the laryngeal area? Why was it performed? Describe the operation. Has his voice been any different since the operation? Has he ever had pain or a sense of pressure around the larynx? Does food ever lodge in the throat causing coughing?

History of Adolescence

Has the child gone through voice change? Describe the voice during this period. Describe any pitch breaks. If a girl, has she started menstruating? At what age did she begin? What is the length of the cycle? Is periodic hoarseness related to the menstrual cycle? Has the child ever worked? Was it in a noisy place? A dusty place? Does he smoke? How much? When did he start smoking?

Voice Therapy History

Has he had a previous voice or speech examination? Where? When? By whom? What were the findings? Has he had any remedial voice or speech work? What kind? Where? When? By whom? How long was it continued? Describe the results. Why was it terminated?

SUMMARY

The management of voice problems requires the coordinated efforts of many specialists. A voice team approach is an efficient and effective method for examination, consultation, treatment, and follow-up. Close contacts must be kept between the speech pathologist and the various specialists. Each child with a voice problem should receive a complete head and neck examination including indicated radiological examinations. A general case history of the child's growth and development and a specific history of his voice are done as one of the first steps in an evaluation. The findings of these examinations serve as a guide to the speech pathologist in selecting special rating scales and tests for each child.

SIX

Examinations: II

Examinations by the Speech Pathologist

The speech pathologist is responsible for conducting detailed examinations of voice problems. Nation and Aram (1977, p. 286) suggested listening to only one voice component at a time, listening carefully for disturbed vocal characteristics, and describing the voice characteristics in perceptual terminology not causal terminology (e.g. hypernasality not cleft palate speech). Pitch and loudness are studied. Voice quality is defined and described as accurately as possible. Vocal abuse must be detected and evaluated. Undue muscular tensions are noted. Breathing habits are checked. Posture is noted, especially in relation to the position of the head and neck. The speech pathologist may use special speech tests and oral breath pressure measures to evaluate velopharyngeal competence. The voice examination includes a brief concentrated therapy session to determine the child's ability to produce a better voice.

The assessment of vocal function is coordinated with the general physical examination, head and neck examination, psychological assessments, hearing evaluations, and other indicated examinations and tests. From the results of the examinations a plan is formulated for the voice therapy program and a prognosis of recovery potential is made.

GROUP PLAY OBSERVATION

It is necessary to obtain voice samples under various speaking conditions. Samples of voice should be obtained under two conditions, when the person knows he is being tested and when he is unaware of being tested (Milisen, 1971, p. 655). Observations in small informal gatherings, a regular school class, and in large groups reveal use of voice (Irwin, 1965, pp. 85–86). Many aspects of vocal behavior may not appear in a one-to-one relationship of an adult with the child. Observation of children in informal but carefully planned play situations gives excellent samples of voice use when they are unaware and when they are aware of being tested. We call this type of evaluation *group play observation*. Many times group play observation can be done by people other than the speech pathologist. In a college or university it may be a student speech pathologist, in a hospital or community clinic it may be a volunteer worker, or in the schools it may be a teacher or a teacher aide. If observers other than qualified speech pathologists are used it is necessary to instruct these assistants on observation techniques. It is not essential for the observer to be a participant in the group play situation; however, it is advisable for him to participate as much as possible to allow him to direct the activities and encourage children to talk so he can observe the various parameters of voice usage. In the Jacksonville, Florida, Child Guidance and Speech Correction Clinic on diagnostic days we used group play observation with much success to evaluate children's voices as well as other aspects of their behavior.

Group play observation can be easily set up in schools and clinics. A 45-min group play period can be scheduled. Children are grouped according to age so activities appropriate to the children's ages can be conducted. These may range from group games for nursery age children to baseball for teenagers. Children are encouraged to engage in all types of play ranging from quiet to very loud noisy activities. A relatively small room can be used for groups of three to six children. If the groups are large or if much activity is desired large rooms, gym areas, and outdoor playgrounds may be used.

Group Play Observation Form

The form to use for group play observation is shown in Figure 18. The form is based on one developed at the clinic in Jacksonville, Florida. With younger children we like to get

Name_____ Birth Date_____ Age_____

Place of Observation: Playroom, gym, playground, other_____

Observer_____ Date_____ Length of Observation_____

1. *Preliminary Behavior and Attitude:*
2. *Activities:* Use of toys, equipment, need for help, destructiveness.
3. *Relationships:* Adults and children.
4. *Learning Ability:* Level of operation observed.
5. *Hearing:* Response to noise and speech.
6. *Speech:* Amount, intelligibility, articulation, rhythm, use of gestures to communicate.
7. *Language Level:* Reception, expression, grammar.
8. *Voice:* Pitch, loudness, voice quality, resonance, pitch breaks, monotone: Do these aspects vary under different conditions?
9. *Vocal Abuse:* Shouting, screaming, cheering, excessive talking, strained vocalizations, reverse phonation, explosive vocalizations, abrupt glottal attack, throat clearing, coughing.
10. *Physical Coordination:* Gross and fine. Walking, running, skipping, kicking, catching, block building, drawing, cutting, writing.
11. *Overall Impression:* Speech, language, and voice.
12. *Recommendations:*_____

Fig. 18. Group play observation.

a description of the child's behavior and attitude as he is being separated from his parents or taken from the classroom and invited to go to a playroom, a gym, or a playground. Item 1 is a description of the child's preliminary behavior and attitude. The more secure and cooperative child will easily separate from the parent or teacher. An insecure child who is reluctant to leave the parent or classroom may later present a problem in establishing rapport during voice therapy. Item 2 is a description of the child's various activities during the period, his appropriate use of toys and equipment, his need for help, and his destructiveness. The third item deals with the child's relationship to adults and to other children. Item 4, the level of the child's operation, may reveal information about his learning ability. The observer may note under Item 5 the child's responses to noise and speech which reveal information about his listening abilities.

Item 6 is concerned specifically with a child's speech. Careful observations should be made of the amount of talking, intelligibility of speech, general accuracy of articulation, rhythm of speech, and use of gestures to communicate. Item 7 deals with the child's language level. How well does he understand what is said to him? Can he put his ideas into words in a manner appropriate to his age? Is

his use of grammar consistent with his age level? For Item 8, voice, the observer should listen very carefully to the child's voice. The pitch of his voice should be noted. Is it appropriate to his age and sex? What happens to it when the voice increases in loudness? Does the pitch rise appropriately as loudness increases? What is the general level of loudness? How much loud talking does he do? Is the quality of his voice breathy, harsh, or hoarse? Is the resonance hypernasal or hyponasal? If any differences in pitch, loudness, quality, or resonance have been noted the observer should listen carefully to see if these deviations vary under different conditions. For example, what happens to a hoarse voice with an increase in loudness? Does the quality get worse or does it seem to clear up? Any pitch breaks and monotonous use of voice in the group play situation should be noted.

Item 9, vocal abuse, is a particularly important item in group play observation. Various types of vocal abuse to be noted include shouting, screaming, cheering, excessive talking, strained vocalizations, reverse phonation, explosive vocalizations, abrupt glottal attack, throat clearing, and coughing. Definitions of these are given on page 87. Item 10 requires observation of the child's physical coordination—gross coordination, such as walking, running, skipping, kicking, and the finer coordinations required for catching, block building, drawing, cutting, and writing. Items 11 and 12 include the observer's overall impression of the child and recommendations for special testing based on the observation.

VOICE RATING SCALES

The speech pathologist uses rating scales to evaluate voice in its various parameters. Each child is rated to establish baselines of vocal behavior.

Establishing Baselines

Baselines are descriptions of behavior a person exhibits. Rating scales can be used to describe such behavior. A child's use of voice is rated before any treatment is started to enable the speech pathologist to know the level of vocal behavior and the aspects which should be improved.

Behavior must be correctly identified and reliably measured (Brookshire, 1967). Therefore, the speech pathologist in measuring any type of vocal behavior or speech behavior for establishing baselines must be sure the measurements are consistently and reliably made. Our examination and evaluative procedures include establishment of baselines for deviant voice behavior through the use of rating scales such as the rating of vocal abuse practices. Brookshire (1967) emphasized the necessity for establishing baselines in varying situations. For example, some children may shout only to a moderate degree in one situation, while in another situation shouting may be extremely loud, and in still other situations he may not shout at all. Brookshire (1967) pointed out that the establishment of specific baselines and their exact identification and measurement " ... forces the clinician to define specific observable behaviors of concern prior to initiation of therapy." These baselines then become the foundation from which improvement can be measured as therapy progresses, with final ratings made at the conclusion of therapy. These final ratings are compared with ratings made when children are seen for follow-up evaluations to check effectiveness of carryover.

Rating Scales

The equal-appearing intervals rating scale is the most frequently used scale in speech pathology. Sherman and Moodie (1957) compared four different methods of scaling articulation defectiveness of children's speech, and Sherman and Silverman (1968) reported on three scaling methods for rating language development. The results of both studies indicated the method of equal-appearing intervals was the most satisfactory scale. We recommend the use of this type of scale for voice evaluations. This scale usually includes three to seven points. A disadvantage of the equal-appearing intervals scale is called the "end effect" (Cullinan and Counihan, 1968), that is a judge's tendency to refrain from using the extreme ends of a scale. The speech pathologist should keep this tendency in mind and use the end ratings whenever indicated.

The number of intervals used on a scale is determined by the characteristics and complexities of the item to be rated. For example, three points can be used for some scales while more points are desirable for others. Three points can be used in describing the amount of certain vocal characteristics such as shouting, with *1* meaning little shouting, *2* frequent shouting, and *3* excessive shouting. Three points are also satisfactory for rating the degree of vocal effort. For example, rating throat clearing can be done with *1* indicating a mild degree of effort or force, *2* a moderate degree, or *3* a severe degree, that is very hard, forceful, and loud throat clearing. In rating other vocal attributes, hoarseness for example, it is desirable to use a 7 point scale with *1* indicating a slight deviation and *7* a severe deviation.

Reports on ratings of voice by speech pathologists show varying reliability. We know that to be a reliable and valid rater a judge has to be trained specifically for that task. Having experience in speech and voice therapy is not sufficient background for precise judging of voice. Villarreal (1950) found a low percentage of agreement among judges in rating voice quality. Bradford, Brooks, and Shelton (1964) also found unreliable ratings were made by both inexperienced and experienced speech pathologists who were not comprehensively trained specifically for the task of rating hypernasality. Schulz, Heller, Gens, and Lewin (1973) reported interjudge reliability was 0.94 for judges using a 7 point nasal resonance scale, and Lewin, Heller, and Kojak (1975) found interjudge reliability among three trained speech pathologists was 0.91 in judging hypernasality on a 5 point scale of severity. Wynter (1974) found that speech pathologists, using a 3 point scale of deviancy, appeared to be in accord in judging pitch deviations and to be in reasonable agreement over hoarseness and stridency. However, they had low agreement in judging breathiness, and even lower agreement in judging nasal resonance.

Speech pathologists should prove their competency in judging various aspects of voice. This can be done through judging types and severity of voice deviations and correlating the ratings with those of other speech pathologists (Wilson and Rice, 1977, p. 2). Reliability or consistency in rating can be determined by comparing the results of periodic ratings of the same samples. When the ratings of several judges are pooled into one rating, either the mean or median value on the equal-appearing intervals scale may be used; Sherman (1970) found this to be true when 7 point scales were used to judge four aspects of cleft palate speech: nasality, articulation, language, and general defectiveness.

Developing terminology to use in voice profiles is difficult. Isshiki, Okamura, Tanabe, and Morimoto (1969) and Isshiki and Takeuchi (1970) in an attempt to objectify terminology in voice did a factor analysis of hoarseness using Osgood's semantic differential technique. They arrived at four factors for describing voice: *Factor R* (rough), the adjectives that characterized this factor were dull, thick, heavy, broad, cloudy, rough, and bad. *Factor B* (breathy), the adjectives describing this factor were dry, hard, excited, pointed, cold, choked, rough, cloudy, sharp, poor, and bad. *Factor A* (asthenic), the adjectives describing this factor were thin, sickly, poor, light, and bad. *Factor N* (normal or only slightly hoarse), the adjectives describing this factor were good, clear, soft, calm, free, and rich.

Voice Screening Form

The Voice Screening Form (Fig. 19) can be used by the speech pathologist when screening large groups of children for voice problems. The following items are suggested for use during voice screening: (1) counting from 1 to 10, (2) a 1 min sample of connected speech, (3) a 1 min sample of reading, and (4) prolonged vowels for 5 sec each: /ɑ/, /ɛ/, /i/, /u/, /ɔ/. A rating on any *one* item of *2* or *3* means the child should be seen later for checking on chronicity and need for further attention. This form is based on one suggested by Boone (1973; 1977, p. 69) in which he suggested a 9 point scale for rating pitch, phonation quality, loudness, and resonance quality.

General Voice Profiles

The special voice profile system described by Connelly, Wilson, and Leeper (1970), Wilson (1972), and Wilson and Rice (1977) is an excellent profile to use both for screening and for rating various parameters of voice to discover the aspects of voice needing attention and to establish baselines at the beginning of a therapeutic program. The profile includes a 7 point rating scale on which the speech pathologist rates the overall severity of the voice problem. A rating of *1* means the voice is normal, while *7* indicates a severe voice problem. The profile includes the maximum phonation time for sustaining /ɑ/. For individuals having voice problems originating in the laryngeal cavity, the voice profile includes a rating of pitch and a rating of the degree of vocal cord closure. Pitch is rated *1* if normal, *+2* for too high, and *−2* for too low. A pitch rating of *+3* (high) or *−3* (low) means the pitch of the voice is such that sexual identity

	School_____	Date_____
Name_____		
Examiner_____	Grade_____ Teacher_____

	Normal	Mild	Moderate	Severe
1. *Laryngeal Tone* (Breathy, harsh, hoarse)	N	1	2	3
2. *Voice Pitch* (Modal level, breaks)	N	1	2	3
3. *Resonance* (Hypernasality, hyponasality)	N	1	2	3
4. *Loudness* (Soft, loud)	N	1	2	3
5. *Overall Voice Efficiency*	N	1	2	3

COMMENTS:

Fig. 19. Voice screening.

is lost. On the open-closed rating a -4 indicates the vocal cords are open and there is complete aphonia since no vocal cord vibration is present. A rating of $+3$ indicates the cords are in a tightly closed position during attempted phonation with the phonatory effort being definitely spastic. The resonating cavity is rated 1 for normal, with $+2$, $+3$, and $+4$ for varying degrees of hypernasality, and -2 for a hyponasal rating. The form also includes a check regarding whether the disturbed vocal parameters are constant or variable. Intensity is rated as too loud, normal, or too soft; and vocal range as a monotone, normal, or too variable in pitch. Starr and Wilson (1976) found this profile system can be used most reliably by both experienced and inexperienced raters for tasks that require the rater to determine whether voice features are normal or deviant. However, they found reliability was reduced when the task required rating the severity of deviant voice features.

Perello and Tosi (1974) presented a method of describing voice diagnosis as well as charting progress in voice therapy. The items measured are vocal intensity at 3 meters (9.84 feet), maximum duration of phonation, vocal range in tones, rating of hoarseness in Yanagihara (1967a; 1967b) units (see pp. 75–76), time in hours before vocal fatigue is reported by the person, and the difference in cubic decimeters between the maximum air expiration with the nostrils open and occluded.

Buffalo Voice Profile

We use the Buffalo Voice Profile in rating voice problems and as a guideline for voice therapy (Fig. 20). Special rating scales for specific voice problems are also used and will be presented later. The scales of the Buffalo Voice Profile contain seven equal-appearing intervals with 1 meaning a slight deviation and 7 a severe deviation. This profile consists of 12 major aspects: laryngeal tone, laryngeal tension, vocal abuse, loudness, pitch, vocal inflections, pitch breaks, diplophonia, resonance, nasal emission, rate, and overall voice efficiency. The speech pathologist circles the appropriate descriptive term listed under each item. For example, pitch may be rated as normal, high, or low. If pitch is rated normal it requires no further rating. If it is rated either high or low the speech pathologist must circle one of the numbers on the deviation scale for that item. Check marks

should not be placed between the numbers. The same procedure is used for all 12 items.

The Speech Anxiety Scale

Ratings of speech anxiety should be done during the appraisal of a voice problem. It may prove useful in establishing therapy goals in many types of voice problems including the speech anxiety manifested in children with vocal nodules and hysterical dysphonia. We base our scale (Fig. 21) for this on the work of Mulac and Sherman (1974) who did a factor analysis of the characteristics of speech anxiety. Mulac and Sherman used a 10 point equal-appearing intervals scale. We have adjusted this rating scale to a 7 point scale with 1 and 2 meaning slight speech anxiety, 3, 4, and 5 moderate, and 6 and 7 strong speech anxiety. They studied 18 variables and found four factors to be significant of 18 variables in describing speech anxiety: *Factor I, rigidity*, includes hypertension of various parts of the body, such as rigid or tense arms and hands, tense face muscles, grimaces, twitches, lack of motion, and lack of appropriate gestures. *Factor II, inhibition*, manifested by a monotonous voice with lack of vocal emphasis, a "deadpan" facial expression, and a too-soft voice. *Factor III, dysfluency*, includes hunting for words, speech blocks, quivering or tense voice, nonfluency, stuttering, halting, breathing heavily, and vocalized pauses. *Factor IV, agitation*, includes fidgeting, swaying, pacing, shuffling feet, lack of eye contact, and extraneous eye movements.

TYPES OF VOICE SAMPLES

In studying the various aspects of voice the speech pathologist should obtain several types of speech samples. These samples should include connected speech, oral reading, isolated speech sounds, and counting. All samples of voice or speech should be tape recorded for further use and study.

Connected Speech

A sample of connected speech can usually be obtained by asking the child to tell a story about a picture. Action pictures of various types are especially useful. Another way to get samples of connected speech is to ask the child to talk about a specific topic such as a vacation with the family or his favorite sport or hobby.

Name_____ Birth Date_____ Age_____ Sex_____

Rater _____ Date _____ Time of Day _____ Place_____

1. *Laryngeal Tone*
   Normal
   Breathy
   Harsh
   Hoarse   1 _____ 2 _____ 3 _____ 4 _____ 5 _____ 6 _____ 7

2. *Laryngeal Tension*
   Normal
   Hypertense
   Hypotense   1 _____ 2 _____ 3 _____ 4 _____ 5 _____ 6 _____ 7

3. *Vocal Abuse*
   No
   Yes   1 _____ 2 _____ 3 _____ 4 _____ 5 _____ 6 _____ 7

4. *Loudness*
   Normal
   Too loud
   Too soft   1 _____ 2 _____ 3 _____ 4 _____ 5 _____ 6 _____ 7

5. *Pitch*
   Normal
   High
   Low   1 _____ 2 _____ 3 _____ 4 _____ 5 _____ 6 _____ 7

6. *Vocal Inflections*
   Normal
   Monotone
   Excessive   1 _____ 2 _____ 3 _____ 4 _____ 5 _____ 6 _____ 7

7. *Pitch Breaks*
   None
   Amount   1 _____ 2 _____ 3 _____ 4 _____ 5 _____ 6 _____ 7

8. *Diplophonia*
   None
   Amount   1 _____ 2 _____ 3 _____ 4 _____ 5 _____ 6 _____ 7

9. *Resonance*
   Normal
   Hypernasal
   Hyponasal   1 _____ 2 _____ 3 _____ 4 _____ 5 _____ 6 _____ 7

10. *Nasal Emission*
    No
    Yes   1 _____ 2 _____ 3 _____ 4 _____ 5 _____ 6 _____ 7

11. *Rate*
    Normal
    Fast
    Slow   1 _____ 2 _____ 3 _____ 4 _____ 5 _____ 6 _____ 7

12. *Overall Voice Efficiency*
    Adequate
    Inadequate   1 _____ 2 _____ 3 _____ 4 _____ 5 _____ 6 _____ 7

Circle the appropriate descriptive term under *each* item. For each item *not* normal or adequate, circle a number on the scale for that item. Do *not* mark between numbers.

Key: 1 = slight deviation   4 = moderate deviation   7 = severe deviation

COMMENTS:_____

Fig. 20. Buffalo Voice Profile.

Name_____ Birth Date_____ Age_____ Sex_____

Rater_____ Date_____ Time of Day_____ Place_____

I	*Rigidity*							
	No							
	Yes	1	2	3	4	5	6	7
II	*Inhibition*							
	No							
	Yes	1	2	3	4	5	6	7
III	*Dysfluency*							
	No							
	Yes	1	2	3	4	5	6	7
IV	*Agitation*							
	No							
	Yes	1	2	3	4	5	6	7

COMMENTS:

INSTRUCTIONS:
A. Circle *yes* or *no* under each item for presence or absence of the factor.
B. For each item rated *yes*, circle a number on the scale for that item.
Do *not* mark between numbers.
Key: 1, 2   = slight anxiety
3, 4, 5 = moderate anxiety
6, 7   = strong anxiety

Fig. 21. Speech Anxiety Scale. Based upon Mulac, A., and Sherman, A. R. (1974). Behavioral assessment of speech anxiety, *Q. J. Speech 60:* 134–143. Approved and used courtesy of Drs. Mulac and Sherman.

Oral Reading

If the child is old enough to read, it is desirable to get an oral reading sample. For children of approximately third grade reading level and above we use a passage which we devised several years ago titled "The Trip to the Zoo." The same passage should be used for all children old enough to read so when listening judgments are made the speech pathologist is not distracted by an unfamiliar passage but can concentrate on evaluating the voice and its attributes. For this reason this same passage should be used when checking progress in voice therapy. If the child's reading level is below third grade his own reading book should be used to get as smooth a sample of reading as possible.

The Trip to the Zoo

Last Sunday Bob went to the zoo with his mother and father. His sister Mary and his brother George went along too. Mother packed a big basket full of good things to eat. Father took the car to the service station to get gas and to have the oil checked. The family left the house at 11 o'clock and got to the zoo at 12 o'clock. You can see that they didn't have far to go.

At the zoo they saw monkeys, tigers, lions, bears, elephants, and lots of beautiful birds. The monkeys put on a special show in their cage. They jumped from one swing to another and pulled each other around in little red wagons. The elephants put on a show too. They stood up on their hind legs and danced with each other.

After the shows the family found a nice cool place under a tree. Mother put a table cloth on the grass and unpacked the lunch. The family ate the lunch and talked about the good time they had seeing all the animals at the zoo.

Isolated Speech Sounds

A sample of isolated vowel production should be obtained on the following vowels, /i/, /ɪ/, /e/, /ɛ/, /æ/, /ʌ/, /u/, /U/, /o/, /ɔ/, /ɑ/. Each sound should be sustained for at least 5 sec and repeated three times. Selected voiced continuant consonants, for example /m/, /n/, /r/, /l/ should also be recorded.

Counting

It is desirable to record a child counting from 1 to 10. Have him count twice, first slowly and carefully and then again as rapidly as possible but still saying each number carefully. This should be done under three levels of loudness: soft, average, and loud; and at three voice pitch levels: low, modal, and high. The contrast between the countings may exaggerate or even reveal pitch and loudness misuse, vocal abuse, defective laryngeal tone, or resonance problems. Mason and Grandstaff (1972) suggested having a hypernasal speaker count from 60 to 100 to obtain samples of varying phonetic contexts ranging from nasal to nonnasal. They also suggested checking to see if hypernasality is reduced as a person counts from 1 to 10 while exaggerating anterior articulatory movements. If it is reduced it can be assumed that habitual inactivity of the anterior articulators is a factor related to velopharyngeal incompetency.

ANALYSIS OF PITCH AND LOUDNESS

Kent (1976) reviewed the research on developmental changes in fundamental frequency from birth to adulthood. The fundamental frequency drops slightly during the first 3 weeks of life and then rises until about the 4th month, and then stabilizes for approximately 5 months. When the child is 1 year old the fundamental frequency lowers rapidly until he is about 3 years of age. Then the pitch level gradually lowers to the point of onset of puberty at 11 or 12 years of age. Fundamental frequency levels begin to be distinguishable by sex at about 11 years and very dramatically by the age of 13 years. In girls the fundamental frequency lowers little more than an octave from birth to adulthood; in contrast boys' fundamental frequency lowers about 2 octaves. The age periods of most rapid change in fundamental frequency levels are: the first 4 months, the years 1 to 3, and years 13 to 17.

Many times it is necessary to teach children to use pitch levels which are adequate and nontraumatizing; therefore, it is necessary to make a careful analysis of the child's use of pitch and loudness before planning voice therapy. This includes determining modal frequency level and comparing it to standards for his age and sex.

When examining a child's use of pitch he should be observed under various voice intensity conditions. We know pitch becomes higher with an increase in the intensity of a person's voice from normal to loud; likewise, a lowering of pitch occurs when a person goes from normal to soft speech. A study of a child's pitch when talking at loud levels may reveal information on the misuse of the vocal mechanism.

If the basal pitch level is used to calculate a child's optimal pitch level, measurements should be taken at various times of day over a period of 2 or more days. Cooper and Yanagihara (1971) studied basal pitch variation in a group of 13 normal-speaking adults, six males and seven females ranging in age from 21 to 50 years. Each person was asked to produce /ɑ/ three times for about 5 sec at the lowest most comfortable basal pitch. This was done for 2 days, morning, noon, and late afternoon. In nearly all individuals the basal pitch varied from 1 to 3 semitones during the day, with a continual daily rise in some individuals and a continual daily lowering in others. For some subjects there was a rise of the basal pitch at noon and then a lowering of pitch in the late afternoon. A similar study was done by Austin and Leeper (1975) using normally-speaking boys and girls, seven boys and eight girls, ranging in age from 9 years 2 months to 10 years 11 months. Each child was instructed to produce the vowel /ɑ/ for 5 sec at the lowest possible most comfortable pitch (basal pitch) for three consecutive trials during each of the testing sessions, which were on 2 consecutive days, morning, noon, and afternoon. The results of their study suggest that the basal pitch level in children varies from time to time within a day and from one day to the next. The basal pitch level of individual boys varied up to 2 semitones from day to day and across time periods in a day. For girls as a group there was a pitch drop from noon to afternoon on any one of the days tested, with the basal pitch of individual girls varying as much as 4 semitones from day to day and as much as 3 semitones from time to time within 1 day. The pattern in basal pitch levels varied for different children and was not always the same from day to day for any one child.

Further, both loudness and modal pitch levels can vary when we ask a child to talk or read at a "comfortable effort level." Brown, Murry, and Hughes (1976) reported on day to day variability of vocal intensity and pitch levels in a group of adult speakers. The speakers repeated vocal and speech utterances at the same time of day plus or minus ½ hour for 5 successive days. Subjects were asked to sustain /ɑ/ and /i/ three times for approximately 5 sec and they were also asked to repeat the phrase "say /ɑ/ again" and "say /i/ again" three times, with the only instruction being to produce the speech materials at a "comfortable effort level." The results indicated that from day to day vocal intensity varied as much as 25 dB and the modal frequency level as much as 4 semitones. These were the extremes of variability in certain speakers; other speakers were quite consistent from one day to the next for both vocal parameters.

It appears to us, therefore, that voice intensity and pitch level testing of children done only once on a certain day may not be the most representative sample for that child. We suggest taking voice intensity and pitch level samples at various times of day over a period of several days to determine intensity and pitch variation and stability.

The study of a child's pitch should be made with knowledge of the results of his laryngeal examination. The pitch level used by children with certain pathologies such as vocal nodules may be quite crucial. A too-high or too-low modal frequency level is sometimes a contributing factor in the formation of vocal nodules. A detailed pitch analysis may not be necessary if pitch usage seems appropriate and there are no laryngeal pathologies thought to be connected with pitch use. There is no need to be unnecessarily preoccupied with pitch manipulation (Brodnitz, 1962).

Pitch Analysis

Pitch analysis can be made using a musical instrument, pitch pipe, or pitch meter. A piano, guitar, or other musical instrument can be used. However, many times a musical instrument is not available and a pitch pipe may not have enough notes to give variety and range to the study of a child's use of pitch. Instruments for pitch analysis in the

clinical situation are available.* With this type of instrument the speech pathologist does not have to be familiar with the musical scale to determine the child's modal frequency level. The child's use of pitch inflections can be studied using a pitch indicator. Direct readings in Hertz can be obtained from the meter on the front of the instrument. Some instruments are designed to use lights to indicate correct and incorrect use of pitch.†

The modal frequency level can be determined with a pitch indicator following Fairbanks' technique (1960, p. 126). Give the child a reading selection of about 180 words. Place vertical lines after about the first 60 words and the second set of 60 words. Have the child read the first third of the passage with normal inflections. When he reaches the first pair of vertical lines have him begin to compress his range gradually until he is chanting in a monotone at his modal frequency level by the time he reaches the second pair of vertical lines. Let him finish the third section of the passage on this pitch gradually changing to humming or singing the note equal to his pitch level. For younger children who cannot read fluently have them repeat a familiar nursery rhyme or poem several times. Hand gestures can be used to signal for compression of pitch. During this process the speech pathologist watches the pitch indicator readings carefully, finally ending up with a definite reading during the third section of the reading passage. As the child compresses his pitch the needle on the pitch indicator will barely fluctuate. The average of the observable fluctuations will be the modal frequency level. The whole procedure should be repeated several times at different times of day on several different days to determine accuracy of measurement. The same method can be used with a piano or musical instrument. Next compare the pitch indicator readings or the musical note for his modal frequency level with the acceptable limits for his age (Tables 1 and 2).

The pitch charts (Tables 1 and 2), including all ages, are presented to give the speech pathologist standards to use in checking the appropriateness of a child's modal frequency level. The pitch charts are based upon the

* Fundamental Frequency Indicator, Special Instrument, Stockholm, Sweden. United States Distributor: SI America, 255 South 17th St., Philadelphia, PA 19103.

† Florida I, Saber, Inc., Cocoa Beach, FL 32931 (controls both pitch and loudness levels).

TABLE 1
Composite Pitch Chart—Boys

Age	Fundamental Frequency (Hz)	Acceptable Limits of Fundamental Frequency (Hz)	Nearest Musical Note to Fundamental Frequency	Acceptable Limits of Fundamental Frequency in Musical Notes
1 & 2	445	370–525	A_4	$F\#_4-C_5$
3	400	340–460	G_4	$F_4-A\#_4$
4	375	320–425	$F\#_4$	$D\#_4-G\#_4$
5	350	300–390	F_4	D_4-G_4
6	325	280–365	E_4	$C\#_4-F\#_4$
7	295	260–330	D_4	C_4-E_4
8	295	260–330	D_4	C_4-E_4
9	260	220–300	C_4	A_3-D_4
10	235	195–275	$A\#_3$	$G_3-C\#_4$
11	225	185–260	A_3	$F\#_3-C_4$
12	210	170–245	$G\#_3$	F_3-B_3
13	195	155–230	G_3	$D\#_3-A\#_3$
14	190	155–220	$F\#_3$	$D\#_3-A_3$
15	165	130–195	E_3	C_3-G_3
16	150	120–180	D_3	$A\#_2-F\#_3$
17	135	110–170	$C\#_3$	A_2-F_3
18	125	100–155	B_2	$G_2-D\#_3$

TABLE 2
Composite Pitch Chart—Girls

Age	Fundamental Frequency (Hz)	Acceptable Limits of Fundamental Frequency (Hz)	Nearest Musical Note to Fundamental Frequency	Acceptable Limits of Fundamental Frequency in Muscial Notes
1 & 2	445	370–525	A_4	$F\#_4-C_5$
3	380	335–475	$F\#_4$	$E_4-A\#_4$
4	355	310–450	F_4	$D\#_4-A_4$
5	335	290–425	E_4	$D_4-G\#_4$
6	315	270–395	$D\#_4$	$C\#_4-G_4$
7	280	245–310	$C\#_4$	$B_3-D\#_4 \ (F_4)^a$
8	290	245–350	D_4	B_3-F_4
9	275	235–335	$C\#_4$	$A\#_3-E_4$
10	265	225–320	C_4	$A_3-D\#_4$
11	265	220–310	C_4	$A_3-D\#_4$
12	260	220–310	C_4	$G\#_3-D_4$
13I[b]	260	235–295	C_4	$A\#_3-D_4$
13II[b]	245	210–295	B_3	$G\#_3-D_4$
14	235	195–270	$A\#_3$	$G_3-C\#_4$
15	220	185–260	A_3	$F\#_3-C_4$
16	215	185–260	A_3	$F\#_3-C_4$
17	210	175–245	$G\#_3$	F_3-B_3
18	205	175–245	$G\#_3$	F_3-B_3

[a] Preferred upper limit.
[b] 13I = premenarche; 13II = postmenarche.

research studies given in Table 3. The *italicized figures* in the pitch charts are from the research studies. The fundamental frequency is either that in the one study in Table 3 for that age or an average of the fundamental frequencies in all the studies for that age. The figures in bold type present values hypothesized by drawing curves of best fit according to inspection. The pitch charts were devised for use with either a pitch indicator or musical instrument. Column 1 lists the ages; Column 2, the fundamental frequency in Hertz; Column 3, the acceptable limits of the fundamental frequency in Hertz; Column 4, the nearest musical note to the fundamental frequency; and Column 5, the acceptable limits of the fundamental frequency in musical notes. Acceptable limits are plus and minus 1 standard deviation. Fundamental frequencies and acceptable limits in Hertz were rounded to the nearest 5 Hz for convenience in using a pitch indicator. The Westphal Chart (Westphal, 1952; in Luchsinger, 1965, p. 36) was used in establishing relationships between musical notes and Hertz values.

TABLE 3
Pitch Table: Results of Research

Age	Fundamental Frequency [a] Hz	Standard Deviation in Tones	Number of Subjects	Reference
			Males	
1 & 2	443.3	1.70	6	McGlone, 1966
7	294	1.1	15	Fairbanks, Wiley, and Lassman, 1949
8	297	1.0	15	Ibid
10	263.5	1.19	6	Curry, 1940
	210.2	1.90	6	Hollien and Malcik, 1962
	235.4	1.48	6	Hollien, Malcik, and Hollien, 1965
	226.4	1.82	6	Hollien and Malcik, 1967
14	232.7	1.70	6	Curry, 1940
	158.2	1.20	6	Hollien and Malcik, 1962
	185.8	1.66	6	Hollien, Malcik, and Hollien, 1965
	184	1.32	6	Hollien and Malcik, 1967
18	133.1	1.79	6	Curry, 1940
	121.9	1.42	6	Hollien and Malcik, 1962
	115.9	2.21	6	Hollien, Malcik, and Hollien, 1965
			Females	
1 & 2	443.3	1.70	6	McGlone, 1966
7	281	1.0	15	Fairbanks, Herbert, and Hammond, 1949
8	288	1.4	15	Ibid
11	266	1.34	6	Duffy, 1970
13I	260	1.22	6	Ibid
13II	245	1.72	6	Ibid
15	237	1.33	6	Michel, Hollien, and Moore, 1965; Hollien and Paul, 1969
	215.7	1.53	89	Ibid; Ibid
16	213.9	1.48	185	Ibid; Ibid
17	211.5	1.67	193	Ibid; Ibid

[a] Note: All fundamental frequencies are means. The studies by Curry (1940) and Hollien and Malcik (1962) presented fundamental frequencies using medians. We took the mean figures for use in our table from Hollien, Malcik, and Hollien (1965) because they had converted the medians in these two studies to means. The children in McGlone's (1966) study included both boys and girls ages 1 and 2 without differentiating age or sex. In Duffy (1970) 13I indicates premenarche and 13II postmenarche.

A study of the voice fundamental frequency in 5- and 6-year-old boys and girls done by Weinberg and Zlatin (1970) is being reported separately because the mean voice fundamental frequencies are definitely lower than those reported for other age groups in earlier studies. Some of these were presented in Chapter 2. The authors stated the method used to elicit speech may have been a reason for the lower voice fundamental frequencies because voice fundamental frequency is lower during spontaneous speech compared to oral reading. Most older studies used reading, but this study used spontaneous speech. The results were as follows: Fifteen 5-year-old boys had a mean voice fundamental frequency of 252.4 Hz with a standard deviation of 1.45 tones. Fourteen 6-year-old boys had a mean of 247.4 Hz, standard deviation: 1.35 tones. Eighteen 5-year-old girls had a mean of 247.6 Hz, standard deviation: 1.45 tones; and nineteen 6-year-old girls had a mean of 247.0 Hz, standard deviation: 1.65 tones.

Mutation

When examining an adolescent the speech pathologist should note mutational changes in the voice. A boy's voice may lower as much as an octave during the period of mutation and a girl's voice may lower 3 or 4 semitones. During mutational changes huskiness or excessive voice breaks may be noted. However, voice breaks may appear in both girls and boys as young as 7 or 8 years of age (Fairbanks, Herbert, and Hammond, 1949; Fairbanks, Wiley, and Lassman, 1949).

A practical test to use on male adolescents with delayed or incomplete mutation is Gutzmann's (1910) pressure test as described by Brodnitz (1958a). This test is especially useful in psychogenic mutational voice problems. Ordinarily, pressure on the thyroid cartilage during phonation produces an initial lowering of pitch in the normal voice. Brodnitz, however, found in psychogenic falsetto voices, pressure on the thyroid cartilage produced an initial pitch rise instead of the usual lowering. With training such cases usually begin to show the ordinary response of a lowering of the pitch of the voice with pressure on the thyroid cartilage.

Basic Pitch Abilities

If we decide to change the child's modal frequency level, Van Riper (1963, pp. 467–468) recommended determining a child's basic pitch abilities as follows. (1) Assess the child's ability to discriminate pitch. The speech pathologist hums, whistles, or sings pairs of notes one tone apart to see if the child can determine if the first note is higher or lower. (2) Check the child's ability to imitate a given pitch. The speech pathologist hums at various pitches (low, middle, and high) and asks the child to match the tones. (3) See if the child can carry a simple tune either in unison or alone. (4) Test the child's ability to follow upward and downward inflections. If the child performs poorly on these tasks he will need a concentrated program in pitch discrimination.

Loudness Analysis

How loud should a child talk? He should talk loud enough to be heard according to the situation and the background noise but not so loud as to be unpleasant to listeners. Rubin (1964) indicated the use of excessive volume over a prolonged period of time has a detrimental effect even when the voice is used efficiently. When loudness control is a problem the results of the hearing evaluation should be reviewed.

The following studies were done with adults, but until there is more information on the loudness ranges and levels of children's voices we will make inferences from these studies. The measurement values vary according to the distance of the speaker from the sound level meter. Fletcher (1953, pp. 76–77) stated the range of face-to-face speech at a distance of 40 in is 46 to 86 dB. Black (1961) defined the range from soft to loud speech as spanning about 30 dB, that is, about 70 dB for soft speech to 100 dB for loud speech at a distance of 18 in from a sound level meter. Yanagihara, Koike, and von Leden (1966) measured vocal intensity of adults when the microphone was approximately 8 in from the outlet of a pneumotach tube attached to a facial mask. The average vocal intensity of the male subjects was 67 dB and for females 64 dB.

Subjective estimates of the loudness of a child's voice can be made as he engages in various activities ranging from relatively inactive play to very active play. Van Riper and Irwin (1958, p. 282) suggested the speech pathologist note the loudness level in the expression of emotion and during various kinds of physical activities. If a sound level meter is available objective measurements of the loudness of a child's voice can be made. However, most loudness evaluations are made subjectively and rated on the voice profile. Attention to the loudness level should be incorporated into the voice therapy program if parents, teachers, and the speech pathologist agree a child has an excessively loud or soft manner of talking.

EXAMINATIONS OF QUALITY

Voice quality needs to be studied and rated carefully. First we study the quality of individual phonemes. We usually find some sounds have little or no voice deviation while others have much deviation. Van Riper (1963, p. 470) stated, "All vowels are seldom equally bad, and usually only a few need remedial work." Voice training can begin with discrimination training by comparing sounds which are relatively clear and free of the undesirable voice quality with those sounds that have a significant amount of vocal deviation.

It is profitable to compare a child's voice quality on sustained isolated vowels with the results of certain research studies. Although these studies were done on adults we are applying them to children. Research results do not always coincide or agree exactly but the findings indicate a tendency for some vowels to be more harsh or hoarse than others. For example, Sherman and Linke (1952) found that a passage containing mainly the high vowels /i/, /u/, /ɪ/, /ʊ/ was perceived by the judges as *less harsh* than a passage with low vowels /æ/, /ɔ/, and /ɑ/. The passage with lax vowels /ɪ/, /ʊ/, /ɛ/, /æ/, /ɑ/ was perceived as *less harsh* than the one containing tense vowels, /i/, /u/, /e/, /o/, and /ɔ/.

Rees (1958) analyzed hoarseness on vowels. Her results indicated the following order from least harsh to most harsh /i/, /u/, /ɪ/, /ʊ/, /ʌ/, /ɛ/, /æ/, /ɑ/, and /ɔ/. This corresponds closely to Sherman and Linke's comparison of high and low vowels. Emanuel, Lively, and McCoy (1973) combined the data from two previously reported studies (Sansone and Emanuel, 1970; Lively and Emanuel, 1970) and found in rating vowel productions of both adult males and females the high vowel /u/ tended to be rated least rough and the low vowel /æ/ the most rough. The average ratings for /i/, /ʌ/, and /ɑ/ were between these extremes.

Coleman (1976) advised the use of the vowels /i/, /u/, /ɛ/, and /ɑ/ because they are representative of extreme tongue positions during production. In contrast, Kasprzyk and Gilbert (1975) found no differences in mean frequency perturbation as a function of tongue height on the vowels /i/, /u/, /ʌ/, /æ/, and /ɑ/. Thus we can see there is not complete agreement on deviations of selected vowels. However, we do need to evaluate the quality of isolated vowels and voiced continuant consonants for guidelines in voice improvement. Some speech pathologists prefer to rate each sound on a 3 point scale with *1* a mild deviation, *2* moderate, and *3* severe. Rontal, Rontal, and Rolnick (1975) suggested voice spectrography for objective evaluation of vocal pathology before and after medical, surgical, and/or voice management. This method provides an objective permanent record and can be used to show improvement or lack of improvement in vocal rehabilitation. We recommend rating each sound according to the amount of acoustical noise present following Yanagihara's spectrographic classification. Perello and Tosi (1974) have used Yanagihara's four degrees of hoarseness classification for clinical ratings.

Yanagihara (1967a; 1967b) in a sound spectrographic study of hoarseness found noise elements more evident in the vowels /ɑ/, /ɛ/, and /i/ than in vowels /u/ and /ɔ/. We use a practical test based upon Yanagihara's findings. We follow his instructions by asking the child first to glide from /ɑ/ to /ɔ/ and from /ɔ/ to /ɑ/ and then sustain each of the five vowels used in his study for at least 5 sec. The speech pathologist listens carefully to any additional noise components heard as the child performs. The types vary in added amount of noise from Type I where only a small amount of added noise is present, to Type IV where there is almost complete replacement of the laryngeal tone by noise. Noise components may be heard as breathiness, harshness, or hoarseness present during voiced sound production. Some vowels will have additional noise components; others may be quite free of the noise components. Each vowel is rated on the scale from I to IV following Yanagihara's (1967b) classification which follows:

"Type I: The regular harmonic components are mixed with the noise component chiefly in the formant region of the vowels. Type II: The noise components in the second formants of /ɛ/ and /i/ predominate over the harmonic components, and slight additional noise components appear in the high frequency region above 3000 Hz in the vowels /ɛ/ and /i/. Type III: The second formants of /ɛ/ and /i/ are totally replaced by noise components, and the additional noise components above 3000 Hz further intensify their energy and expand their range. Type IV: The second formants of /ɑ/, /ɛ/, and /i/ are replaced by noise components, and even the first formants of all vowels often lose their periodic components which are supplemented by noise components. In addition, more intensified high frequency additional noise components are seen."‡ Rating laryngeal tone according to amount of noise components heard is a useful test once the speech pathologist becomes experienced with this type of rating.

Vocal fry is apt to be noted when assessing quality of the voice. If so, according to Erickson (1974), the following areas should be investigated: (1) the frequency of occurrence of vocal fry during speaking and reading, (2) the average length of vocal fry productions, (3) the occurrence of fry at the beginning or at the end of a word, or at the beginning or end of a phrase or sentence, (4) how frequently fry occurs during an uninflected phonation compared to upward and downward inflections, (5) the occurrence of fry during a series of productions of representative sounds in isolation, and (6) the occurrence of vocal fry when phonation is produced at a pitch higher than modal frequency level.

MEASUREMENT OF PHONATION TIME

A child should have an adequate supply of air and be able to maintain steady phonation sufficient for effective speech communication. The measurement of maximum phonation time is an index of this ability. Research has been conducted on maximum phonation time of adults and children. Ptacek and Sander (1963) using 40 men and 40 women, found the maximum phonation time for men averaged about 25 sec and for women about 17 sec. Yanagihara et al. (1966) and Yanagihara and Koike (1967) measured maximum phonation time in normal adults. Phonation time was reported at three different vocal

pitches, low, medium, and high. Phonation time was reduced at high pitch levels for both men and women. The figures for men were 28.4 sec for low pitch, 30.2 sec for medium pitch, and 23.7 sec for high pitch. The figures for women were 21.7 sec for low pitch, 22.5 sec for medium pitch, and 16.7 sec for high pitch.

Studies of maximum phonation time of children present some conflicting information as to length of phonation time. No doubt this is due to the methods used in obtaining maximum phonation time. Olsen, Perez, Burk, and Platt (1969) found the average maximum phonation time was 12.8 sec and the mean flow rate was 106 ml per sec for 28 normally speaking boys and girls between 5 and 10 years of age, with a mean age of 7 years 6 months. Bless and Saxman (1970) studied maximum phonation time in boys and girls aged 8 and 9 and found the maximum phonation time for girls was 19 sec and for boys 16 sec. Launer (1971) measured maximum phonation time for /ɑ/, /i/, and /u/ on 179 children (95 females and 84 males) aged 9 through 17 years. There were no statistically significant differences between the three vowels. Phonation time increased with age increase and boys had longer sustained phonation time than girls. Averaged phonation times, averaged standard deviations for the 3 vowels, and the number of children in each age group are shown in Table 4. The results of a study by Cunningham-Grant (1972) are presented in Table 5. Inspection of the table indicates that the maximum phonation time for the 6-, 7-, and 8-year-old girls was considerably higher than those found for older girls by Launer (1971). However, the 6-, 7-, and 8-year-old boys fairly well fit into the developmental standard of Launer's boys. Olsen et al. (1969) reported on three girls and four boys with vocal nodules, approximately 7 to 9 years of age with a mean age of 8 years 4 months. Their mean flow rate was 192 ml per sec and their maximum phonation time was 10.1 sec.

A significant reduction below normal levels can be related to inadequate voice production. Sawashima, Totsuka, Kobayashi, and Hirose (1968) cited Sawashima's study (1966) published in the *Japanese Journal of Logopedics and Phoniatrics* showing that phonation lengths below 15 sec in adult males and below 10 sec in adult females should be

‡ From Yanagihara (1967b). Quoted with permission.

TABLE 4
Averaged Maximum Phonation Time in Sec for /ɑ/, /i/, and /u/ [a]

Age	Females			Males		
	Time	S.D.	N	Time	S.D.	N
	sec			sec		
9	8.8	3.6	8	11.4	5.9	5
10	9.4	2.8	7	10.4	4.2	7
11	11.5	2.7	8	12.8	7.2	8
12	12.2	3.7	9	12.2	5.3	13
13	11.0	3.5	11	12.3	4.4	15
14	13.3	6.2	12	17.6	7.2	11
15	12.4	5.2	20	18.9	6.0	10
16	12.9	2.9	10	17.8	4.5	6
17	13.5	2.9	10	16.9	8.0	9

[a] Adapted from Launer, P. G. Unpublished master's thesis, State University of New York at Buffalo, 1971.

TABLE 5
Averaged Maximum Phonation Time in Sec for /ɑ/, /i/, and /u/ [a]

Age	Females			Males		
	Time	S.D.	N	Time	S.D.	N
	sec			sec		
6	11.17	2.82	11	11.74	3.27	10
7	10.57	2.50	12	11.77	3.55	11
8	15.27	2.89	12	12.97	3.03	13

[a] Adapted from Cunningham-Grant, J. D. S. Unpublished master's thesis, State University of New York at Buffalo, 1972.

ends when his voice changes to a whisper. Time him on several productions until he is following instructions exactly. The maximum phonation time is the longest sustained phonation on any one of the three vowels.

The following is an example of a child with inadequate respiratory function.

> Joan, an 8-year-old girl, suffered brain damage as a result of an automobile accident. Her respiratory function was reduced so she had insufficient air flow for phonation. The first task of the speech pathologist was to develop sustained phonation ability. Initially, even after many attempts, she was able to sustain phonation for only 2 or 3 sec. After 3 weeks of voice therapy with a coordinated program in physical therapy her maximum phonation time had increased to approximately 10 sec. Breathing exercises and a modified version of Froeschels' pushing technique (see Chapter 8) were used to increase phonation time and improve the quality of phonation.

ANALYSIS OF BREATHING HABITS

In most instances it is not necessary to evaluate breathing habits of children with voice disorders. No two persons breathe exactly alike and we should not attempt to force a universal pattern of breathing on everyone (Brodnitz, 1971a, p. 103). A brief analysis of breathing to make sure proper breathing is being used during speaking is usually all that is necessary. In most cases if a person can breathe adequately for physiological purposes breathing during phonation is normal.

regarded as pathological. Gould (1975) stated maximum phonation time gives an indication of the overall status of laryngeal functioning and of tension in the larynx, and of any neuromuscular disability. A short phonation time with a large air escape suggests a neuromuscular deficit such as laryngeal nerve paralysis. Gould added a sharply fluctuating air flow may suggest an unstable voice. Iwata, von Leden, and Williams (1972) stated higher mean air flow rates reflect a laryngeal hypotensive status as in unilateral laryngeal paralysis; lower mean air flow rates are suggestive of hypertensive conditions found in constricted strident voices.

To measure maximum phonation time have the child practice sustaining one of the vowels /ɑ/, /i/, or /u/ at constant pitch and loudness levels. Be sure he takes a deep breath before sustaining a vowel. Have the child follow the hand on a stop watch with the instruction to keep phonation going as long as possible. Make it a game so that he takes a maximal inhalation, tries to "beat" the watch hand, and does not stop phonation until exhalation of air is complete. Timing begins with the initiation of phonation and

We do not need a large supply of air or high subglottic air pressure to initiate and maintain adequate vocalization (Curtis, 1967, p. 196). However, it is necessary to analyze breathing habits for special types of voice problems such as a child with cerebral palsy (Murphy, 1964, p. 97) or cases of extremely inefficient respiratory habits. Attention should be paid to breathing if there is something unusual about a child's physiological breathing habits. Clavicular breathing may cause spreading of tension to the throat, promote vocal constriction, and reduce vital capacity (Perkins, 1971, p. 522). Abnormal breathing habits during speaking should also be noted. Gould (1975) suggested pulmonary function should include tidal volume (the quantity of air breathed in and out during quiet breathing), inspiratory capacity (the maximum quantity of air taken into the lungs at the end of a period of quiet respiration), and expiratory reserve volume (the quantity of air exhaled at the end of a quiet respiration). Vital capacity is also measured (the greatest amount of air expelled following maximum inspirational effort). A child with improper breathing habits or pulmonary dysfunction affecting his voice should be referred for medical consultation.

EXAMINATION OF RESONANCE

Children and adolescents who have defects of resonance should be given special tests by the speech pathologist before a remedial voice program is planned. Two types of problems are of interest here: hypernasality, which is most noticeable on consonants requiring high oral breath pressure and vowels, and hyponasality specifically on the /m/, /n/, and /ŋ/ sounds. Examinations for resonance problems by the speech pathologist include: (1) ratings of various parameters of resonance using a resonance profile, (2) special articulation tests, and (3) oral pressure measurements. The examiner should not let the disfigurement of a cleft lip and nares influence an objective assessment of hypernasality and the need for voice therapy (Podol and Salvia, 1976).

Buffalo Resonance Profile

The Buffalo Resonance Profile (Fig. 22) is used as a supplement to the Buffalo Voice Profile. Schulz et al. (1973) found interjudge reliability was 0.94 on a resonance scale. The directions for using this special profile are similar to the voice profile. The speech pathologist first determines whether the voice is hypernasal (Item 1) or hyponasal (Item 2) remembering, however, both characteristics can be present in one person. If so, ratings are made on both items.

On the appropriate scale the speech pathologist then rates the defective resonance with 1 indicating a slight deviation and 7 a severe deviation. The defective sounds reflecting the resonance problem are listed. The severity of nasal emission of sounds (Item 3) is rated on the 7 point scale and the sounds nasally emitted are listed. Item 4 deals with facial grimaces which usually are seen in constrictive action of the nares and occur during sounds which require increased oral breath pressure (Rise, 1966). Facial grimaces are rated on a 7 point scale and a description of the grimaces included. Item 5 is used to rate articulation defectiveness and to list defective sounds other than those listed under other items. Item 6 is for rating speech intelligibility. This is included on the profile because Subtelny, Van Hattum, and Myers (1972) found intelligibility to be an independent variable in rating the speech communication of children with cleft palate.

Articulation Tests for Hypernasality

Children with hypernasality should be given special articulation tests to determine adequacy of velopharyngeal closure (Morris et al. 1961). Shelton, Brooks, and Youngstrom (1965) evaluated several methods used to measure velopharyngeal closure in children. They concluded a carefully administered articulation test is a better measure of palatopharyngeal adequacy than simple measures of nasal air escape or oral breath pressure. A combination of articulation score and lateral x-ray rating, according to Van Demark, Kuehn, and Tharp (1975), appears to be the best predictor for secondary treatment of cleft palate. They found treatment was correctly predicted for 96% of a group of 75 subjects.

The results of the articulation tests will answer Morris and Smith's (1962) questions about the speech production of a person with a velopharyngeal insufficiency, "Does the speaker misarticulate those consonants ... [fricatives: /s/, /z/, /ʃ/, /f/; plosives: /k/, /g/, /t/, /d/, /p/, /b/; affricate: /dʒ/] ... which have been demonstrated to require high intraoral breath pressure? Do the mis-

Name_____ Birth Date_____ Age_____ Sex____

Rater_____ Date_____ Time of Day_____ Place_____

1. *Hypernasality*   1   2   3   4   5   6   7
    No
    Yes
    Hypernasal sounds
2. *Hyponasality*   1   2   3   4   5   6   7
    No
    Yes
    Hyponasal sounds
3. *Nasal Emission of Sounds*   1   2   3   4   5   6   7
    No
    Yes
    Sounds emitted
4. *Facial Grimaces* (including nares constriction)   1   2   3   4   5   6   7
    No
    Yes
    Describe_____
5. *Articulation Defectiveness*   1   2   3   4   5   6   7

    List defective sounds (in addition to those listed above)
    _____

6. *Intelligibility*   1   2   3   4   5   6   7
    Normal
    Poor
COMMENTS:
INSTRUCTIONS:
    A. Circle the appropriate descriptive term under each item.
    B. For each item *not* normal or adequate, circle a number on the scale for that item. *Do not* mark
       between numbers.
       Key: 1 = slight deviation
               4 = moderate deviation
               7 = severe deviation
    C. List sounds where indicated.

Fig. 22. Buffalo Resonance Profile.

articulations ... involve audible nasal emission? Are there evidences of facial contortion during the production of these consonants? Does occluding the nostrils (preventing an air leakage) result in normal production of them?"

A standard articulation test and the Iowa Pressure Articulation Test (IPAT) (Morris et al. 1961; Templin and Darley, 1969) should both be given. The latter test consists of 43 words containing sounds which require oral pressure for correct production and discriminates between speakers who have adequate velopharyngeal closure and those who do not. Each item is scored correct or incorrect, with the per cent of correct responses reflecting the

severity of the velopharyngeal incompetence. We also score the IPAT by making a distinction between errors accompanied by nasal emission and errors which are not accompanied by nasal emission (Lubker, Schweiger, and Morris, 1970). Thus the final score shows not only the percentage of correct responses, but also the percentage of errors with nasal emission and those without it.

Van Demark et al. (1975) arbitrarily defined three categories of correct articulation scores for classifying IPAT competency levels: (1) above 50%, (2) between 50% and 34%, and (3) below 34%. Van Demark and Morris (1977) reported on 278 children aged 4 to 10 on whom 1248 IPAT's were available.

A comparison of results of these tests to the norms established by Templin and Darley (1969) showed that at no age level between 4 and 10 did more than 9% of the children achieve the mean on the IPAT without secondary management. Their examination of the "risk rates" indicated by these data showed the IPAT to be a very useful tool in predicting the need for secondary management, i.e., children who scored 0 on the IPAT at 4½ years of age had a 96% risk of needing secondary palatal management.

A list of the test words with the test sounds in decreasing order of their importance in discriminating between good and poor velopharyngeal closure is shown in Figure 23. The mean scores for the 43 item test are shown in Table 6. The articulation tests should include checking the child's responses to stimulation, both auditory and visual, on all sounds incorrectly produced on the tests. The amount of improvement reveals the potential for adequate velopharyngeal closure for speech (Morris and Smith, 1962).

The reading passage "The Picnic" using the 43 words from the Iowa Pressure Articulation Test should be recorded. In this way the production of the test words in reading can be evaluated. The test words are in *italics*. Be sure the words are not italicized in the copy the child reads.

The Picnic

Mother told the *twins*, Jimmy and Susie, to *jump* out of bed and get *dressed*. Mother and Susie wore pink *dresses*. Jimmy lost one *shoe* and both *socks* as he came down the *stairs*. Mother put clothes in the *washer*. The children brought *string, scissors, paper*, and *crayons*. *Two blocks* from home they saw a circus parade. A *tiger* and a *wolf* were in cages on

TABLE 6 [a]
Mean Scores on 43 Item Iowa Pressure Articulation Test by Age for Boys and Girls

Age	Boys (N = 30)		Girls (N = 30)	
	Mean	S.D.	Mean	S.D.
3	26.4	12.5	23.6	11.6
3½	28.8	12.5	32.9	9.6
4	35.1	9.7	33.5	8.8
4½	34.1	9.4	35.0	8.8
5	33.8	11.2	37.5	8.6
6	35.5	10.3	39.5	6.5
7	39.6	5.7	41.6	3.0
8	42.0	3.3	41.7	2.9

[a] From Templin, M. C., and Darley, F. L. *The Templin-Darley Tests of Articulation— A Manual and Discussion of Articulation Testing.* Ed. 2. Iowa City: Bureau of Educational Research and Service, University of Iowa, 1969.

Discrimination Levels	Sounds	Words
1	/s-, sk-/	sun, *skates*
2	/-k-, sm-, -sm, sn-, str-/	pocket, *smoke*, po*ssum*, *snowman*, *string*
3	/ʃ-, -z-, -kɚ, st-/	shoe, scissors, cra*cker*, *stairs*
4	/-s-, -ʃ-, kr-/	dresses, dishes, crayons
5	/-g-, -s, sp-, tr-, gr-, -gɚ, -ɚk, -pt, kl-, gl-, -mps/	wa*gon*, mou*se*, spoon, *tree*, *grass*, ti*ger*, *fork*, sto*pped*, *clown*, *glasses*, sta*mps*
6	/k-, g-, -g, -ʃ, dʒ-, -ʃɚ, bl-, -ks/	cat, *girl*, dog, fish, *jump*, wa*sher*, *blocks*, so*cks*
7	/-k, br-, dr-, tw-/	truck, *bread*, *drum*, *twins*
8	/t-, f-, -f, -pɚ, pl-, -lf/	two, tele*phone*, knife, pa*per*, *planting*, wo*lf*

Key: Level *1* most discriminating, Level *8* least discriminating. Sounds are shown according to position in word, e.g., initial /s-/, medial /-s-/, and final /-s/.

Fig. 23. Iowa pressure articulation test sounds and words in order of decreasing discrimination levels. Discrimination levels from Morris, Spriestersbach, and Darley (1961). Words from Templin and Darley (1969).

a *wagon*. A *clown* rode in a funny *truck*. Whenever he *stopped* he ate a *cracker* and *smoke* came out of his *pocket*. A *girl* clown talks on a *telephone* and *stamps* her feet in time with a *drum*. Another clown on *skates* looks like a *snowman* wearing *glasses*. Mother gave everyone *dishes* and a *knife, spoon, fork, bread,* and *fish*. They sat in the *sun* and saw men *planting grass*. They saw a *cat* run after a *mouse*, and a *dog* chase a *'possum* up a *tree*.

Hypernasality on vowels should also be checked. Spriestersbach and Powers (1959) had judges rate on a 7 point equal-appearing intervals scale the amount of hypernasality on certain vowels in children with cleft palate speech. The vowels from *least nasal* to *most nasal* were: /ɑ/, /ʌ/, /æ/, /o/, /ɛ/, /u/, and /i/. Carney and Sherman (1971) also found that cleft palate speakers on the average showed least hypernasality on /ɑ/ and most on /i/ and /u/. Moore and Sommers (1973), in studying cleft palate speakers, found the order of perceived hypernasality from *least* to *most* severe was /ɔ/, /ɑ/, /ɛ/, /æ/, /u/, and /i/. Borlak and Moller (1976), also studying cleft palate speakers, tested four vowels and found that hypernasality was judged to be less severe on the low vowels /ɑ/ and /æ/ and more severe on the high vowels /i/ and /u/. These four studies are in agreement that the most hypernasal vowels in cleft palate speakers are the high vowels /i/ and /u/, and they are in fairly good agreement on the least hypernasal vowels being low vowels, specifically /ɑ/.

The specific vowels that are hypernasalized are different when the hypernasality is functional. Lintz and Sherman (1961) studied nasality on vowels of adults with functional hypernasality, having judges rate the nasality in a manner similar to Spriestersbach and Powers (1959). They found the order from *least nasal* to *most nasal* was /u/, /ʊ/, /ʌ/, /i/, /ɛ/, /ɑ/, and /æ/. Carney and Sherman (1971) showed similar results, with hypernasal speakers without cleft palate showing, on the average, less hypernasality on the high vowels (/i/ and /u/) and most on the low vowel /ɑ/ (the reverse order from their comparative group of cleft palate speakers). Lintz and Sherman (1961) found certain consonant environments tended to influence the amount

of nasality rated on vowels. From *least* influence to *most* influence were /z/, /v/, /d/, /g/, /f/, /s/, /t/, and /k/. It would seem, therefore, that nasality on vowels should be studied in these consonant environments.

Bloomer and Wolski (1968) suggested obtaining samples of sounds, words, or sentences not containing /m/, /n/, or /ŋ/. For example, have the child say "Buy baby a bib," "Zippers are easy to close," "Go get a bigger egg," the numbers 2, 3, 4, 5, 6, or /i-o/. Each sample should be said under two conditions: with the nares unoccluded and then occluded. Hess (1976) recommended the nasal flutter test described by Weiss (1974) in which the speech pathologist rapidly and repetitively closes and opens the child's nares to see if there is a discernible change in nasal resonance. Any nasal resonance present will be exaggerated on the occluded performance because of the cul-de-sac effect. With normal velopharyngeal functioning the resonance on both productions will be normal.

The speech sample should include a study of sound confusions often found in cases of velopharyngeal insufficiency. Shupe (1968) used the following words in studying sound confusions in cleft palate subjects: bake/make, rib/rim, dine/nine, mad/man, wig/wing, and bag/bang. In a person with velopharyngeal insufficiency both sounds are hypernasal; for example, the bake/make pair sounds like make/make.

The following is an example of submucous cleft palate.

Sharon, 6½-year-old first grader, was brought to the speech clinic by her mother because she had a severe articulation problem and according to the mother, "Talks like she has a cleft palate." These problems had always been present but a recent head and neck examination had not been done. A tonsillectomy and adenoidectomy were performed when she was 4½ years of age because of repeated ear infections and the operation had no adverse effect on voice resonance. The child's general health was good.

The speech examination confirmed the mother's description of speech as resembling that of a child with cleft palate. Hypernasality was present on vowels and nasal emission of air occurred on the stop sounds /p/, /b/, /t/, /d/, /k/,

/g/, and on most fricative sounds including /f/, /s/, /z/, and /ʃ/. Nasality was rated 6 on a 7 point scale, nasal emission 5, and intelligibility 4.

An examination of the oral cavity revealed a palatal condition often found in those with a submucous cleft. There was a midline notching of the uvula which looked as if it had been sutured together. The soft palate appeared thin and tight although there was adequate movement. The hard palate was high and narrow and appeared thin and weak. The nasopharynx appeared capacious. Contact of the velum with the posterior pharyngeal wall was not observed upon phonation of /a/. When the child swallowed, liquids came through the nose. She could not blow up a balloon. Sharon was referred to the cleft palate team and the voice team for evaluation.

Oral Pressure Measurements

Various types of physical measurements are used to evaluate velopharyngeal closure and oral breath pressure. A simple method is to have a child blow up a balloon with the nares open and compare this effort with that used when the nares are occluded. A carnival blower or other similar toy can be used.

A quick clinical test to determine whether a child has the capability of adequate velopharyngeal closure is a modified tongue-anchor technique described by Fox and Johns (1970).This test is advised because some children can puff up their cheeks and hold the air pressure by humping the tongue against the intact portion of the palate. The child is asked to puff up his cheeks while the speech pathologist demonstrates. Then the child is asked to stick out his tongue, which is held by the speech pathologist with a sterile gauze pad. The child is then asked to puff up his cheeks again as he did during the first trial. The speech pathologist occludes the child's nose. The child is then asked to hold the air in his cheeks after the pressure has been released on the occluded nose. If there is no escape of air as the nostrils are released it can be concluded that velopharyngeal seal is adequate. Several trials should be done to verify the presence or absence of air escape. Hess (1976) recommended this test be included in determining velopharyngeal adequacy.

A spirometer can be used to measure amount of air and an oral manometer§ to measure pressure in the oral cavity. On the oral manometer an air pressure of 8 ounces per square inch is necessary to close the nasopharynx to produce acceptable speech (Spriestersbach and Powers, 1959). Various types of pressure gauges‖ have also been used. Measurements on these instruments should be taken under two conditions, with the nares open and occluded.

The oral manometer is commonly used. After several practice trials on this instrument, measurements are made for each condition. Moore and Sommers (1973) recommended that oral manometer readings be made with the bleed condition and that subjects undergo a four trial examination for each condition. Measurements may be taken during positive (blowing) and negative (sucking) conditions, and with the tongue tip outside the mouth. The readings are averaged and a ratio between the two nares conditions calculated. For example, if the unoccluded reading on the oral manometer is 5 and the occluded reading is 10 (5/10), the ratio is obtained by dividing the numerator by the denominator, giving a ratio of 0.50. If velopharyngeal closure is achieved the readings will be the same when the nares are open as when they are occluded and the ratio would be 1.00 (10/10). The ratio may be confusing in a child with velopharyngeal insufficiency who cannot or does not increase the pressure with the nares occluded; if the child has very low pressure readings with the nares occluded and a similar low reading with the nares unoccluded the ratio would be a misleading 1.00 (Quigley, 1968). This problem can be avoided by making sure a child exerts full effort when the nares are occluded. Subtracting the negative from the positive ratio score gives the manometer difference score.

Morris (1966) suggested conservative use of the oral manometer as an indicator of velopharyngeal competence. He felt manometer ratios are useful in predicting adequacy of velopharyngeal function for speech when used along with other test findings.

In a study of 75 cleft palate individuals ranging in age from 6.9 to 20 years with a mean age of 12.67 years, Van Demark (1970)

§ Hunter Oral Manometer, Hunter Manufacturing Company, Iowa City, IA 52243.
‖ Emerson Resuscitator, J. H. Emerson Company, Cambridge, MA 02140.

divided the individuals into the three groups designated by Spriestersbach, Moll, and Morris (1961) (See Table 7). He found that with only one exception subjects with high manometer ratios achieved the highest articulation test scores, the marginal closure group was next, and the poor closure group was lowest. Other studies have also shown a positive relationship between manometer ratios and articulation skill. Pitzner and Morris (1966) studied children who had cleft palates. Those who had adequate manometer ratios had articulation skills comparable to normal children. However, children with inadequate ratios had poor articulation skills on plosives, fricatives, affricates, vocalic /r/, and /l/. Barnes and Morris (1967) found performance on the oral manometer was a good predictor of articulation skills.

Bernstein (1967) used the oral manometer to determine manometer ratios before and after pharyngeal flap operations in patients with velopharyngeal incompetence. He found only 6% of the patients had a manometer ratio of 0.90 or greater before the operation but after the operation they reached this ratio in 86% of the cases.

A few cautions about the use of certain types of measures for assessing velopharyngeal competency are in order. Van Riper (1972, p. 367) noted the inadequacy of testing velopharyngeal competency by ability to suck liquids up a straw, various blowing exercises, or visually observing uvular movement. Studies indicate little if any relationship of nonspeech blowing activities to velopharyngeal closure during speech. Calnan and Renfrew (1961) compared x-rays of velopharyngeal closure when blowing on a carnival blower with x-rays of velopharyngeal closure during the production of the sound /i/. They concluded during blowing certain compensating muscular mechanisms were used that either did not occur or were ineffectual during the production of /i/. Prins and Bloomer (1965) in studying 10 children with velopharyngeal insufficiency concluded pressure gauge readings taken during blowing activity appeared unrelated to speech intelligibility or nasality. Moll (1965) as a result of cinefluorographic investigation of 10 normal subjects and five subjects with cleft palate, concluded ability to suck liquid through a straw or to puff the cheeks does not reflect ability to achieve velopharyngeal closure because both of these

tasks can be done with only tongue-palate valving.

Air flow has been measured in evaluating velopharyngeal competence during speech. For example, Hixon, Saxman, and McQueen (1967) described a technique which could be used for the clinical evaluation of velopharyngeal competence. A person wears a face mask divided into oral and nasal sections so that transmission of air between the two is impossible. The speaker may be asked to repeat /tʌ/, /kʌ/, /sʌ/, /ʃʌ/, and /fʌ/, count from 1 to 10, repeat sentences, or use connected speech under three speaking conditions, soft, normal, and loud. The amount of air emitted orally and nasally is fed separately into a device to measure the amount of nasal and oral air flow.

Velopharyngeal competency should be evaluated as objectively as possible. The conservative use of spirometer¶ or oral pressure measures is suggested as part of the battery of tests and examinations for velopharyngeal insufficiency.

Oral Breath Pressure Ratios

The following three studies can be used as comparative guides by the speech pathologist in assessing oral breath pressure ratios obtained on children (Table 7).

Spriestersbach et al. (1961) compared articulation test scores and oral breath pressure measurements on a group of cleft lip and/or palate children aged 3 years 6 months to 16 years 11 months. The articulation scores were the percentage of consonants correctly articulated on the Templin-Darley Diagnostic Test of Articulation. Oral breath pressure ratios were found by dividing readings on the wet spirometer nares open by readings with the nares closed.

Weinberg and Shanks (1971) reported on perceived hypernasality ratings and various oral manometer ratios in 100 persons with cleft palate aged 3 to 20 years with a mean age of 9.65 years. They were divided into three groups, normal resonance, mild hypernasality, and moderate-severe hypernasality. Three pressure ratio measures were derived— positive, negative, and the manometer difference score. Brennan and Leeper (1974) reported on four oral breath pressure measures for 75 persons with cleft lip and palate who

¶ Propper Dry Spirometer and Hutchinson Wet Spirometer, C. H. Stoelting Company, Chicago, IL 60624.

TABLE 7
Oral Breath Pressure Ratios

The Spriestersbach, Moll, Morris Study (1961)	
Mean Percentage of Correct Consonants	Oral Breath Pressure Ratios
81.40	0.90 or more
61.00	0.51 to 0.89
57.91	0.50 or less

The Weinberg and Shanks Study (1971

Resonance Condition	Positive		Negative		Difference Score	
	Mean	S.D.	Mean	S.D.	Mean	S.D.
Normal resonance	0.989	0.03	0.942	0.15	0.05	0.15
Mild hypernasality	0.894	0.21	0.487	0.20	0.41	0.25
Moderate-severe hypernasality	0.471	0.25	0.437	0.16	0.03	0.28

The Brennan and Leeper Study (1974)

Resonance Condition	Positive		Negative		Difference Score		Tongue out of Mouth	
	Mean	S.D.	Mean	S.D.	Mean	S.D.	Mean	S.D.
Normal balance	0.98	0.033	0.97	0.048	0.0148	0.0486	0.97	0.039
Mild imbalance	0.91	0.104	0.77	0.164	0.1413	0.1648	0.85	0.174
Moderate-severe imbalance	0.52	0.281	0.55	0.297	−.0383	0.3785	0.57	0.248

had histories of velopharyngeal incompetence. The ages ranged from 4 years 6 months to 24 years 5 months, with a mean age of 10 years 10 months. The subjects were rated for severity of judged resonance imbalance—normal, mild imbalance, or severe imbalance. The manometer measures were positive, negative, difference scores, and tongue-tip-outside the mouth ratios. The findings indicated that the negative manometer ratio, the manometer difference scores, and tongue-tip-outside the mouth ratios are more sensitive measures for evaluating resonance imbalance than is the positive ratio. The positive ratio may not be a valid way of predicting velopharyngeal incompetence because a person may employ tongue-palate valving. However, using the tongue-tip-outside the mouth technique prohibits this. Persons who employ tongue-palate valving, according to Brennan and Leeper (1974), can be recognized clinically as follows: (1) back of tongue sounds may be substituted for front of tongue sounds, (2) during phonation of low vowels tongue humping may be observed, (3) in the presence of hypernasal speech a person may exhibit high manometric ratios, and (4) mylohyoid

activity (muscle from the region of the lower molar teeth to the hyoid bone) may be observed or palpated during the administration of the test.

The results of the three studies which can be used as guides when relating resonance to oral breath pressure ratios are shown in Table 7.

Here is an example of the testing and management of a child with velopharyngeal insufficiency revealed after tonsillectomy and adenoidectomy.

Nancy was 7 years old when we first saw her. Her speech and voice had been normal until after a tonsillectomy and adenoidectomy at 3 years because of chronic secretory otitis media. Her speech was hypernasal to the point of being almost unintelligible. The soft palate raised but appeared short on phonating /ɑ/, the pharynx appeared capacious, and the lateral pharyngeal wall showed vigorous mesial movement. Ratings on the Buffalo Resonance Profile were: hypernasality, 6; nasal emission, 6; especially on /s/, /z/, /k/, /g/, /ʃ/, /t/, and /d/; facial grimaces, 4; articulation, 6; and intelligibility, 6. The IPAT score was 35 (4$^1/_2$ year level). Lateral still x-rays of velopharyngeal opening while at rest measured 10.00 mm and 3.45 mm while producing /s/. We classified her as a Morris Group II, with closure almost but not quite achieved (Morris, 1972, pp. 152–154). We felt inclined toward supporting a recommendation for physical management but the parents requested a trial period of speech and voice therapy to determine results of behavioral management. We therefore placed Nancy in a concentrated 6 week program. Therapy averaged 4 hours daily both individual and group. The goals were to improve oral pressure sounds and decrease the hypernasality. Results were only minimal. Soon thereafter a pharyngeal flap operation was performed. We saw Nancy 1 month later. Her profile ratings were: hypernasal, 4; nasal emission, 3; facial grimaces, none; articulation, 5; and intelligibility, 4. Her IPAT score was 37. Speech and voice therapy was resumed and after a 3 month period of therapy, three 1 hour sessions weekly, her intelligibility improved from the original rating of 6 to 2. The hypernasality and nasal emission of sounds improved from 6 to 1 and the other ratings were normal. The IPAT score was 40 (6 year level). Additional therapy over the next year at school yielded positive results with acceptable speech and voice.

Tests for Hyponasality

Hyponasal speech, in contrast to hypernasal speech, shows an absence of nasal resonance on the /m/, /n/, and /ŋ/ sounds. Other consonants remain undisturbed but there may be slight alterations in the vowels because the normal nasal transients before and after nasal sounds are not present (also called assimilation nasality) (Arnold, 1965, p. 685).

The examination of hyponasality should include sentences that have many /m/, /n/, and /ŋ/ sounds, such as "Mamma made some lemon jam" (Bloomer and Wolski, 1968). When there is definite hyponasality present the /m/ may sound like a /b/, the /n/ like a /d/, and the /ŋ/ like a /g/. The pairs of words used in testing for hypernasality can be used here (bake/make, rib/rim, dine/nine,

mad/man, wig/wing, bag/bang) (Shupe, 1968). The sound substitutions, however, would be reversed. For example, the bake/make pair would be produced bake/bake. Hyponasality remains constant whether or not the nares are occluded.

VOCAL ABUSE

Vocal abuse must be identified and analyzed carefully. Vocal abuse as a cause of voice problems was presented in Chapter 3. Traumatizing vocal abuses center at the level of the larynx and result in a disruption of the normal physiological activity of the vocal cords. The analysis of vocal abuse is particularly important in a child with laryngeal dysfunction. It includes evaluating muscular tensions during the use of the abuse. Tension may appear in various muscles of the larynx, the pharynx, and the neck. Excess tension not only in the laryngeal area but in almost any area of the body may affect the voice. Van Riper (1972, p. 146) stated, "Tension in any area of the body tends to flow toward and focus in the larynx." According to Isshiki and von Leden (1964) vocal nodules, laryngeal edema, and other problems causing an incomplete approximation of the vocal cords cause a person to attempt to overcome this imperfect closure by contracting the laryngeal muscles with greater force; this continued forceful contraction starts a "... vicious circle of laryngeal hyperfunction" which is a contributing factor in voice disorders. This problem is represented by the following child.

Joyce, a 13-year-old girl, was referred by her teacher to the school speech pathologist. She had a hoarse voice rated 7 on a seven point scale. She talked with great effort, taking excessively deep breaths with a raising of the shoulders. When she talked she strained so hard to phonate her face reddened and the muscles in her neck stood out, reflecting the amount of hyperfunction in the neck and shoulder areas. The laryngeal examination revealed bilateral vocal nodules at the junction of the anterior and middle thirds of the vocal cords. The nodules were approximately 2 mm. Complete approximation of the cords was hampered by the large nodules thus accounting for the extreme effort required for talking. The nodules appeared newly formed and voice therapy was recommended.

The speech pathologist should determine

whether the external laryngeal muscles or swallowing muscles are used in phonation. Zerffi (1939; 1948; 1952) recommended using Kenyon's (1928) finger palpation technique as the testing method. This is done by placing a finger above the larynx at the angle of the chin and asking the person to swallow. The upward movement of the larynx and muscle contractions reveal the normal cooperation of the external laryngeal muscles. Then still keeping the finger in place ask the person to speak or sing. If there are any muscular movements or upward movement of the larynx like those noted during swallowing, it reveals an unnecessary involvement of the external laryngeal muscles. This indicates the vocal cords are being brought together with greater force than their muscles can tolerate causing irritation of the free edges of the vocal cords. This results in a weakening of the vocal muscles.

Buffalo Vocal Abuse Rating Scale

Vocal abuse is identified through the use of a special rating scale. The Buffalo Vocal Abuse Rating Scale (Fig. 24) contains various kinds of vocal abuses with a rating of the amount and degree of each. The rating scale includes 11 of the most common types of vocal abuses. The child should be observed in many different situations in order to assure a complete inventory of vocal abuses. These situations should include the classroom, the structured group play observation, gym, outdoor playground, and an interview with the speech pathologist. Parents can be instructed in the use of the vocal abuse rating scale and asked to rate the child during various activities at home, when playing outdoors, and in other after-school activities. Talking in noise should be especially noted and rated.

The *0* for none is circled if the vocal abuse is not observed, and no other rating is then made for this item. If an abuse is observed the amount and degree of each one should be carefully rated. The observed amount of each vocal abuse is indicated on a 3 point scale as follows: *1* little used, *2* frequently used, or *3* excessively used. The degree of severity of each vocal abuse is also rated on a 3 point scale: *1* mild, *2* moderate, or *3* severe. Let us look at coughing as an example. A child may cough very seldom (rating *1* in amount), but he does it in a very loud and strained manner to a severe degree (rating *3* in degree). Another child may cough very frequently (rating *3* in amount) but he does it in a mild degree (rating *1* in degree). Thus

---

Name_____ Birth Date_____ Age _____ Sex_____

Rater_____ Time of Day_____ Date_____

Length of Observation _____ Place Observed_____

		Amount			Degree		
1. *Shouting*	0	1	2	3	1	2	3
2. *Screaming*	0	1	2	3	1	2	3
3. *Cheering*	0	1	2	3	1	2	3
4. *Excessive Talking*	0	1	2	3	1	2	3
5. *Strained Vocalizations*	0	1	2	3	1	2	3
6. *Reverse Phonation*	0	1	2	3	1	2	3
7. *Explosive Vocalizations*	0	1	2	3	1	2	3
8. *Abrupt Glottal Attack*	0	1	2	3	1	2	3
9. *Throat Clearing*	0	1	2	3	1	2	3
10. *Coughing*	0	1	2	3	1	2	3
11. *Talking in Noise*	0	1	2	3	1	2	3
Other:							

Circle appropriate numbers.
Key: Amount: 0 = None; 1 = little; 2 = frequent; 3 = excessive
     Degree: 1 = mild; 2 = moderate; 3 = severe

Fig. 24. Buffalo Vocal Abuse rating scale.

it can be seen that all combinations of amount and degree ratings are possible.

Shouting, Screaming, Cheering

Shouting is extremely loud talking sometimes reaching 90 to 100 dB in intensity. A shout is "a loud burst of voice" (Webster, 1963). In contrast to shouting, screaming means "to voice a sudden sharp loud cry . . . to produce harsh high tones . . ." which has " . . . a vivid startling effect" (Webster, 1963) on listeners. Cheering is heard at sports events, on the playground, and in the gym. It is essentially " . . . a shout of applause or triumph" (Webster, 1963).

Excessive Talking

Excessive talking simply means talking a lot. Some children talk day and night. This is especially detrimental when combined with other vocal abuses. Children with vocal nodules are about three times more talkative than their peers without nodules (Wilson, 1971).

Strained Vocalizations

Strained vocalizations include vocal imitation of cars, trucks, and airplanes during a child's play or when he is talking about noise sources.

Reverse Phonation

Reverse phonation consists of vocalizing on the intake of air. It does not occur frequently during regular conversation or reading but usually during play and strenuous activities. Children typically do this as they play or imitate sounds of trains or trucks (Wilson, 1968).

Explosive Vocalizations

Explosive release of vocalizations occurs most often during play but is sometimes heard during quiet talking. It consists of building up air pressure in the subglottic area with the vocal cords tightly closed, followed by a sudden opening of the cords as a raucous vocalization is made. Many children build up excessive air pressure against the under surfaces of the vocal cords as they speak (West and Ansberry, 1968, p. 216) resulting in a staccato type of talking.

Abrupt Glottal Attack

The abrupt glottal attack is referred to variously as the hard attack, hard vocal attack, harsh vocal attack, coup de glotte, glot-tal stroke, firm glottal attack, or glottal stop. It is the most commonly found faulty vocal production (Flower, 1959). The mechanical aspects of the abrupt glottal attack are essentially the same as an explosive release of vocalization. That is, in abrupt glottal attack there is a buildup of pressure and then a sudden release of the sound, but this is usually quite subtle compared to the loud explosion of sound in an explosive type of release.

The trained ear can detect even the slightest degree of abrupt glottal attack (Luchsinger, 1965, p. 85). Isshiki and von Leden (1964) found no air flow observable before the onset of phonation in the abrupt glottal attack. Werner-Kukuk and von Leden (1970), using high speed motion pictures, studied vocal cord vibrations during hard vocal attack. The vibratory movement was first seen in the median part of the vocal cords, followed a few cycles later in the anterior, and last in the posterior section. The amplitude of the vibratory cycle increased rapidly at the beginning of the hard initiation, which indicates there is a quick rise in the intensity of the phonation and also an early establishment of the vibratory pattern typical of hard initiation. There was very limited amplitude of the vibratory movement in the posterior portion of the cords. This portion remained tightly closed during the alternating vibratory cycles. In the anterior two-thirds the vocal cords opened rapidly with the median part showing the widest lateral excursion.

Erickson (1974) suggested the hard glottal attack be analyzed according to its frequency of appearance during 1 min of oral reading, in 1 min of spontaneous or free speech, and during the speaking of a series of representative vowels in isolation.

Coughing and Throat Clearing

Habitual, excessive, and hard coughing and vigorous and excessive throat clearing are common vocal abuses (Greene, 1972, p. 124; Peacher, 1952, p. 9; Wilson, 1966).

Talking in Noise

As we know, both vocal abuse and vocal misuse occur when a person talks in the presence of high level noise. These situations include listening to rock music, riding in automobiles, sports machines, and garden and farm equipment.

EXAMINATION OF RATE

The rate at which a child talks should be measured during the appraisal since we know that a too-fast rate may interfere with or influence other variables of speech and voice. Calvert and Silverman (1975, pp. 36–37) stated the conversational speaking rate of most adults is about 270 words per min with 5 to 5.5 syllables per sec, and the oral reading rate is 168 to 180 words per min. Kelly and Steer (1949) measured the talking rate of university students giving an extemporaneous speech in a beginning public speaking course. They measured (1) the total number of words spoken in a particular time interval and (2) the average number of words a minute spoken in a sentence. The number of words spoken in the total elapsed time of an extemporaneous speech was 159 words per min. When they checked the number of words a minute in sentences, the mean rate was 208 words per min. Kelly and Steer stated the actual speed of utterance is more accurately described as 208 rather than 159. Reading rates of 140 and 185 words per min are usually considered the limits for desirable oral reading rate (Franke, 1939, cited in Hanley and Thurman, 1970, p. 148).

In evaluating the rate at which a child talks, it should first be noted on the Buffalo Voice Profile whether the rate is normal, fast, or slow as the speech pathologist observes the child in various speaking situations. To obtain the number of words per minute, a 60 sec sample can be designated from the audiorecording of connected speech, and the number of words counted. If there are no samples of connected speech of that length, time a sentence, count the words in it, and multiply by whatever is necessary to make the time equivalent to a minute.

The speaking rate of a child with a severe hearing impairment should be noted by analyzing a tape-recorded sample of his speech. Often the too-slow rate and the altered duration of syllables affect voice quality as well as speech intelligibility. Ling (1976, p. 160 and p. 163) recommended checking the mean number of syllables per second and rating the duration of vowels and of consonants by noting whether they are sustained, brief, or varied. Colton and Cooker (1968) recommended assessing the speaking rate of hearing-impaired children with hypernasality to determine if increasing the rate might result in reduced hypernasality.

Rate should be checked when there is a voice problem associated with a motor speech disorder. For example, rate should be evaluated in patients with myasthenia gravis to determine deterioration of rate over a period of time. Darley et al. (1972) recommended determining the effect of multiple sclerosis on motor speech through the measurement of oral reading rate, oral diadochokinetic rate, evaluating the precision of consonant articulation, and also examining prosodic aspects of speech to determine any impairment of emphasis.

EXAMINATION PROCEDURES FOR THE HEARING IMPAIRED

Prior to initiating voice therapy for a child with a hearing loss, his voice should be evaluated carefully to determine the areas needing attention. The speech pathologist should be on the alert for voice problems typically found in hearing-impaired children. These problems include undesirable resonance, improper use of pitch, inappropriate loudness, defective laryngeal tone, and inadequate rate. Typical resonance problems are hypernasality, hyponasality, and a hollow muffled quality usually referred to as cul-de-sac resonance. Pitch may be too high, too low, and monotonous. Vocal intensity may be too soft or too loud. Laryngeal dysfunction may be present causing the voice to sound breathy, harsh , or hoarse. The rate of speaking may be slow and monotonous.

Ling (1976, Ch. 9) emphasized the importance of analyzing these aspects of the speech of a hearing-impaired child. For young children who cannot imitate speech well enough to take a formal speech test, he recommended making a tape recording of at least 50 representative utterances. These can be analyzed not only for the articulatory aspects but also for voice. Ling (1976, pp. 160–169) used a form which includes the specific items of pitch, intensity, breath control, intonation, and duration of vowels and consonants. For older children a more detailed voice analysis should be done. Not only is the child's ability to produce a stimulus syllable noted, but also whether he can produce it in a loud voice, a quiet voice, or a whisper, and whether he can vary the pitch over 8 semitones during its production. Ling also included a check list for noting common voice problems of hearing-impaired children, such as hypernasality, breathiness, and harshness. Berg (1976, pp. 199–228) described and discussed instrumentation used in analyzing the voice aspects of the speech of a hearing-impaired child. Some of these instruments are not available to most speech pathologists, others are discussed elsewhere in this book.

The examination procedures described in this chapter for use with normal hearing children can be used or adapted to hearing-impaired children. Ratings to assess vocal parameters should be made at the beginning of training to establish baselines and then repeated periodically to chart progress. All items of the group play observation chart (Fig. 18) give useful preliminary information. The use of the Buffalo Voice Profile (Fig. 20) is essential; any items not rated normal should be evaluated in more detail. For example, if a child has improper use of pitch, his modal frequency level should be determined and compared with norms in Tables 1 and 2. It may be necessary to evaluate the child's use of loudness carefully. If resonance appears to be a problem, the Buffalo Resonance Profile (Fig. 22) should be completed. Children with hypernasal voices should be given the Iowa Pressure Articulation Test and appropriate oral and nasal air flow measures. If vocal abuse is noted, it should be carefully evaluated using the Buffalo Vocal Abuse Rating Scale (Fig. 24). Irwin (1965, p. 255) stated problems of voice quality in hearing-impaired children often appear to be related to pathologies of the nose, throat, or ear. Streng, Fitch, Hedgecock, Phillips, and Carrell (1958, p. 228) indicated breathy, harsh, or hypernasal voices found in children with hearing losses are not necessarily related to the loss. Ling (1976, p. 138) stated he has observed that about 5% of hearing-impaired children have some abnormality of the oral peripheral structures which could interfere with acquiring speech. He added that compensatory adjustments are often more difficult for a hearing-impaired child than for a normal-hearing child.

The results of audiological evaluations should be available to the speech pathologist. It is necessary to know the child's hearing ability without a hearing aid and particularly a detailed analysis of the improvements resulting from hearing aid use. The report should include speech reception thresholds and speech discrimination scores without and with a hearing aid, and the results of any special auditory tests.

STIMULABILITY EXAMINATION

A voice stimulability test should be given each child as he nears the end of his diagnostic examinations. The question to be answered is: Can the child improve his voice after being presented with correct models? Each deviant voice parameter should be tested and the results checked on the Buffalo Voice Profile. The ability to produce a clear voice upon stimulation does not mean the problem will resolve itself without training; rather it means voice therapy has a good chance of being successful. Thus a child who can produce a better voice under clinical stimulation should not be eliminated from voice therapy (Webster, Perkins, Bloomer, and Pronovost, 1966).

All stimulability tests should include vowels and voiced consonants in isolation, in nonsense words, words, and sentences. For example, for disturbances in laryngeal tone all of the sustainable vowels should be used in isolation, then combined into CV (consonant-vowel) or CVC combinations, and then into words and sentences. Counting from 1 to 10 should also be used. The best procedure is to have the child listen carefully as the speech pathologist presents the stimulus three times, and have the child immediately imitate the speech pathologist. The procedure should be repeated up to four times if the child does not succeed on the first three trials. Pitch deviations are similarly checked.

Van Demark (1971) described a stimulability evaluation for children with resonance problems. Each item missed on the IPAT is retested but using another picture. The speech pathologist then repeats the item twice and the subject responds immediately. Stimulation is then provided for the item in isolation, in nonsense syllables (initial, medial, and final positions), and in words. We suggest adding a sentence also. Following this stimulation, Van Demark suggested again showing the subject a picture containing the missed item. The child should be made aware that this word contains the stimulated sound, and he should attempt to produce the word correctly. The subject then reads a word and then a sentence containing the stimulus sound.

We use the Miami Imitative Ability Test described by Jacobs, Philips, and Harrison (1970) in determining level of stimulability responses in children with velopharyngeal insufficiency. The test is designed to evaluate a child's ability to imitate both acoustic production and the articulatory placement of consonants. Twenty-four consonant sounds are used in the initial position only, followed by the neutral vowel /ʌ/. The child is instructed to "watch and listen" as the speech pathologist repeats each stimulus three times; this gives the child an adequate opportunity to observe and hear the stimulus. Then the child is instructed, "Now you do it" and two separate scores are given for the response: (1) the ability to imitate articulatory placement, and (2) the accuracy of the acoustic production. The score values are: One point if correct, ½ point if questionable, or 0 if incorrect. For correctness of articulatory placement visible sounds are scored by direct observation, and where articulatory placement is not easily seen the speech pathologist judges the articulatory placement on what can be seen supplementing the evaluation by the acoustic production.

Van Riper (1963, pp. 470–471) listed several types of stimulation as follows. Use two or three of the most deviant sounds and vary the position of the tongue and lips to see if this results in improved quality. These same deviant sounds can be used to investigate the effect of different pitch levels on the quality of the voice. This can be tried with continuous speech as well as isolated vowels. The same sort of trial can be made by varying the loudness of the voice to determine whether a louder voice or a softer voice reveals better quality. Van Riper and Irwin (1958, p. 282) suggested noting differences in voice quality when a child sings and hums. Thus, through these types of stimulation we find those sounds and situations in which the voice quality is at its worst and those in which it is at its best.

INDICATIONS FOR VOICE THERAPY

After all recommended diagnostic examinations including medical, psychological, audiological, and voice are completed, decisions can be made regarding rehabilitation procedures for the child. These decisions may be made in a formal type of team staffing as described under Stage II of the voice team or they may take place as a less formal type of consultation between the specialists involved.

Voice therapy may be indicated for a child either as a procedure of choice or in coordination with other forms of treatment. It is the procedure of choice under the following circumstances: (1) to determine if a laryngeal pathology can be alleviated through voice therapy prior to consideration of other treatment, (2) for adaptation to congenital or acquired anomalies, or (3) for nonorganic cases. Voice therapy is used in coordination with other treatment: (1) preceding an operation or prosthesis, (2) following an operation or prosthesis, or (3) in combination with other treatment such as medication or psychotherapy (Wilson, 1966; 1968). These indications may be followed individually or in various combinations.

Voice Therapy as the Procedure of Choice

Alleviation of Laryngeal Pathology

Voice therapy may be indicated to determine if a vocal pathology can be alleviated before other methods of treatment are considered. Laryngeal pathologies likely to respond favorably to voice therapy include vocal nodules, vocal fold thickening, diffuse polypoid conditions, hyperkeratosis, and chronic nonspecific laryngitis. This is especially true in cases where vocal misuse and vocal abuse are felt to be the cause of the laryngeal pathology. Most children with continued hoarseness due to chronic laryngitis because of vocal abuse respond favorably to improvement in speech habits (Murphy, 1967).

Voice therapy is the treatment of choice for children with simple vocal nodules (Arnold, 1962; Brodnitz, 1971a, p. 86), particularly if the nodules seem to be soft, quite newly formed, and not fibrotic. Levbarg (1939) suggested voice therapy as the treatment of choice for vocal nodules to improve the muscular tonus of the vocal cords. Brodnitz (1971a, p. 86) stated vocal nodules in children should not be touched as they are reversible lesions which respond well to voice therapy. Withers and Dawson (1960) recommended voice therapy as the treatment of choice in certain vocal nodule cases and other times following surgical removal of the nodules. Brief voice rest followed by voice therapy may be suggested (Holinger et al. 1952; Levbarg, 1939). However, Brodnitz and Froeschels (1954) stated inactivity is diametrically opposed to good principles of modern rehabilitation and there is danger of muscular atrophy because of the inactivity during voice rest. Peacher (1952, p. 16) stated voice rest is not indicated in the treatment of vocal nodules but vocal education should commence immediately upon diagnosis. Peacher recognized a reduction in the amount of speaking for a time may be necessary. Cooper (1973, p. 60) stated in some rare instances vocal rest may be used for 7 to 14 days at the beginning of voice therapy if the person's voice is so hoarse that the optimal pitch cannot be determined. We sometimes, in consultation with the laryngologist, recommend voice rest or very limited voice use for periods up to 10 days. This is usually for children rated 6 or 7 on laryngeal tone; laryngeal hyperfunction, and vocal abuse, and who have marked swelling and reddening of the vocal cords either in isolation or associated with a vocal pathology. A short rest period often results in marked reduction of the condition and an improved voice. This demonstrates to the child the deleterious effects of the vocal abuse and lays the foundation for successful voice therapy.

Voice therapy to determine if a pathology can be alleviated must be given a good trial. Often after this trial period laryngeal conditions caused by vocal misuse and vocal abuse are definitely reduced if not absent. Even very young children can be taught to handle their voices with care and avoid flagrant vocal abuse if they are given various types of exercises appropriate for their age and interests (Wilson, 1961).

Adaptation to Anomalies

Voice therapy may be indicated to improve a child's voice in the presence of congenital or acquired anomalies. According to Moore (1971a, p. 561) if the vocal mechanism is permanently altered in some way there are three compensatory objectives: (1) obtain the greatest possible use of the remaining structures; (2) develop physiological compensations; (3) help the child and his parents adjust to the different voice. Anomalies include velopharyngeal insufficiency in the absence or presence of an overt cleft palate, vocal palsy, paralysis of one or both vocal cords, ventricular dysphonia, and stenosis of either the pharyngeal area, the glottis, or of both. Anomalies may also be present following various types of laryngeal operations, for example scarring of the edges of the vocal cords following removal of nodules, cysts, polyps, papillomas, or laryngeal webs. Laryngeal injury may result from intubation during an operation. A few children have voice problems due to structural anomalies as a result of accidental injury to the larynx.

In marginal cases of velopharyngeal insufficiency, preliminary voice therapy sessions are indicated to see if the undesirable voice and speech habits can be eliminated. Children with velopharyngeal insufficiency who show inconsistent results on speech examinations are good candidates for voice therapy as the primary treatment. The inconsistencies may be the result of fluctuating palatopharyngeal closure associated with neuromuscular dysfunction (Owsley, Chierici, Miller, Lawson, and Blackfield, 1967) or they may be related to marginal velopharyngeal competency (Morris and Smith, 1962). In marginal competency a speaker may produce a good plosive but nasalize a fricative, or he may produce an acceptable pressure consonant in isolation but not in connected speech (Morris and Smith, 1962). In either condition the child may respond well to voice therapy. Voice therapy should be initiated if hypernasality persists following an operation for removal of the adenoid (Berner, 1962; Weiss, 1948). However, a child with a marked velopharyngeal incompetency will not respond favorably to voice therapy without surgical intervention or a prosthesis. Therefore, attempts to eliminate hypernasality through voice therapy should be initiated only when examinations and tests indicate anatomical and physiological potential for velopharyngeal closure (Casper, 1972).

Nonorganic Problems

Voice therapy may be the preferred procedure for nonorganic problems, that is when nothing can be found wrong with the child physically. For example, hypernasality or a mutational voice problem may be seen in the absence of positive medical findings or anomalous conditions. Voice problems due to imitation and faulty learning are included here. Our goal under this indication is to teach new vocal habits to improve voice.

Voice Therapy in Coordination with Other Treatment

Preceding an Operation or Prosthesis

Voice therapy should begin preceding an operation (Brodnitz, 1971a, p. 87). For example, when vocal nodules are long-standing and appear hard and fibrotic an operation may be necessary. The child should be given several sessions of voice therapy before the operation for the purpose of introducing him to the principles of good voice use. This paves the way for continuation of voice therapy following the operation. For these same reasons voice therapy is sometimes recommended in cases of velopharyngeal insufficiency preceding an operation or the insertion of a prosthesis. Owsley et al. (1967) pointed out speech improvement following surgical correction of velopharyngeal incompetence is more rapid in children who have had some preoperative speech therapy.

Following an Operation or Prosthesis

If surgical and medical procedures can provide normal or near normal structures, the speech pathologist can attempt to establish adequate voice production (Moore, 1971a, p. 561). Gould (1975) stated the immediate postoperative result after surgical procedures involving the larynx is usually not the restoration of a "normal" voice, but rather reestablishing conditions which may permit the normal or preoperative vocal ability to be regained. Training in good use of voice following surgical procedures is usually necessary (Levbarg, 1939) to restore normal voice by breaking down acquired bad habits (Tarneaud, 1958), to avoid a recurrence of the condition (Clerf, 1952, p. 16), and to assure proper use of the voice (Loré, 1950). This is especially true when vocal misuse and vocal abuse are thought to have caused the original pathological condition (Brodnitz, 1955; Moore, 1955). Arnold (1962) felt nodules will return after being removed if vocal abuse and vocal misuse are continued. Holinger et al. (1952) stated surgical removal of small nodules may be postponed because they tend to disappear during puberty when the larynx increases in size and the stresses and strains of phonation change with the new pitch. However, if the vocal nodules do not resolve and are removed voice therapy is of great benefit following the operation. Voice training should also follow surgical removal of some hematomas and thickened vocal cord tissues (Moore, 1955), polyps, and polypoid thickening.

The laryngologist decides when a patient is ready for vocal rehabilitation after an operation. Some laryngologists recommend a period of voice rest, others do not. Billeaud (1971) stated that if voice rest is recommended for a patient the speech pathologist should understand the negative psychological stresses involved in requiring voice rest. Billeaud reported on a study with college students with normal voice who were assigned 12 hour or 24 hour voice rest periods. Reactions reported by the subjects included physical stress, laryngeal stress, depression, anger, frustration, guilt feelings, and self pity. Brodnitz (1971a, pp. 87–88) suggested voice rest during healing with no whispering for a few days up to longer periods. He stated the periods of voice rest vary according to pathology. Vocal nodules and small pedunculated polyps require a few days to a week, sessile polyps require about 2 weeks, and larger polypoid thickenings may require a longer period. He recommended voice therapy be initiated immediately after voice rest. Loré (1973, p. 716) stated following vocal cord stripping, the procedure he prefers for most lesions involving the vocal cords, the patient should be allowed to talk immediately after the operation but with certain restrictions. He should not be allowed to talk excessively, whisper, shout, or sing for a period of 3 to 5 weeks.

In a few cases postoperative voice therapy may be indicated because the child clings unnecessarily to his defective manner of speaking. A hoarse voice may persist after successful surgical procedures because it sounds natural to the child.

In cases of velopharyngeal insufficiency voice therapy is indicated following surgical procedures (Goda, 1966) or insertion of a prosthetic speech aid. Berner (1962) also suggested if good speech is not regained following adenotonsillectomy it may be necessary to consider palate lengthening and pharyngoplasty; these surgical procedures may be performed alone or in combination. Voice therapy may be recommended following such procedures.

In Combination with Other Treatment

Sometimes voice therapy is conducted concurrently with other treatment such as psychological-psychiatric, medical, and physical therapy.

Psychological-Psychiatric. Emphasis should be placed on psychological factors as well as physiological factors in a person with a vocal disturbance (Brodnitz, 1971a, p. 85; Moore, 1955). Many patients with voice problems need psychiatric consultation and treatment, some need only guidance and the solution of minor problems, but others need psychiatric referral (Alfaro, 1960; Lewy, 1963). A psychological approach freeing the patient of problems through sympathetic understanding may be necessary (Brodnitz, 1958b). Vocal rehabilitation should not be based only upon the condition of the larynx; the speech pathologist must also have an understanding of the personality of the client (Bloch, 1960). Psychiatric help may be indicated in cases of vocal nodules when excitement, worry, fear, and anxiety are detrimental to good voice use (Levbarg, 1939). Psychotherapy is indicated in some cases of infantile personality where there has been a continuation of high pitch levels into and through adolescence (Van Riper, 1972, pp. 145–146). Psychotherapy should be part of the treatment of incomplete mutation because of the frequent accompanying emotional disturbances (Luchsinger, 1965, p. 194). Psychotherapy may be an adjunct to voice therapy in ventricular phonation (Luchsinger, 1965, p. 320). Psychotherapeutic measures may be indicated if a child needs better adjustment and a less aggressive personality (Arnold, 1962; Luchsinger, 1965, p. 184; Mosby, 1970; 1972).

People with laryngeal dysfunction are apt to be gregarious, talkative, and physically active (Moore, 1955). Vocal nodules will often recur after removal in the overly active shouting boy if his personality remains unchanged (Holinger et al. 1952). Hysterical dysphonia or aphonia in adolescence is of concern to the laryngologist, the psychiatrist or psychologist, and the speech pathologist. A child with long-standing hysterical aphonia may need direction and instruction in good voice production. For example, Wolski and Wiley (1965) reported the successful treatment of functional aphonia in a 14-year-old boy who had become aphonic 6 months previously following laryngitis. Voice therapy was coordinated with psychiatric treatment with a normal voice the result.

Medical. Many children with laryngeal dysfunction are overly active. The physician may recommend placing a child on medication during voice therapy. We have seen such children become much more vocally manageable when receiving proper medication. Medication in some cases produces a favorable atmosphere and relaxation of physical tensions; tranquilizers may be indicated, hormonal treatment may be used in metabolic deficiences, and corticosteroids may reduce allergic conditions (Brodnitz, 1958b). Hormonal treatment may be indicated in cases of incomplete voice mutation where slight endocrine deficiencies are found (Luchsinger, 1965, p. 194).

Physical Therapy. In cases of ventricular phonation, physical therapy including heat and vibratory massage of the neck along with voice therapy is sometimes suggested (Luchsinger, 1965, p. 320). In the hands of a physician or properly qualified person a weak electric current may relax muscles for better production of voice while a stronger current may stimulate muscular activity if stimulation is necessary for better voice (Brodnitz, 1958b). Shelton (1963) in discussing therapeutic exercise and speech pathology concluded the speech pathologist "... should concentrate on the development of speech skill and leave remediation of the speech mechanism to physicians." The coordination of both aspects may result in facilitating voice improvement.

PROGNOSIS IN VOICE DISORDERS

Prognosis, the prediction of the outcome of voice therapy, depends upon the individual child and his particular problem. A prognosis is based upon the cause of the problem, examination results, indications for therapy, and the planned therapy procedures. We recognize a prognosis for an individual child cannot be made until the treatment plan has been formulated. However, the speech pathologist should keep a tentative prognosis in mind while formulating therapy plans. Therefore, we are discussing prognosis before presenting material the speech pathologist will use in making specific plans for therapy.

A prognosis may be *favorable, unfavorable,* or *guarded.* A favorable prognosis indicates that a child upon completion of his therapy program will have a much improved or corrected voice. An unfavorable prognosis means the opposite, that is the outlook is negative regarding the end result of voice therapy. A guarded prognosis indicates a question about improvement in voice for many reasons including cooperation of child and parents, associated physical or psychological problems, or the very nature of the voice problem itself.

Motivation to improve voice is a special problem with children. Motivation must be stimulated to a high degree; we must carefully assess the degree of motivation in a child to improve his voice; progress with some children who state they want to change their voice habits may be slow because of unconscious resistance to therapy (Van Riper and Irwin, 1958, pp. 274–275). Motivation is not too difficult if we plan a therapy program carefully and then present it to the child in clear-cut step-by-step fashion so he knows what is wrong with his voice and what is going to be done to help him improve it.

A favorable prognosis for therapy is indicated if we can get a better voice from a child during the stimulability test and during a brief teaching period. Van Riper and Dopheide (1966) recommended the inclusion of a trial period of therapy during diagnostic evaluations. They stated even a 20 min period may reveal much about a person's motivation, cooperation, and difficulties. We feel, therefore, during the trial therapy administered during the evaluation procedure, the speech pathologist should determine if a child can achieve correct vocal production without going through a complete discrimination program. For example, Williams and McReynolds (1975) showed that production training as the first step in therapy for articulation training was effective in changing both articulation and discrimination ability in children. They found that discrimination training administered without production training was effective only in changing discrimination ability.

Prognosis depends to a large degree upon the amount of therapy time available. It is more favorable if a child can be seen on a regular basis. If possible a child should be seen daily during the first week or two. After this the sessions should be scheduled so he is seen for 20 to 40 hourly sessions of voice therapy during a 12 week period to see if the pathology can be alleviated and the voice improved. For functional voice problems a marked progress in improved voice should be charted. Frequent brief periods of practice are often recommended. For laryngeal dysfunction Peacher (1952, p. 10) recommended 2 to 5 min practice sessions about 20 times a day for the initial week or two of therapy. Moore (1971a, p. 564) suggested frequent short practice sessions avoiding overuse of the voice. He recommended only 3 min an hour gradually increasing the length of practice sessions until an occasional practice session of 30 min might be attempted. After a 12 week period the child may be rechecked

by the laryngologist or seen by other members of the voice team. The total voice therapy time is usually 4 or 5 months in cases of vocal nodules (Peacher, 1952, p. 16).

Prognosis for laryngeal dysfunction depends upon many factors and in most cases is favorable. Van Riper and Irwin (1958, p. 189) stated, "Prognosis in voice cases where vocal nodules are present depends upon the location and size of the nodules, their duration, and the necessity for surgery, and the case's ability to change his habits of phonation." When hoarseness is a result of excessive use of the voice, improvement will be proportionate to the success in correcting the vocal abuse (Orton, 1951). The prognosis for children with vocal nodules depends upon controlling vocal abuse and helping the child develop a less aggressive pattern of vocal expression through voice therapy (Luchsinger, 1965, p. 186). Vocal nodules should show a reduction in size within 3 months of voice therapy (West and Ansberry, 1968, p. 218). Children with hoarseness because of chronic laryngitis occasionally require prolonged voice therapy (Murphy, 1967). Inflammation due to hyperkinetic dysphonia usually improves as speech habits normalize and vocal abuse is reduced (Greene, 1972, p. 153). Saunders (1956) stated the prognosis in dysphonia plicae ventricularis usually should be guarded as some patients remain hoarse despite all efforts to help them. However, Luchsinger (1965, p. 32) stated generally the prognosis is quite favorable in ventricular phonation unless there is a serious neurosis present.

Prognosis can be exemplified by Baynes' (1967) program. Fourteen children with vocal nodules and vocal cord thickening had small group therapy 2 hours a week for a period of 8 weeks. The children were reexamined by a laryngologist 12 weeks after the initiation of the program. Seven of the children exhibited normal vocal cords without any pathology remaining. Four of the children showed a definite decrease in the amount of vocal cord thickening but three of the children did not continue in the program throughout this period. It was found as voice quality improved pathology diminished.

If the aim is to adjust to structural anomalies, in most cases the prognosis must be quite guarded (West and Ansberry, 1968, p. 216). This is especially true with anomalies of the laryngeal area and with velopharyngeal insufficiency. These conditions may require extensive therapy often lasting many months. In cases of velopharyngeal insufficiency Barnes and Morris (1967) suggested the speech pathologist should recheck sounds incorrectly produced on the articulation test to see if the child can produce the sounds correctly after stimulation. If the child can this indicates a potential for good velopharyngeal competence and gives a favorable prognosis. Van Gelder (1974b) reported that patients with hypernasality following adenoidectomy and tonsillectomy got more satisfactory results from speech therapy with a velopharyngeal distance of not more than 5 mm for vowels and 2½ mm for consonants.

In nonorganic cases the prognosis must be guarded since it depends in part upon unknown factors. Overall exposure time to voice therapy varies. The prognosis varies according to the child and the presenting problem in children with functional voice problems. These problems include hypernasality in the absence of structural deviations, problems of hoarseness with no organic basis, pitch deviations, and problems of loudness. The prognosis for persistent falsetto in the young male is especially favorable (Aronson, 1973, p. 58; Luchsinger, 1965, p. 197; Weiss, 1950).

When voice therapy is coordinated or combined with other treatment the prognosis is dependent to a large extent on the prognosis for the other treatment. In cases in which an operation or prosthesis is necessary the prognosis is always better if the child is given several sessions of voice therapy before these procedures. Brodnitz (1955) recommended beginning with two or three sessions a week following removal of cord lesions with the average length of voice therapy about 2 months. Progress in psychotherapy may determine progress in voice therapy. Medication may relieve physical conditions contributing to the voice problem. Physical therapy may improve the balance of muscular tonus. Progress in other therapies speeds progress in voice and improves the voice prognosis.

SUMMARY

Examination by the speech pathologist is a major responsibility since the results form the foundation for voice therapy goals and techniques. Baselines for vocal parameters and behavior are established from the results of the examinations. The baselines are used later to measure observable changes toward target behaviors. Children are seen in many situations ranging from informal play activities to standardized testing situations. Detailed ratings and descriptions are made of a child's use of voice quality and resonance, his misuse and abuse of the physical mechanisms used in talking, his pitch level, his rate of speaking, and his speech anxiety. Many of the test results are expressed in rating scale units and test scores; other results are in terms of the measures made by instruments such as a pitch indicator, an oral manometer, or a sound level meter. All of the results are coordinated, reports written, and therapy plans carefully structured.

SEVEN

Voice Therapy:
Some Basic Approaches

We have seen that each child with a voice problem needs special appraisal and diagnostic methods specifically designed for him. In this chapter we will present some basic approaches to voice therapy; later we will present procedures for specific voice problems. We will discuss the fundamental 10 step voice therapy outline and listening training, procedures which are basic to approaches for all types of voice problems. The use of negative practice in voice therapy will be explained, and methods of charting speech behavior will be explored. Special approaches to voice therapy will be described, including operant conditioning, client- and communication-centered therapy, psychotherapy, and reciprocal inhibition.

During the initial part of the voice therapy program the child should be taught how voice is produced and given basic facts about his voice problem (Wilson, 1961; 1962c). The level and detail of instruction are dependent upon the age and intelligence of the child. Having a basic understanding of vocal function and malfunction enables him to understand therapy procedures and serves to motivate him to improve his voice. A young child can be given a simplified explanation of how the larynx functions and how the laryngeal tone is resonated and articulated to form meaningful speech communication. The cause of his defective voice can be explained without elaborate detail. A young child responds best to drawings made by the speech pathologist as the child's problem is discussed. For example vocal nodules can be compared to calluses on the hands or merely called "bumps" on the vocal cords. Older children and adolescents benefit not only from drawings but also from carefully selected charts from anatomy books and models (Irwin, 1965, pp. 188–189). Care should be taken to avoid drawings that might be considered too detailed or too pathologically ori-

ented. These explanations are particularly beneficial when the child must be given reasons for modifying or eliminating vocal abuse and vocal misuse (Wilson, 1962b).

Children are seen individually and in groups organized according to type and severity of voice problems. Thurman (1977, p. 234) suggested the speech pathologist keep the child informed about the therapy program and the reasons for using specific procedures. This can be done by presenting a brief statement of objectives at the beginning of a voice session, explaining the specific procedures and the purpose of each as it is used, and giving a summary at the end of the therapy session. We have found this can be carried out very nicely by having each child use a personal voice notebook. A description of each session is placed in the notebook, including objectives, procedures, a summary of what was accomplished, and outside assignments.

Generally we approach a voice problem first in a segmental way, choosing the one aspect that needs primary attention and has been rated amenable to change on the stimulability examination. We then attempt, as Perkins (1977, p. 391) suggested, to merge the segmental and overall approaches into a unified whole. We will see, therefore, that our approaches to vocal rehabilitation include overall approaches, such as breathing exercises, chewing exercises, and relaxation procedures. At the same time we work on segmental aspects of voice that need attention, such as vocal abuse or pitch.

The basic program for improving voice follows a 10 step voice therapy plan and includes the following: (1) listening training, (2) teaching correct voice use, and (3) habituation of new vocal patterns. Elimination or modification of vocal abuse and vocal misuse is important with many voice problems. The role of the family during all stages of vocal rehabilitation is stressed. Consideration is given to emotional and social problems of the child with a voice problem. Throughout a therapy program the speech pathologist must keep detailed records of each session and write periodic progress reports.

TEN STEP VOICE THERAPY OUTLINE

Therapy procedures for modifying vocal behavior are carefully structured. The 10 step outline shown in Figure 25 is used for dealing with each major aspect of a voice problem. This outline can be used to modify all vocal parameters needing attention. The 10 steps can be arranged so they resemble a ladder to be climbed with the first step at the bottom and the final step, complete carryover, at the top. The outline is followed carefully. (1) The child is first taught the correct standard or rule about a specific vocal parameter. (2) He is then taught to identify in others an inadequate or incorrect vocal habit, and (3) to recognize in others the corresponding correct use. (4) The child begins to modify and control his own vocal behavior by learning to recognize an incorrect vocal production in himself, and (5) to differentiate it from his correct vocal production. (6) Then he identi-

1. I KNOW THE RULE ABOUT MY VOICE.
2. I CAN TELL WHEN OTHER PEOPLE USE THEIR VOICES INCORRECTLY.
3. I CAN TELL WHEN OTHER PEOPLE USE THEIR VOICES CORRECTLY.
4. I CAN TELL WHEN I USE MY VOICE INCORRECTLY.
5. I CAN TELL WHEN I USE MY VOICE CORRECTLY.
6. I KNOW THE PLACES WHERE I USE MY VOICE INCORRECTLY.
7. I KNOW THE PLACES WHERE I USE MY VOICE CORRECTLY.
8. I CAN USE MY VOICE CORRECTLY *SOME* OF THE TIME.
9. I CAN USE MY VOICE CORRECTLY *MOST* OF THE TIME.
10. I CAN USE MY VOICE CORRECTLY *ALL* THE TIME.

Fig. 25. The 10 step voice therapy outline. From Wilson, D. K. (1977). Voice problems of children and teenagers. In M. Cooper and M. H. Cooper, eds., *Approaches to Vocal Rehabilitation*. Courtesy of Charles C Thomas, Springfield, Illinois.

fies the situations and places where he uses undesirable vocal behavior and (7) the situations where his vocal behavior is acceptable. Carryover comprises the last three steps where the new vocal habit is used (8) *some*, (9) *most*, and (10) *all* the time (Wilson, 1977, p. 263).

LISTENING TRAINING

A key to attaining almost all the goals of voice therapy is the application of carefully programmed listening training procedures. As the term listening training implies the child is the listener. He is given experience in distinguishing between good voice use and poor voice use. He listens as the speech pathologist demonstrates good and poor voice. He listens to other children with voice problems (Moore, 1971a, p. 562), and sometimes to recordings of his own voice. Through these types of listening activity his ability to identify defective aspects of voice, including vocal misuse and vocal abuse, is developed and refined.

Since the use of a tape recorder is frequently recommended throughout the voice therapy program the speech pathologist should exercise a certain amount of care in asking children with voice disorders to listen to their own voices. Even though most children have heard their voices on a tape recorder at school or at home, those recordings were usually made for fun in an uncritical situation. It is not a good idea to have a child with a severe voice problem listen to himself on a tape recorder during the first therapy session. Without proper preparation a child may be upset by the way he sounds, often refusing to listen to himself by putting his hands over his ears. The speech pathologist should make tape recordings just for fun before doing listening training or voice analyses with a child (Pronovost and Kingman, 1959, p. 114). The speech pathologist explains how a tape recorder works and what he will hear. He is told his voice may not sound as pleasant as he would like but the use of a tape recorder will help him improve his voice.

Listening material can be live or prerecorded. In our program of listening training we constantly contrast optimum performance with inadequate performance. The speech pathologist selects one defective aspect present in the child's voice for initial listening training. If vocal abuses are present, elimination or modification of these abuses should be approached early in therapy; or listening training could start with too-high pitch level, overly loud voice, hoarseness, hypernasality, or hyponasality. The speech pathologist simulates specific parameters of the child's voice problem during the therapy session, or they may have been prerecorded. In either case all productions should be consistent from sample to sample.

It is best, as Van Riper (1972, p. 164) stated, to be careful in selecting the terms used to describe a deviant voice or to express the amount of deviation from normal. For example, instead of saying something is *bad,* the speech pathologist can say it is *farther* from a goal; instead of *good,* it can be described as *closer* to a goal. Andrews (1975) suggested avoiding negative terms such as wrong, bad, or unpleasant, with the term *different* as preferable. Once a child begins to improve his voice we use *cloudy* for the old voice and *clear* for the new voice. Andrews (1975) also recommended the judicious use of instruments such as a sound level meter where numbers represent various levels of loudness rather than using the terms *too soft* or *too loud.*

The Three Steps of Listening Training

The three steps of listening training for a child with a voice deviation are (1) awareness of differences in others, (2) gross discrimination of differences in others, and (3) fine discrimination of differences in others.

Awareness of Differences in Others

In this step the child becomes aware of the defective aspect. The speech pathologist demonstrates the defective aspect and points out the identifying features. The speech pathologist then produces sounds, syllables, words, and sentences with the defective aspect on some. The child signals the occurrence of the defective aspect; for example the child indicates when the speech pathologist's voice is hoarse. A scoring system should be devised to enable the child to tabulate his own responses. For example, the speech pathologist reads a passage where previously underlined vowels are hypernasalized while the child listens carefully, underlining on his copy of the passage the words he heard hypernasalized (Van Riper, 1972, p. 161). Rewards for correct responses may be appropriate.

Black (1970, p. 10) suggested the following activity (played on a "Simon Says" basis) which we consider an introductory type of listening training. The speech pathologist demonstrates different types of voices, hypernasal, breathy, strident, and pleasant. The children are told they are to do certain things such as stand up or touch their nose when Simon says to do so in a pleasant voice. They are not to move if Simon talks in a deviant voice.

Baynes (1967) developed awareness of differences in children by teaching them differences between various voice qualities by listening to each other. Brief recordings were made of each child in the group. They then listened to an unidentified recording of a member of the group and were asked to identify the person from the recording. In a like manner, children were taught to distinguish loud from soft voices and high-pitched voices from low-pitched voices. Each child was immediately rewarded for correct responses by receiving a point after his name listed on a chart.

Skelly et al. (1971) reported using listening training for hypernasality with groups of children. The speech pathologist demonstrated hypernasality by playing previously prepared audiotapes of hypernasality samples of children in the group. The children learned to detect the hypernasal sounds as they heard them in other children and then were able to apply discrimination to hypernasal resonance in their own voices.

Gross Discrimination of Differences in Others

The second step in listening training is gross discrimination of differences. The speech pathologist explains the identifying features of two levels of voice production, the correct and incorrect. The child is then asked only to discriminate between the two productions, using the same-different technique. That is, pairs of the speech pathologist's vocal productions are judged by the child as being the same or different. Some pairs have two correct vocal productions, other pairs have one correct and one defective production, and other pairs have both defective. This can be done live or recorded. The speech pathologist can record many pairs on language master cards. The child can run the cards through the language master and stack the cards in appropriate piles— same or different.

In listening training with the same-different technique the material at first should contain more different than same pairs. It takes a longer time to determine if two identical stimuli are the same than to determine if two dissimilar stimuli are different (Bindra, Williams, and Wise, 1965). Thus a child can experience more success initially if he is asked to discriminate between pairs that are different.

The speech pathologist should be cautious about using a same-different discrimination task with children under 6 years of age. Beving and Eblen (1973) asked three groups of children, whose mean ages were 4½ years, about 6 years, and 8 years, to perform two tasks with pairs of nonsense syllables. They were to identify the pairs as *same* or *different,* and at another time were asked to repeat the pairs. All three age groups were about equal in ability to repeat the pairs accurately, but the youngest group (4½ years) was significantly poorer on the same-different task. Apparently they were not yet familiar with this concept.

Next the child identifies the vocal characteristics of each inadequate or adequate production in the pairs previously used for the same-different task. For example he listens to pairs and identifies the first one in the pair as cloudy and the second one clear, both productions as clear, or both as cloudy. Eisenson and Ogilvie (1977, pp. 323–324) stated a child can learn to recognize nasal resonance as it normally occurs by listening for nasal resonance in word pairs and sentence pairs. One word or one sentence of each pair should contain /m/, /n/, and /ŋ/ which normally have nasal resonance. Nasal resonance, normal and deviant, are explained and demonstrated to the child. Then the speech pathologist uses pairs of words with one word containing a nasal consonant, for example, moo-two, me-bee, no-go. Paired sentences such as those suggested by Fairbanks (1960, p. 173) are next presented:

"The pup was stuffed full of toast."
"Dan's gang changed my mind, Sam."

"Sue roasted a duck for supper."
"Ten men came in when Jane rang."

If a child has difficulty with discrimination it may be helpful to use sentence pairs of the type used by Lichtenberg (1966); paired sentences accompanied by pictures were used where only one phoneme in the sentence is different. For example, we use:

Jerry likes to read.
Mary likes to read.

See the beet.
See the meat.

Fine Discrimination of Differences in Others

The third procedure in listening training is fine discrimination of differences. At least three levels of vocal performance are selected for the child to discriminate. The differences between the levels are reduced as the child becomes more proficient, requiring him eventually to discriminate very fine differences. The three levels are demonstrated by the speech pathologist and their identifying characteristics explained. For example the speech pathologist records three vowels on a language master at different pitch levels, high, middle, and low. Other cards can be recorded with the order scrambled. The child must designate which productions are high, which middle, and which low. For hypernasality the speech pathologist uses excessive hypernasality, moderate hypernasality, and normal resonance. For hoarseness, the child is asked to discriminate between a voice that has moderate hoarseness, one with mild hoarseness, and one with no hoarseness. The child listens to the three productions and identifies each one according to the descriptions provided by the speech pathologist.

We have found listening training can be more effective when auditory stimuli are accompanied by visual stimuli. Huffman and McReynolds (1968) found learning was facilitated when a visual stimulus was presented simultaneously with an auditory stimulus. Karlovich (1968) asked young adults to judge sensation levels of pure tones when the tones were accompanied by a light flash. He found simultaneous presentation of a visual stimulus and a standard auditory stimulus caused the auditory stimulus to be perceived as louder by the subjects. Siegel and Allik (1973) included kindergarten, second, and fifth graders in a study of short-term memory. They found that stimuli presented only visually produced a higher percentage of correct responses than when stimuli were presented only auditorially. Therefore, when only the auditory stimulus is given in discrimination training, the child may not benefit maximally. Accompanying visual stimuli for younger children can be simple drawings. For older children sounds or words can be written on language master cards to reinforce the auditory input.

Andrews (1975) suggested using nonauditory representation for the loudness parameter, for example, by providing a visual feedback through pictures where the size of the picture represents the loudness level. Andrews and Madeira (1977) also found many normal children under 8 years of age were not able to discriminate pitch levels unless the task was especially constructed and free of relational language such as *low* and *high*. They used pictures of two barns, one big and one small, and of two animals, one big and one small, to represent low and high pitch. Tones an octave apart were presented to children by the speech pathologist, either using a pitch pipe or by saying the animal sound at approximately the same frequency as the pitch pipe. The child was shown that the lower pitched tone or animal sound was to be paired with the big animal and the big barn and the higher pitched tone or animal sound was to be paired with the small animal and the small barn. The child moved the animals to the appropriate barns in steps according to the pitch level indicated by the animal sound or pitch pipe. A variety of animal sounds can be used; Andrews and Madeira used "oink" for pigs of two sizes. We like to use "baa" with a lamb and a sheep.

For a very young child, 3 or 4 years of age, listening training for loudness should include pairs of words where the first of the pair is louder than the second. Carter, Ricker, and Corsini (1972) studied relational judgment of sound intensity in children aged 3, 4, and 5 years. Paired stimuli similar to white noise, each having a duration of 2 sec and separated by a 1 sec interval, were used. In all, three pairs were presented, the first pair had sounds at 40 dB and 59 dB, the middle pair sounds at 50 dB and 77dB, and the third pair 70 dB and 82 dB. A child indicated which sound was *louder,* or *softer,* by pointing to one of two loudspeakers. The pairs were presented twice. The first time the child was asked to indicate which sound was louder, and the second time to indicate which of the two sounds was softer. The 3 and 4 year olds had more difficulty making the judgment when the first of the pairs was softer than the

second, than when it was louder than the second. The group of 5 year olds had no difficulty with the task at all. Thus, in teaching loudness discrimination to very young children under 5 years of age, the louder stimulus should be given first.

In summary of listening training, it is important to remember the child is the listener and judge and the speech pathologist is the performer. The main objective is to teach the child to become a discriminating judge of the voices of others so he can later apply this ability to his own voice. Listening training has three basic steps: (1) awareness of differences in others, (2) gross discrimination of differences in others, and (3) fine discrimination of differences in others.

NEGATIVE PRACTICE

Negative practice is a most useful method in teaching good use of voice. It is the conscious use of an undesirable habit for the purpose of gaining voluntary control over it. Dunlap (1932, pp. 78–80, 94–96) termed this method the *Beta* hypothesis and advocated it as an *unlearning* procedure for undesirable habits. We find it especially useful in modifying or eliminating vocal abuse and misuse, improving voice quality, and establishing proper oral-nasal resonance balance. Other speech pathologists have described its usefulness in voice therapy. For example, Skelly et al. (1971) found negative practice helpful in reducing hypernasality in children with scoliosis.

There are two steps in the use of negative practice: gross differences negative practice and fine differences negative practice. These two steps enable a child to gain conscious control of the undesirable habit and to reject the undesirable and assume the desired behavior. The undesirable habit is always contrasted immediately with the desired production.

Gross Differences Negative Practice

The child uses two types of voice production, the desired and the undesired. For example in pitch problems the levels are very high pitch *versus* normal pitch or very low *versus* normal pitch. Other examples are very hypernasal *versus* normal resonance, too loud *versus* normal loudness, and very hoarse *versus* no hoarseness.

Fine Differences Negative Practice

When the child can do gross negative practice with control he is ready to do fine differences negative practice. Here three or four levels are used, for example mild, moderate, and severe hoarseness, and a clear voice. When a child can gain this type of control over a faulty vocal habit contrasted to a desirable vocal habit the elimination of the undesirable one becomes a conscious choice.

The Use of Negative Practice

Negative practice is used conservatively and in limited amounts to bring undesirable vocal practices to a conscious level. It also demonstrates kinesthetic and auditory sensations of incorrect vocal production so the child can eliminate the incorrect production more easily and rapidly. Negative practice is ordinarily used only within the therapy situation. Except for special cases we do not recommend asking a child to do voice negative practice in outside situations. This must be made very clear to a child because unsupervised negative practice may lead to overuse of this technique. When consulting with physicians about voice therapy for a child, the speech pathologist should always ask about restrictions on voice therapy. Voice therapy procedures including negative practice should be explained in detail to the physician. The speech pathologist must be sure it is not harmful for a child to use even limited amounts of negative practice. Negative practice may be contraindicated for some children with vocal cord pathology. There may be a psychological basis for not using negative practice; it may reawaken old problems and reactions in both the child and his family (Flower, 1959). However, we feel carefully supervised negative practice is not harmful physically or psychologically with most types of children's voice problems. We rarely have been requested not to use it.

When a child is first seen in therapy we gather information about his likes and dislikes to use in negative practice. LeSaz (1973) suggested a favorite and unfavorite item inventory. We use the unfavorite item for negative practice and the favorite item for positive practice. The following categories were listed by LeSaz: " ... color, game, sport, story, song, pet, wild animal, bird, flower, tree, season, month, day, time of day, word, number, city, state, foreign country, car, movie, TV program, friend, teacher, man, woman, sandwich, ice cream, candy, gum, meat, dessert, building, material, vacation, school subject, and job ... " adding any other categories suggested by the child.

A child is ready to begin negative practice when he can produce the desired vocal behavior. By now he has had training identifying both the desired and the undesired aspects in recordings of his own voice. For example, if we are working on a vocal abuse such as abrupt glottal attack, negative practice can begin the moment he can consciously control the abuse. He is asked to use an abrupt glottal attack on a word and then produce the word without it.

Creative dramatics and role playing including the use of hand puppets are useful in therapy (Hahn, 1955). During the portrayal of a character we can control various aspects of a child's voice, such as loudness, pitch, and quality, and pay special attention to vocal abuse. We use role playing in which a child assumes a character in his environment, especially one who may be a loud talking vocal misuser and vocal abuser. In this way a child's attention is focused on the undesirable aspects of voice production making him aware of undesirable habits. The undesirable is replaced with more desirable habits which the speech pathologist teaches as the child continues role playing.

Here is an example of the use of negative practice:

John, a 6½-year-old boy, had bilateral vocal nodules. His frequent use of explosive release of vocalizations was our first target for elimination. Negative practice was essential to this elimination. In his notebook we pasted pictures of things he liked and things he did not like (see Fig. 26). For example pictures of asparagus and ice cream were placed side by side. He did not like asparagus so an explosive release of vocalization was used in saying this word, while his favorite food, ice cream, was to be produced easily and smoothly. This was the first step of negative practice with only two levels used. For fine differences negative practice John used four levels for the explosive release of vocalizations—severe, moderate, mild, and normal. These types of negative practice demonstrated to John how he could control this vocal abuse and he soon eliminated it.

CHARTING

Some type of charting of vocal behavior is necessary. There are three basic purposes of charting voice behavior: (1) to establish baselines at the beginning of a voice therapy program; (2) to measure changes from the baselines during the program, at the end of the program, and during follow-up appointments; and (3) to analyze the therapeutic process. Programmed instruction in voice therapy requires careful charting by both the child and the speech pathologist. Such programs have been described by Deal et al. (1976) in a program for children with vocal nodules, by Drudge and Philips (1976) in modifying vocal behavior in college students with vocal nodules, by Johnson (1976) for reducing vocal abuse, and by Wilson and Rice (1977)* for children with hyperfunctional and hypofunctional voice problems.

The speech pathologist should use a systematic method of charting. Speech pathologists initially will want to chart specific occurrences of vocal abuses, such as throat clearing or abrupt initiation of tone. For example, abrupt initiation of tone may be tabulated as occurring 50 times during the first therapy session. Then after working on this vocal abuse for a period of time its occurrence is again tabulated to determine decrease in use. Diedrich (1971) suggested the following procedure in counting and charting speech behavior. It is especially suitable for establishing baselines.

1. Engage a child in a 3 min conversation. During this time the speech pathologist talks only when necessary to encourage and maximize the child's talking.

2. The speech pathologist counts the target speech behavior, both incorrect and correct. Diedrich (1973, p. 7) stated counts can be tallied on paper or with a mechanical counter of some kind. Wrist counters† as advocated by Johnson (1976, p. 4), and Landes (1977, p. 128), golf counters, or inexpensive shopping counters can be used.

* Audiotapes, slides, and manual (with M. Rice) on voice disorders by F. B. Wilson are available from Teaching Resources, 50 Pond Park Road, Hingham MA 02043.

† Available from Behavior Research Company, Box 3351, Kansas City, KA 66103.

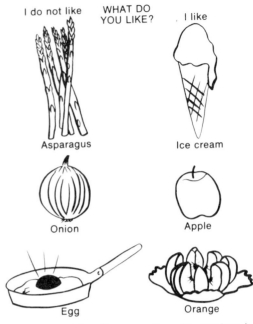

Fig. 26. Negative practice. Illustration by Geraldine Balsam.

3. The correct and incorrect counts are entered on a chart. A 6 cycle 140 day behavior chart† can be used. Figure 27 shows the kind of chart we like to use in voice therapy for tabulating behavior which is to be faded and also for tabulating behavior where the frequency is to be increased. For example, for a 5 min period tally marks are placed in the tally box for the selected date. The tally marks are counted and a star placed after that number in the column above the tally box. After 5 days the stars are connected by lines to make a graph. This type of chart can be used during therapy by either the speech pathologist or the child. Also it can be used by the child himself for tallying during outside assignments and by parents to monitor a child's voice. We suggest having a child chart behavior only 5 out of 7 days—giving him a vacation 2 days a week. The charting days should include those days when he most often engages in the target behavior being charted, for example, shouting while watching a hockey game.

The following procedure was described by Diedrich (1973, p. 4) for counting and charting behavior. We are applying the steps of his program to the elimination of shouting.

1. The behavior to be charted should be carefully and specifically defined. For exam-

Name_____ Date_____ Place_____

Activity_____ Name of Observer_____

12					
11					
10					
9					
8					
7					
6					
5					
4					
3					
2					
1					
Tally					
Dates					

N U M B E R   O F   S H O U T S (vertical label at left)

Fig. 27. Chart for shouting.

ple, shouting should be explicitly defined in its various parameters.

2. The speech pathologist and the child should decide what are to be the criteria for deciding which response is correct and which response is incorrect.

3. The exact amount of time to be used for charting responses should be decided.

4. The frequency of charting behavior should be decided.

5. The means by which the responses will be elicited or provoked should be determined.

6. The places where the charting will be done are determined. Diedrich (1973, p. 6) suggested that if the behavior occurs fewer than 10 times in 3 minutes, it is desirable to increase the length of time or to structure a specific time when there would be at least 10 occurrences to be charted.

The number of correct responses expected during any one therapy session should be determined individually according to the child's ability to use the target vocal behavior. For example, Bennett (1974) stated that requiring hearing-impaired children, even as young as five, to make 100 responses during a session is not unreasonable. He recommended that in speech sessions lasting between 15 and 20 minutes target behavior responses should occur between 100 and 175 times.

Only positive symbols should be used when charting is done with a child for his notebook or for a bulletin board. We prefer to use positive tally marks such as large filled-in circles for correct and small filled-in squares for incorrect rather than plus and minus marks.

Regnell and Thomas (1976) presented a measurement technique for establishing baselines and measuring progress in voice therapy. The authors suggested having a person read a standard passage while two speech pathologists listen carefully and underscore each word which has deviant voice quality in it. We suggest using a standard passage such as "The Trip to the Zoo," or a portion of it. As noted before, seldom are all vowels and voiced consonants deviant. Therefore, in most cases deviant voice quality will be noted by observers on only a certain number of words in the passage. Built into this technique is a per cent agreement between the two observers in order to determine reliability of measurement. The number of deviant words found by each observer is counted. Regnell and Thomas suggested the following formula in calculating per cent of agreement:

$$\frac{SMALLER\ SCORE}{LARGER\ SCORE} \times 100 = \frac{PER\ CENT}{AGREEMENT}$$

Ninety per cent agreement should be obtained before the results can be reliably used. Thus when agreement is 90% or better, the total number of deviant words is the average of the smaller and larger scores. Then the number of deviant words is subtracted from the total number of words in the passage to get the number produced with acceptable quality. We suggest this procedure be used to establish baselines of various types of vocal behavior in children and adolescents. It should be noted the most accurate counting of deviant words can be done when a person is reading; however, a sample of spontaneous talking may also be used especially for children who cannot read. The voice sample should be audiotaped for purposes of a permanent record and for confirming agreement of two observers. It may not be possible to have two qualified observers present at any one time so the second rating of the recording can be done by the second person at a different time. We suggest the recording be replayed several times, each time evaluating a different vocal parameter. For example, the first time may be deviant laryngeal tone, the second time abrupt glottal attack, the next time throat clearing, until all parameters under consideration are carefully tabulated. It is desirable to have such tabulation done frequently; we suggest this type of analysis be done every 2 months. Three typical times should be during either the examination or the first session, approximately half way through the therapy program, and upon termination of therapy. It should also be done during follow-up appointments.

A voice therapy progress chart should be used for each child. Our form for charting changes in vocal behavior is shown in Figure 28. It shows an example of a 9-year-old boy with vocal nodules. The goals for each child as determined during the examination are entered in order of therapy priority on the horizontal axis and the severity rating for each goal checked on the vertical axis. To use the voice therapy progress chart, rating dates are entered in the spaces provided. Letters of the alphabet are used to indicate record dates, with A the first, B the second, etc. This chart is kept in the child's clinic record file, and a copy placed in his notebook. At the beginning of therapy the goals are identified and described and the severity rating explained to the child. Soon children are taught to rate their own progress. The opinions of teachers and parents are often useful in determining goals and progress.

Boone and Prescott (1972) presented a method of analyzing speech and hearing therapeutic processes which we apply to voice therapy. Drudge and Philips (1976) also used this procedure in voice therapy. Boone and Prescott (1972) suggested the speech pathologist either videotape or audiotape the middle 20 min of a therapy session and select a 5 min segment of this for analysis. The purpose of this procedure is to analyze the speech pathologist's behavior as well as the behavior of the child, to answer the question, "Do we know that what we do as clinicians does any good?" Following the Boone-Prescott protocol we tabulate responses to ten questions about clinical behavior:

1. Did the speech pathologist adequately describe and explain the goals and procedures of the session?

2. Did the speech pathologist specify what was expected of the child by either modeling behavior or explaining specific requests?

3. Did the speech pathologist objectively evaluate the child's response by verbal or nonverbal approval?

4. Did the speech pathologist evaluate the child's response as incorrect and indicate so by verbal or nonverbal disapproval?

5. Did the speech pathologist engage in behavior not therapy related?

6. Did the child make a response which was correct following the instructions or structured model?

7. Did the child make incorrect responses to instructions or models?

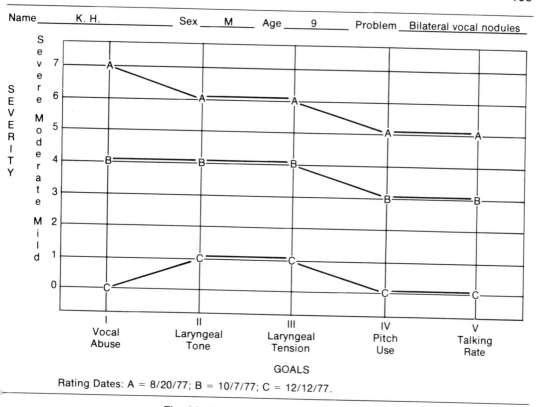

Fig. 28. Voice therapy progress chart.

8. Did the child make responses which were inappropriate for therapy goals?

9. Was the child aware of his correct responses?

10. Was the child aware of his incorrect responses?

We suggest this type of evaulation be done about once a month. After the first analysis to see where the baselines are, we suggest each question be assigned a 4/5 weighting; for example, four out of five times the answer to question 1 should be "Yes," indicating that the speech pathologist adequately described and explained specific goals and procedures of the therapy session. The reverse would be used for incorrect response tabulation—for example only one response out of five— 1/5—would be allowed for inappropriate responses by a child. Diedrich (1973, p. 3) suggested criterion control for most speech behavior be set at a minimum of 75%—for example 3/4.

Costello (1977) advocated that a child make frequent, continuous, overt responses to stimulus material as he is learning. This does two things, it focuses the child's attention on the task and allows the speech pa-

thologist the opportunity to observe whether or not the child is learning. Active participation by a child stimulates interest and makes charting more accurate.

SPECIAL APPROACHES

Many children with voice problems are extremely active, many are overaggressive. A genuine acceptance of children by the speech pathologist will help them understand and modify their own behavior. Some children may need psychotherapy or specific behavior therapy before or during voice therapy.

Operant Conditioning

Operant procedures may be especially useful as a basic method in voice reeducation. These procedures, described by Skinner (1953), can be applied to children with all types of voice problems. They can be used in programming instruction for a child individually or in groups.

In behavior modification it is important to follow shaping techniques, realizing that the desired terminal behavior is usually reached by a series of successive approximations. That is, when we get an initial approximation of the desired vocal response we are satisfied with this attempt and reinforce or reward the child. As therapy progresses, however, our standards become increasingly higher and a child's approximations must come closer and closer to the desired goal.

Holland (1967) described two basic rules regarding approximations, "(1) Begin with a form of behavior which the learner is fully capable of emitting and (2) move rigorously and precisely in small steps from this initial performance, differentially reinforcing each step, to progressively closer approximations of the desired final behavior." She emphasized the use of shaping procedures should not be haphazard but very clearly defined and the steps worked out carefully making certain they are small enough to assure mastery.

Costello (1977) stated a child should not proceed to more difficult material until he has mastered previous material. It is necessary that the child have correct performance on each programmed step before progressing to the following step. Costello also stated if response requirements are increased gradually and the child produces a large number of correct responses, the learning process requires little effort from the child and is a pleasant experience for him.

The desired change may be either in decreasing the rate of occurrence of an undesirable response or increasing the rate of occurrence of a desirable response (Brookshire, 1967). Throat clearing may be used as an example of decreasing the rate of an undesirable response. A speech pathologist may want to establish a change in the number of times a child clears his throat during a specified period. First the baseline is established; for example a child cleared his throat 25 times during a 5 min period. The allowable rate is varied so during specified 5 min periods he can clear his throat 20 times, 18 times, 15 times, and so on. This definite program in reducing the number of times a child clears his throat eventually leads to extinction of this undesirable vocal habit. An example of increasing the rate of occurrence of a desirable response is substituting easy initiation of tones for abrupt glottal attacks. Here the number of desired responses is gradually increased in the time period designated.

Brookshire (1967) stated, "Operant conditioning, in its simplest sense, is the process whereby consequences . . . occur relative to a response so that the rate of the response is controlled." He presented the basic procedures in operant conditioning: (1) positive reinforcement, (2) negative reinforcement, and (3) punishment which takes two forms, presentation of an aversive stimulus and removal of a positive reinforcer. Brookshire (1973) stated that reinforcers and punishers may affect behavior for two different reasons. First, consequences may serve to motivate a child and thus lead to increased response rates and increased energy expenditure. Second, they may provide information to the child regarding the appropriateness, correctness, or accuracy of his responses.

When reinforcers are used they are never delayed but are made immediately following the response (Brookshire, 1967; Holland, 1967). Costello (1977) stressed the necessity of immediate knowledge of results with some form of immediate feedback to the child. Each appropriate response is acknowledged. Waiting until the end of a therapy session to place a star beside a child's name on a chart gives him little reward for any specific accomplishment other than just coming to the therapy session. Bennett (1974) advocated that sessions for the hearing-impaired child should be approached as work periods. A child must work for rewards; emphasis should be placed on the fact that these are not bribes but "paychecks" for good work.

Positive reinforcement is the use of a reward for a desired response. Material consequences (soft drinks, candy, small toys, cereal, or points toward the winning of a toy) are often given for approximating or producing the desired behavior (McReynolds, 1970). Holland (1967) preferred not to use these types of rewards; rather the reinforcers should be transitory so the child's attention is not distracted by eating, drinking, or playing with small toys. She preferred winning points in a game, the pleasant noise of a door chime, or other immediate, clearly distinguishable but transitory reinforcers. The child should not be so overloaded with material rewards that they become meaningless. The speech pathologist accompanies the act of material reinforcement with the word "Good," gradually decreasing the number of times material reinforcement is used and continuing to say "Good" so that later this verbal reward is substituted for material reward. Gradually all rewards are given less frequently. This gradual withdrawal, termed fading, makes the child less dependent upon constant and frequent rewards. In this way his own modified behavior becomes the reward. Costello (1977) stated that in the early steps of a sequence many models, prompts, and cues are given to insure correct responses. These are gradually reduced until at the end of the program a child's responses are evoked by stimuli that are relevant and natural. For example, an improved voice may be rewarded by the positive comments of friends, teachers, and parents.

Negative reinforcement is removing an aversive or undesirable stimulus upon production of the desired response. A child is presented with a continuous undesirable stimulus which is then removed when he responds acceptably. A continuous white noise (McReynolds, 1970), a bright light, or a blindfold can be used. Negative reinforcement should be used sparingly and with care so children are not uncomfortable or even frightened by them. The speech pathologist can use the continuous moderately intense ringing of a cowbell or buzzer either operated manually or recorded on a tape loop with the noise removed when the undesirable vocal habit is stopped or a desirable habit begun.

Punishment is the presentation of an aversive stimulus whenever undesirable behavior or responses occur. Examples of punishment are sudden bursts of noise or a flashing light. This type of reinforcer can be useful in working with vocal abuse habits such as coughing and throat clearing which have no substitute behavior. Reinforcing the desired response is a better method for eliminating an undesired response with the emphasis on what to do and how to behave rather than on what not to do.

Removal of a reward is the fourth type of reinforcement. This can take two forms, either time out from positive reinforcement or response cost (McReynolds, 1970). Time out from positive reinforcement is used when the child does not respond appropriately. Reinforcement is merely stopped; no response is made by the speech pathologist.

We have found *time out* from positive reinforcement can be used effectively in working with children with voice problems. For example, if a child momentarily slides upward into the old high pitch we do not give a reinforcer. Response cost can be used when a child has accumulated a certain number of material things in the way of reinforcers. When undesirable behavior occurs the accumulated material things can be taken away one at a time. When children are accumulating points in a game, incorrect responses are charged by removing points.

We generally use time out rather than response cost. McReynolds and Huston (1971) found that operating under a no-token-loss condition with two boys aged 6 and 7 was more effective in decreasing incorrect responses in language and articulation than when taking away tokens for incorrect responses. We suggest that when working with children accumulated rewards should not be taken away.

Operant conditioning methods have definite applications for structured programs in voice rehabilitation of children and teenagers. There are many aspects of vocal rehabilitation which lend themselves to operant conditioning and programmed instruction methodology. The main advantage is that the speech pathologist as well as the child then knows exactly what is expected and how to reach the goal in achievable and logical steps. As we discuss vocal rehabilitation for various types of pathology we will point out how operant conditioning can be programmed into the ongoing therapeutic regimen.

Client-Centered Therapy

Client-centered therapy (Rogers, 1942; 1951) is a useful approach for helping children understand themselves (Martin, 1963). Thorn (1947) described the use of this procedure for voice and personality problems. She stated psychological tensions, inadequate adjustment to interpersonal relationships, feelings of insecurity in social situations, long-established patterns of reacting characterized by feelings of inadequacy, and extreme self-consciousness may contribute to unacceptable voice patterns. This approach allows permissiveness and directs the child to the appropriate goals. The speech pathologist sets limits on behavior. For example, a child is not allowed to break toys but the speech pathologist recognizes the child's desire to do so with understanding.

Placing responsibility directly on a child to set therapy goals and to determine therapy procedures is a modified approach to client-centered therapy. Freedman and Garstecki (1973) described a method for treating voice problems which they called child-directed therapy. Basically their approach includes helping a child recognize and understand the aspects of his behavior to be changed, and then supporting his motivation to assume responsibility for the therapy goals. Freedman and Garstecki suggested during the first session the speech pathologist define and describe the vocal parameters to be modified or changed—for example, modal frequency level, voice quality, and loudness. A rating scale concept is described to the child. These authors used a 10 point scale, but we suggest making the task easier by using a 3 point scale with *1* representing good use of voice; *2,* average use of voice; and *3,* poor use of voice. An audiotape is then made and the child rates the specific vocal parameters that are listed for modification or change. One of these parameters is selected by the child as the goal for the next session and a therapy plan is outlined. Each session then consists of an audiorecording, rating specific voice parameters, and selecting those to be included in the next session. Once parameters have been defined, explained, and demonstrated by the speech pathologist, a child can successfully identify those parameters which need improvement. We feel it is important for a child to assume as much responsibility in therapy as possible and this suggested procedure is a good way to do it.

Communication-Centered Therapy

Communication-centered speech therapy as described by Low, Crerar, and Lassers (1959) combines learning principles and therapy techniques drawn from numerous areas of human behavior. The basic tenet is the concept that communication is the nucleus for the learning of speech and the basic motivation for learning speech is to communicate not to imitate. Motivation is derived from group relationships with five general aspects which may proceed as a group begins to work together: (1) determine group and individual needs; (2) unify the group through integrating activities; (3) plan activities which include verbal and nonverbal expression; (4) plan activities requiring new speech patterns and different behavior; (5) practice specific speech behavior in context, if necessary re-move it from context for practice but always return it to the original context for further practice. If we apply communication-centered therapy to a group of children with vocal nodules, the five general aspects can be sequenced as follows: (1) define the need of the group to modify or eliminate vocal abuse identifying specific vocal abuses in each group member; (2) the group is then unified through activities such as listening training to become aware of various types of vocal abuse used by group members; (3) arrange activities which evoke communication on the vocal as well as nonvocal levels (a game in the gym or on the playground practicing controlled vocal and nonvocal communication could be arranged with the vocal abuses beginning to come under control); (4) arrange an activity requiring specific adjustive behavior on the part of the child (for example, decreased shouting would require him to adjust his behavior to a more quiet level by getting closer to people to whom he talks); (5) practice new shouting techniques in group activities as much as possible with special practice for the children who do not show adequate control of shouting in the group. Soon these children would be returned to the group situation for actual control of loudness in the original context such as a ball game.

Buck, Gallant, and Freshley (1973) described a communication therapy program as being especially useful for children who exhibit excessive withdrawal, hyperactivity, aggressiveness, anxiety, negativism, passivity, regression, distractibility, lack of effort, or depression. Children meet in groups of five to eight for a 1 hour weekly session. Children are grouped according to chronological age and language level disregarding behavioral styles. The theoretical rationale for a communication therapy program is that it must include certain developmental concepts and hypotheses regarding communication as follows: (1) Speech cannot be separated from the total personality. (2) Individual functioning must be approached within the context of the family. (3) The family must be understood within the context of the particular hearing and speech facility. Under the supervision of a consulting psychologist, speech pathologists are trained as group leaders and observers. The main emphasis is to provide an environment within which a child can grow in a self-directed way. This is the only general direction of the group. Maximum opportunity is given the children to direct their own activities and work out their own interpersonal relationships. Emphasis is placed on active listening by the speech pathologist who in turn does not overtly react to negative aspects of a child's behavior. Mirroring a child's feelings and centering on activities in order to get children to understand themselves better is helpful.

We can apply these concepts to a group of children who manifest vocal abuse and misuse. In order to modify their vocal behavior according to the communication therapy program, when a child screams we would ask, "Why are your screaming?" instead of ordering him not to scream. This would help the child explain his own behavior and lead him to his own solution of his screaming problem. Limits would be set in the group regarding a child's behavior so that he would not become overly aggressive vocally.

Psychotherapy

Mosby (1970) suggested psychotherapy may be a preferred approach for some children whose behavior does not permit them to benefit from regular voice therapy. Mosby presented a case study of a boy 10 years 11 months with vocal cord nodules with a severe voice problem characterized by hoarseness, stridency, tension, and low pitch. Voice therapy alone did not produce consistent gains. After 20 sessions of psychotherapy the boy's behavior reflected less tension, and aggressive reactions were reduced. The boy was helped by learning how he used his voice as aggressive behavior. Laryngoscopic examination 4 months after psychotherapy ended revealed the vocal nodules were no longer present, and a recheck 13 months after termination of therapy revealed the boy was operating satisfactorily in his environment.

In a later study Mosby (1972) reported on four boys aged 6 to 9 years with voice problems. All had average to superior intelligence. Three of the four boys had vocal nodules and all were below grade level in achievement due to emotional problems. Therapy was psychoanalytic, involving individual play. They were seen for 10 months with an average of 61 sessions per child. At the end of therapy normal voice quality and adequate personality integration were observed.

Hypnosis has been used as a psychothera-peutic approach to control vocal abuse in children. LaGuaite (1976) used hypnosis with 18 children approximately 4½ to 10 years of age with a mean of 6 years 8 months. Seven of the children had vocal nodules, four hypertrophy of the vocal cords, five normal larynges, and two could not be visualized because of an interfering epiglottis. Following a standard induction to hypnotic trance a child was helped to analyze situations where he yelled. Then suggestion was used to reduce the need to yell, which resulted in reduced vocal abuse. Fifteen children completed an average of 10.9 sessions and all but two showed improvement in the appearance of the larynx, with seven of the children showing disappearance of the nodules or the hypertrophy.

Reciprocal Inhibition

Principles and methods of reciprocal inhibition are useful in modifying vocal behavior associated with anxiety. According to Wolpe (1973, p. 17) the reciprocal inhibition principle can be summarized as follows: "If a response inhibiting anxiety can be made to occur in the presence of anxiety-evoking stimuli, it will weaken the bond between these stimuli and the anxiety." Applying this principle to voice therapy, the objective is to teach a child to remain physically and vocally relaxed in situations which usually promote general muscular hypertension resulting in specific laryngeal hypertension and vocal abuse. For example, in some children with vocal nodules it has been noted that being called upon in class when they are not prepared results in general and specific muscular hypertension and promotes hard glottal attacks. These children can be taught relaxation and can learn to remain relaxed in anxiety and tension producing situations so that vocal abuse can be eliminated. Relaxation procedures are presented in Chapter 8.

The theoretical and clinical approach of reciprocal inhibition in treating a 29-year-old woman with vocal nodules as described by Gray, England, and Mohoney (1965) will be presented. We will then outline a therapy program for children who can benefit from this approach. Gray et al. (1965) stated the basic premise of their treatment was that there are certain people in whom benign functional vocal nodules develop as a result of pervasive anxiety. Pervasive anxiety is defined as free-floating anxiety, that is, as more and more cues are associated with the stimulus situation, the anxiety reaction becomes conditioned to a vareity of stimuli which in the past did not evoke anxiety. This type of person moves from one anxiety producing situation to another until he is more or less in a constant state of anxiety or stress even in the absence of anxiety producing stimuli. Emotional over-reaction to situations and misuse of the vocal apparatus due to psychological and physiological stress characterize pervasive, free-floating anxiety.

It should be recognized that activities which are anxiety or stress associated, such as cheer leading or singing, may result in vocal nodules. Anxiety may be evoked in a child when he is exposed to a situation requiring good vocal performance such as giving a report in class. As a result he talks in a constricted, hypertensive manner with an inappropriate voice pitch level. Soon this anxiety which resulted in detrimental voice use spreads to many situations, such as conversations with teachers, reciting in class, and expressing his ideas to peer groups. Thus continual anxiety results in continued vocal misuse and abuse with the end result being the formation of vocal nodules or other vocal pathology. Gray et al. (1965) stated therapy including techniques to remove the anxiety state would lessen vocal abuse and result in vocal nodule remission. They formulated the following voice therapy goals:

1. Develop awareness of bodily tension both in an overall body awareness and in specific muscle groups. Give instruction in the technique of relaxation for thorough general body relaxation and selected muscle group relaxation.

2. Construction of lists of situations which under ordinary circumstances produce anxiety. The items are listed in the order of strength of anxiety arousal. Wolpe (1973, p. 120) discussed this type of scale, called the subjective anxiety scale, with situations rated according to subjective units of disturbance (*sud*). Instructions are given patients as follows: "Think of the worst anxiety you have ever experienced, or can imagine experiencing, and assign to this the number 100. Now think of the state of being absolutely calm and call this zero. Now you have a scale of anxiety. On this scale how do you rate yourself at this moment?" (Wolpe, 1973, p. 120).

Lists are made according to type of situation or subject matter. For example, with children anxiety producing situations might include the school, mother, father, brothers, and sisters. Then for each situation a subjective anxiety scale based on the *sud* unit is formulated.

3. Situations are provided in the clinic and structured around the low anxiety responses from the lists.

4. Expose the person to increasingly difficult anxiety producing responses for desensitization within the clinic situation.

5. Desensitization then is carried out by exposing the person to ever-increasing anxiety producing situations outside the clinic. The person is to keep relaxed and objective so his responses are antagonistic to the anxiety evoked by these stimuli.

The following is a typical sequence for use in systematic desensitization (Wolpe, 1973, pp. 103–140).

1. Training in deep muscle relaxation.

2. Establishing the use of a scale of subjective anxiety (*sud*).

3. Constructing anxiety hierarchies surrounding various nucleus situations.

4. Desensitization is accomplished by presenting anxiety evoking stimuli while the person keeps relaxed.

Phillips (1976)‡ and Phillips and Mordock (1974, Ch. 71) applied this method to children as young as 4½ years. A relaxation training program is developed. Next, scales of subjective anxiety are developed with the child. For a very young child the information must be gathered from the parents or others intimately acquainted with him in order to construct hierarchies of anxiety producing situations. For a child over 10 or 11 years of age information gathering can be done directly with him. Hierarchies are then structured on the 0 to 100 *suds* scale. A typical therapy session starts with a period of muscle relaxation, then the child is presented with anxiety arousing situations and the child is helped to become less sensitive to the anxiety. For example, a child may have listed as an anxiety provoking situation someone calling him a

‡ Phillips (1976) is based on lectures by Dr. Debora Phillips at a seminar "The Practice of Behavior Therapy with Children," January 22–23, 1976, Temple University Medical School, Philadelphia, Pennsylvania. Notes by the author. Used courtesy of Dr. Philips.

"robber." According to Phillips the therapist says, "Imagine Johnny is calling you a robber." After ascertaining the *sud* level the child is asked to relax until he indicates a low *sud* level. This procedure is repeated until the child is so desensitized about the situation that anxiety is not provoked and his *sud* level remains at zero. In this way children can be desensitized so that specific situations no longer provoke anxiety with vocally abusive behavior and vocal hyperfunction.

In vivo desensitization, which is desensitization in the actual situation, not the imaginary situation, is especially useful for young children under 11 years of age. The therapist helps the child gradually approach the anxiety situation with a counterconditioning agent. Here operants can be used as motivators and counterconditioning agents. Food, for example, can be used as a reward. The therapist accompanies the child into a situation and the therapist starts at the bottom of the hierarchy working up to desensitize the child to ever-increasing anxiety-fear provoking situations.

Included in our program for children with hypertensive voice problems with or without pathology is a program of assertive training. According to Phillips (modified by Phillips from Salter (1961)) assertiveness is expressiveness not aggression. It is teaching a child to stand up for his individual rights and it results in bringing about beneficial dividends in a situation for the child. The key to this behavior change is asserting without harming others and expressing feelings and opinions without smothering others. Most important, it should be remembered anxiety is incompatible with assertiveness. Phillips stated that the following types of children need assertive training: (1) the child who has difficulty with his peers, (2) the child who has difficulty with his social environment and who is a nonparticipant in class, (3) a child who is under social criticism, and (4) a child with undesirable aggressive behavior.

We have found that many children with hypertensive voice problems, especially vocal nodules, are those who have difficulty with their peers and difficulty in their social environment. As a result they are under social criticism and fight back with undesirable methods of aggressiveness including vocal abusive practices. The general training program for assertiveness is particularly helpful to these children.

The following assertive training program was suggested by Phillips: (1) Have the child say and write positive things about himself. (2) Have him accept compliments without downgrading himself. How often do we hear people react to the compliment "You are looking good today," by responding, "I don't think I look as good as usual." Rather the compliment should be accepted by replying, "Thank you very much." (3) Teach the child to express his opinion adequately without harming others. (4) Have the child habitually use the word "I" at the beginning of sentences. (5) Allow the child to express his feelings openly but without aggression and without harming others. (6) Teach the child to disagree in an appropriate way when he feels disagreement is warranted.

Many principles and methods of reciprocal inhibition can be used by the speech pathologist in helping selected children who have voice problems.

SUMMARY

Some basic approaches to voice therapy have been presented. Voice therapy procedures are structured around a 10 step outline, an outline which is followed in modifying any aspect of vocal behavior. Listening training enables a child to recognize and discriminate various levels of good and poor voice use as a foundation for improving his own voice. Negative practice is used to bring undesirable vocal behavior to consciousness in order to eliminate the undesirable behavior. Careful charting of behavior is used to eliminate the undesirable and to promote desirable voice use. Teaching children innovative and interesting charting techniques many times results in more rapid voice improvement and helps the child assume responsibility for his own voice improvement. Special approaches to voice therapy include operant conditioning and client- and communication-centered therapy. It is essential to recognize the judicious use of psychotherapy for some children. Use of the principles and methods of reciprocal inhibition is especially effective for children when anxiety evoking situations cause vocal hyperfunction and vocal abuse.

EIGHT

Voice Therapy for Laryngeal Dysfunction: I

Vocal Abuse and Muscular Tonus

Specific voice therapy procedures are indicated for children with laryngeal dysfunction with or without laryngeal pathology. The goals of voice therapy for laryngeal dysfunction are (1) eliminating or modifying vocal abuse; (2) balanced muscular tonus; (3) appropriate loudness; (4) desirable use of pitch; (5) controlled rate of speaking; (6) production of a clear voice.

These goals are adapted to each child with laryngeal dysfunction. Some children with this problem may require all six goals in a therapy program while other children may need only a few of these goals to attain improved voices. The goals constitute an overall program and are not necessarily listed in order of approach. They are the goals of the voice therapy program only and do not include the work of other team members. The basic listening training program described in Chapter 7 is essential to nearly all these goals. In this chapter we will discuss the first two goals, eliminating or modifying vocal abuse and balanced muscular tonus. The other goals will be presented in the following chapter.

VOCAL ABUSE

Vocal abuse must be eliminated or modified to such an extent that it is no longer considered an actual abuse (Wilson, 1961; 1962b; 1962c). It is important to reduce abuse for three reasons, (1) the vocal abuse may be unpleasant and distracting to listeners, (2) modifying or eliminating vocal abuse in the absence of laryngeal pathology is a preventive measure to avoid the possibility of the later development of laryngeal pathology, and most important (3) modifying or eliminating vocal abuse often results in the reduction or elimination of a laryngeal pathology. Aron-son (1973, p. 19) stated that when vocal nodules are small to moderate in size, voice therapy designed to eliminate mechanical abuse to the vocal cords often results in remission or dissolution of the nodules. Modifying or eliminating vocal abuse assumes primacy in the program for children who have laryngeal pathology. When hoarseness is attributed to excessive and improper use of the voice, improvement in voice is in direct proportion to the success in correcting vocal abuse (Orton, 1951).

Rules of Voice Hygiene

Observance of the rules of voice hygiene is basic to vocal rehabilitation. A set of rules should be given to each child according to his particular vocal abuses. All possible vocal abuses were explored during the examination and evaluative procedures by obtaining information about the child's vocal behavior in school and home situations, including sports and outdoor activities. The speech pathologist has this record in the form of rating scales showing how frequently each vocal abuse occurs and how vigorously it is used. Using this record the speech pathologist should select from the list in Figure 29 the rules that apply to a particular child. During the first therapy session these rules are written in a child's notebook in terms he can understand and they can often be illustrated with pictures appropriate for his age. The speech pathologist should explain each item in detail. Some rules must be given simply as orders to follow, for example not talking in noisy places. Cooper (1973, pp. 154–155) stated voice hygiene may involve restricting a child's activities. He advised parents must intervene and remove the child from situations involving vocal abuse. Also, Cooper suggested termi-

1. Avoid shouting, screaming, cheering, and excessive loud laughing.
2. Cough, clear your throat, or sneeze only when you must, and then do it gently and easily.
3. Do not make strange noises with your voice, like using reverse phonation, abrupt glottal attack, or strained vocalizations.
4. Avoid talking in noisy places—around machinery, power lawnmowers, farm equipment, when listening to loud music, or using a hairdryer.
5. Avoid talking while using noisy transportation such as buses, trains, subways, and riding in autos at high speed. Also no talking when riding in snowmobiles, dunebuggies, swampbuggies, motorcycles, motorbikes, and motorboats.
6. Avoid talking when you have an upper respiratory infection such as a cold.
7. You may be requested not to sing, act in plays, or give speeches or oral reports.
8. Talk when you wish but not too much. You may be asked to limit the amount of talking you do.
9. Talk with adequate loudness, at the best vocal pitch for you, and with a good rate.
10. Talk easily, initiate vocal tones smoothly and effortlessly. Hold your head straight when you talk. Do not strain the muscles of the face, throat, neck, and shoulders as you talk.
11. It may be recommended that, if possible, your house have filtered heating and air conditioning, and proper humidity. Avoid breathing through your mouth in very cold weather.
12. Keep in good health. Exercise regularly, but not too vigorously or noisily. Do not smoke. Stay away from smoky or dusty places. See your physician regularly for general check-ups. If you are on regular medications, check to be sure they have no adverse effects on the throat, mouth, and nose.
13. You may be requested to avoid highly spiced foods and to substitute skim milk and ice milk for whole milk and ice cream.
14. Sit in the center of a room so you can be heard easily without talking loudly, and then speak only when others in the room are quiet.
15. Wear seat belts and shoulder straps when riding in autos.

Fig. 29. Rules for voice hygiene. Based on Anderson and Newby (1973, pp. 280–284); Bryce (1974, p. 74); Cooper (1973, p. 128); Fox and Blechman (1975, pp. 61–63); Punt (1974); Wilson (1961; 1962b; 1962c; 1966; 1977, p. 262).

nating choral singing because a child may be singing at traumatic pitch levels or singing too loudly. Other rules will necessitate an organized program for eventual modification or elimination, for example excessive throat clearing. In some instances substitute behavior or activity will be incorporated into the therapy program, such as whistling instead of cheering at a sports event.

Reduce Talking

We recommend reduction in the amount of talking during the first 10 days of a voice therapy program when the voice rating is 6 or 7 for vocal abuse and 6 or 7 for laryngeal tone. This makes a child more aware of how his voice sounds and often reduces inflammatory conditions of the vocal cords. Wilson and Rice (1977, p. 22) suggested if it is possible total voice rest for 4 days to a maximum of 1 week is extremely helpful because a short period of voice rest can produce remarkable changes in vocal characteristics and demonstrates to a child and his parents the effects

of excessive voice use. When total voice rest is not possible or desirable, Wilson and Rice (1977, p. 22) stated the child can communicate with his parents using a very soft whisper without great harm, but any forced "stage voice" whisper should be avoided.

Wilson and Rice (1977, p. 22) gave the following guide lines for helping a child reduce talking time: It is desirable to have a 50% to 75% reduction of vocalization time during a period of 10 days or so. The child must be told he is responsible for changing vocal behavior and his first obligation is to reduce the amount of talking. Specific directions should be given the child: He is told he can talk quietly in the morning before going to school and he should answer questions in school. There should be no talking during recess, lunch, and gym. When he gets home from school he can talk in a very soft voice to his parents for a few minutes, but there should be no more talking until suppertime. During the evening a restricted amount of talking is permitted. Having the child chart his successes with appropriate rewards is useful. Comparison of audiorecordings before and after decreased voice use should show dramatic changes. If not, the continuation of restricted voice use is not indicated.

We recognize that it is most difficult for children to follow an extended program of "Don't do it!" even though they may be able to follow a short-term program of restricted talking. For example, a short period, 4 to 6 weeks, of easy talking with no vocal abuses often results in a dramatic reduction or elimination of vocal nodules. However, resumption of abusive practices may result in a return of the pathology. *Permanent* and *satisfactory* vocal replacements must be structured if a child is to remain free from vocal pathology.

Control of Environment and Activities

One of our goals in controlling vocal abuse is to control the child's activities and environment so the situations are not conducive to vocal abuse. We try to avoid permanently eliminating specific activities in a child's life because they provoke vocal abuse. Rather we prefer to control situations by changing them in some way, giving the child a different role that is more conducive to control of undesirable vocal behavior. Perkins (1971, p. 524) emphasized the importance of determining situational and emotional stress and its effect on vocal production in children before undertaking an organized therapy program. Attention should be directed to circumstances that elicit abusive vocal patterns. Perkins stated attention to the conditions and situations where a child talks should assume primacy rather than centering attention on a child's performance once he is in those conditions. Perkins stated control of situations is especially critical if the child is in poor health, such as having an upper respiratory infection which would make him more vulnerable to tissue damage of the vocal cords. Wilson and Rice (1977, p. 27) also suggested manipulating a child's environment so the need for vocal abuse is decreased. This would include discussing with the child his use of hostile abusive voice when with friends and his brothers and sisters. The speech pathologist should spend considerable time listing each activity classified as vocally abusive and discussing with the child how he can control his vocal abuse while he is in these situations, or how he can use substitute activities. Anderson

and Newby (1973, p. 280) suggested situational control can be obtained by encouraging a child to spend at least a portion of his leisure time in more quiet activities, such as model building, reading, playing quiet non-talking games, listening to recorded music (when not talking or singing), and watching television.

It may be necessary to enlist the cooperation of the child's family to improve his voice environment at home. Bryce (1974, p. 74) discussed ways the family may need to change their vocal behavior at home. He stated parents must assume responsibility for changing undesirable vocal practices of all family members to assure a good voice environment for the child with vocal nodules. Examples he noted that should be changed at home include loud talking to overcome the high output of television and radio, and shouting from one room to another or from one floor to another.

The 10 Step Outline for Vocal Abuse

The following procedure is used for eliminating vocal abuses. It is based on listening training and follows the 10 steps of the voice therapy outline. For each of the child's vocal abuses a chart is placed in his notebook, for example, a chart on shouting is shown in Figure 30. The chart reflects the basic approach for eliminating a vocal abuse. It can be appropriately titled for use with any type of vocal abuse. Progress is noted with each step rewarded as the child moves from Step 1 to Step 10. For young children small picture stickers can be placed after each item as he progresses from one step to another. For older children a written "O.K." is an appropriate reward.

Step 1. I know the rule about my voice. A rule is devised about the vocal abuse. This is done by explaining what the vocal abuse is and why it must be eliminated. The rule almost always is "Don't use the vocal abuse." The vocal abuses are demonstrated by the speech pathologist to show the child the characteristics of each abuse and to stress the importance of their removal. The specific vocal abuse to be approached first should be practiced by the child and the speech pathologist so that the child has a vivid picture of the abuse (Wilson and Rice, 1977, p. 22). Initially it is useful to select a vocal abuse that stands out above the others and also is one where change can be rapidly effected.

1. I KNOW THE RULE ABOUT NOT SHOUTING.   _____
2. I CAN TELL WHEN OTHER PEOPLE SHOUT.   _____
3. I CAN TELL WHEN OTHER PEOPLE ARE NOT SHOUTING.   _____
4. I KNOW HOW MY VOICE *SOUNDS* AND *FEELS* WHEN I SHOUT.   _____
5. I KNOW HOW MY VOICE *SOUNDS* AND *FEELS* WHEN I DON'T SHOUT.   _____
6. I KNOW THE PLACES WHERE I USUALLY SHOUT.   _____
7. I KNOW THE PLACES WHERE I DON'T SHOUT.   _____
8. I CAN KEEP FROM SHOUTING *SOME* OF THE TIME.   _____
9. I CAN KEEP FROM SHOUTING *MOST* OF THE TIME.   _____
10. I DON'T SHOUT ANY MORE.   _____

Fig. 30. Shouting.

Johnson (1976, p. 3) stated it is important to pinpoint the specific abuse behavior which occurs most frequently in a child. The behavior must be observable and countable. Phillips and Mordock (1974, pp. 351–352) in discussing behavior therapy with children stated, "It is usually desirable to focus first on a behavior most readily accessible to change because successful rapid diminution of one obtrusive behavior is extremely reinforcing to both parents and the therapist, and serves to increase their motivation to handle other behaviors." Shouting and screaming are examples that fit these criteria.

The child must be informed that many of his vocal abuses are harmful to him even though other children may not suffer disastrous results from such practices. It is advisable to help the child understand his problem by giving him the basic facts about his voice disorder and explaining the rationale for eliminating the vocal abuse (Wilson, 1961). When appropriate the child is given an acceptable substitute activity.

Step 2. I can tell when other people use their voices incorrectly. The speech pathologist and the child listen to specific vocal abuses in others. This can be done through listening to recordings, or the child and the speech pathologist can go to a playground or gym to observe and tabulate vocal abuse in others (Wilson, 1977, p. 265).

Step 3. I can tell when other people use their voices correctly. Tabulations are made in several situations where vocal abuses are not heard. Typical places to visit are libraries, museums, and art galleries.

Step 4. I can tell when I use my voice incorrectly. Shouting can be used as an example (Wilson, 1977, p. 265). The child is taught to recognize his own undue shouting through learning the auditory and kinesthetic aspects of shouting. First, for listening training, the speech pathologist makes tape recordings as the child engages in shouting activities. These recordings are then played for the identification of the auditory aspects of shouting. Second, the kinesthetic aspects of shouting are combined with the auditory. Here the speech pathologist asks the child to talk and read at various levels of loudness including shouting. The speech pathologist selects five different sentences of about 10 words each. Five levels of loudness are used: soft, normal, raised, very loud, and shouting. Each sentence is labelled in this order and the child is instructed to read or repeat them at these levels. A sound level meter is used to help the child monitor the five levels. With the child 25 to 30 in from a sound level meter, the five levels are approximately 60, 70, 80, 90, and 100 dB. When the child reaches a shout he is asked to describe the auditory feedback and the kinesthetic sensations felt especially in the throat and neck. A page in his notebook can be titled "Do you do these things?" Pictures of his various vocal abuses can be placed on this page. For example a page may contain pictures of people shouting, screaming, cheering, and using other vocal abuses (Fig. 31). The speech pathologist can sometimes bring these types of vocal abuse to the child's consciousness merely by describing them and pointing them out as they occur; other times a tape recording helps him identify his undesirable vocal behavior (Wilson, 1961). Many times a throat microphone is useful in identifying undesirable auditory aspects of laryngeal habits. The microphone is attached to an amplifier and the child listens to his voice through earphones. This method can be used to identify and then modify or eliminate glottal fry, abrupt glottal attacks, excessive breathiness, pitch breaks (Anonymous, 1966), coughing, and throat clearing. A stethoscope is also useful here.

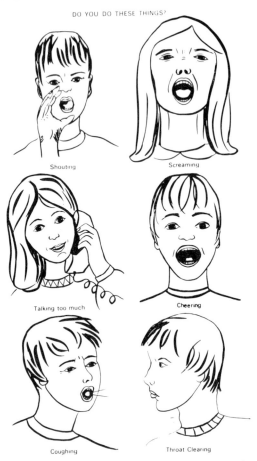

Fig. 31. Typical vocal abuses. Illustration by Geraldine Balsam.

The more flagrant types of vocal abuse are relatively easy to bring to the child's attention but this may be difficult to do with certain types of abuse used involuntarily. For example the child may automatically use abrupt tone initiations as he shows enthusiasm while playing cards. Also when playing with cars, airplanes, and other toys he may automatically and unconsciously imitate the sound of the car or jet plane by producing strained vocalizations. No doubt in the process of teaching the child to identify vocal abuses in others and in himself he began to learn the auditory aspects of abuses. Now for example he more specifically analyzes the piercing quality of his scream and the accompanying muscular tensions in his neck, throat, and shoulders.

Accurate tallying is required for eliminating vocal abuse. Johnson (1976, p. 3) stated self monitoring by using a counter to tally vocal abuse brings behavior to a conscious level and provides countable data to tally daily. Landes (1977, p. 129) suggested having a child tally for a week the number of times he engages in a specific abuse, probably best paying attention to only one abuse at a time. Initially no effort is made to curtail these activities but merely to tabulate their occurrence. Johnson (1976, p. 5) suggested that initially the child count during only one short period of time and then add high probability times such as recess and lunch. This procedure is continued until all high probability situations are included. Johnson (1976, p. 5) stated a careful analysis of the child's daily vocal behavior is necessary to determine high probability time periods when vocal abuses occur most frequently.

Johnson (1976, p. 6) suggested daily phone calls by the speech pathologist to the child should be carefully programmed into the initial therapy sequence. They provide reminder stimuli to the child and underline the interest of the speech pathologist in the child's progress. If a child knows he will receive a phone call at a specified time each evening, he will be prompted to remember to tally his behavior and be ready to report. As the program progresses and the child is satisfactorily collecting his data the calls may be faded (Johnson, 1976, p. 6).

The Vocal Intensity Controller (VIC)* is suggested as a useful way of controlling vocal abuse. Described by Holbrook, Rolnick, and Bailey (1974) and Holbrook (1977, pp. 65–72), it is designed for use in a treatment program to control vocal abuse. This device (4½ × 2½ × 1 in) is worn in daily speaking situations to provide auditory feedback and it can be set according to vocal intensity. A microphone is attached directly to the skin in front of the trachea by means of a stick-on electrodisc. A signal is sent to an earphone providing auditory feedback to the individual. The sensitivity of the instrument can be regulated so that a loud voice activates the feedback tone and warns the individual of potential vocal abuse. Also, the microphone can be taped to the side of the nose to detect hypernasality. Holbrook et al. (1974) described a program with 32 persons using the VIC to decrease vocal abuse and voice intensity. Eleven of the 32 experienced complete resolution of their identified vocal nodules, polyps, or contact ulcers with no need for

* Behavioral Controls, Inc., P. O. Box 480, Milwaukee, WI 53201.

surgical intervention. In eight others there was a reduction in the size and extent of the lesions making surgical intervention unnecessary.

Step 5. I can tell when I use my voice correctly. The child is taught the auditory and kinesthetic sensations of talking at a normal loudness level. These are compared to the sensations noted during soft talking and shouting. A sound level meter is also useful here in demonstrating loudness levels and the accompanying auditory and kinesthetic features.

Step 6. I know the places where I use my voice incorrectly. The speech pathologist and the child discuss and identify the places or situations where the vocal abuse is used. This is a particularly important step if his vocal abuse occurs only under certain circumstances, for example at an athletic event, on the playground, or while playing with certain toys. Recognition of the connection between abusive vocal practices and certain activities can be a big step toward eliminating the abuse.

Step 7. I know the places where I use my voice correctly. At this point the child lists situations where specific vocal abuses do not occur. Shouting, for example, does not occur in the child's classroom, the library, church, school, or while he watches television. Later his list can be expanded to include situations where the child might have shouted but did not.

Steps 8, 9, and 10. Carryover. A program of carryover is planned with the child. One or two situations where he shouts excessively are selected as situations in which shouting is to be avoided. When the child reports success with this amount of elimination more situations are added. The goal at this point is to reduce systematically the occurrence of a vocal abuse and then proceed to eliminate it completely. For example, Landes (1977, p. 129) suggested after tabulating occurrence of a specific vocal abuse during a typical week the child may be instructed to control the vocal abuse by allowing its occurrence only seven times a day, tabulating them on a chart. Then the next week or two the number of allowed occurrences is reduced. As the child succeeds with this amount of control the abuse is further reduced until it is no longer present.

A reward system, especially for children, is many times a motivational factor. Johnson

(1976, p. 6) suggested small weekly reinforcements should be given for bringing in voice data consistently. Activity pictures can be placed on a page in the notebook to reward the child as he begins to gain control of the vocal abuses. For example, if he or the parents report they have been on a picnic and certain vocal abuses were not used, a picture of a family on a picnic titled "I can have fun with my family and not shout or scream" is appropriate. Older children and teenagers, when pictures are not appropriate, can use their notebooks for reporting success in eliminating or modifying vocal abuse. An exact report is required. It is not satisfactory for the child to report, "I guess most of the time I'm not shouting any more." The report should be, "Here is a list of three situations where I shouted and here is a list of ten situations where I might have shouted but did not" (Wilson, 1977, p. 267). Johnson (1976, p. 7) recommended that a substantial final reinforcement be planned early in the program. Johnson emphasized that the final reinforcer is given only when the laryngeal pathology is no longer present. Final reinforcements suggested by Johnson range from model airplanes or games to bicycles.† Additional techniques for carryover are found in Chapter 12.

Each vocal abuse is approached until all have been completely eliminated or so modified and controlled they are no longer traumatizing. With many children progress in the vocal abuse therapy program results in definite reduction or elimination of pathology and return of normal voice.

The general plan outlined above can be adapted to handle the different vocal abuses, shouting, screaming, cheering, excessive talking, strained vocalizations, reverse phonation, explosive vocalizations, abrupt glottal attack, throat clearing, coughing, and talking in noise. Additional techniques for the more common vocal abuses follow.

Throat Clearing and Coughing

Throat clearing and coughing are vocal abuses which must be modified because they cannot be eliminated (Wilson, 1977, p. 266). Training to modify these habits follows the voice therapy outline. After the child has been guided through the first four steps of the

† A 75 min audiocassette and instructional text *Vocal Nodule Reduction Program* by T. Johnson is available from Ideas, P. O. Box 741, Tempe, AZ 85281.

outline, he is ready to learn a modified manner of throat clearing and coughing. He is instructed to clear his throat or to cough in an easy, effortless manner with a breathy initiation. A method of silent coughing and throat clearing was described by Zwitman and Calcaterra (1973), "When the patient has the urge to cough or clear his throat, he is instructed to 'push' air from the lungs in blasts, being careful not to produce sound ... The 'silent cough' appears to reduce the vocal cord tension experienced during the regular cough, to eliminate the duration of the throat-clearing activity, and to lessen the degree of tension."

Cheering

The child or youth should be taught to attain loudness without strain. Cheering by teenagers at sports events is especially difficult to curb. Uris (1962) presented a program to teach the teenager to cheer, taking the major muscular strain off the vocal cords and transferring it to the abdominal muscles which can stand strain. Uris suggested the following exercises to be used with groups of teenagers.

1. Breathe in rhythm and on inhalation take a deep breath. The low abdominal wall, not the chest, should expand on inhalation and then contract on exhalation. The group breathes in unison and upon signal says /hɑ/ several times.

2. Cheer with syllables beginning with /h/: /haɪ/, /ho/, /hi/; /haɪ/, /ho/, /hi/.

3. The /h/ is dropped and the group chants vowels without the /h/, attempting to retain the same release feeling as with the /h/.

4. Each teenager places his hands on his abdomen, takes in an easy deep breath, and then cheers /rɑ/, /rɑ/, /rɑ/. With each /rɑ/ the abdominal wall contracts and then relaxes. "Without any forcing from the throat, the cheer grows more and more vigorous and with enough volume to please the most rabid fan."

Strained Vocalizations

The elimination of the child's use of strained vocalizations to imitate the sounds of cars or planes may require special techniques. Turn on the tape recorder and play a racing car game with the child with car noises represented by strained vocalizations by both child and speech pathologist. Play the recording, teach the identifying features of the abuse, and then have the child tally his own and the speech pathologist's strained vocalizations. Go through the same procedure again but this time substitute the strained vocalizations with easy vocalizations, or a nonvocal substitute. The 10 steps on the chart can be followed to eliminate this abusive practice and achieve carryover of substitute activities.

Explosive Vocalizations and Abrupt Glottal Attack

Special attention must be paid to eliminating explosive vocalizations and abrupt glottal attacks. A soft normal attack should be taught. It should be emphasized that in the soft normal attack the vocal cords gradually begin to vibrate without any breathy sound or without the clicking noise of a sudden release. Clarity of tone depends upon the synchronous action of the expiratory and laryngeal muscles; this synchronous action results in a normal soft attack (Fomon et al. 1966). In the normal soft attack between 30 and 100 cc of air are expelled before the actual start of phonation (Isshiki and von Leden, 1964). Werner-Kukuk and von Leden (1970) observed regular vibratory movements of the vocal cords along their entire length during soft vocal initiation. The frequency of these vibrations was quite stable and the amplitude increased gradually during the first eight cycles of vibration. Measurements made on the anterior, median, and posterior portions of the cords showed closure to be complete at all three measured points. The period of total approximation of the cords was equal for the anterior and posterior parts during each vibratory cycle. At the midpoint the approximation period was somewhat prolonged initially. The amplitude of the excursion of the cords was widest at the posterior portion and narrowest at the anterior portion. The maximum opening was reached quickly, being observed first at the median portion of the cords, and then at the posterior third, and last at the anterior third of the vocal cords.

Leeper (1976) studied vocal initiation characteristics of eight children with bilateral vocal nodules compared with the vocal initiation of eight children with normal voices. The mean age of the children was 9 years 5 months with a range of 7 to 14 years. Each child was taught to produce three types of vocal initiation—hard, soft, and breathy— while saying /p$_a$/, /b$_a$/, and /h$_a$/. Airflow and acoustical analyses indicated children with vocal nodules had more air wastage and unstable phonation than children without nodules during the three types of attack. Leeper concluded that breaking the "vicious cycle of vocal abuse" in vocal nodule children should be a voice therapy goal, with specific attention paid to modifying the hard initiation to a soft vocal initiation. This also requires the child to reduce vocal intensity.

Teaching easy breathing for speech (pp. 126–127) is particularly recommended when abnormal vocal attacks are found in a person who has vocal nodules (Berry and Eisenson, 1956, p. 213; Rubin, 1964; Van Riper and Irwin, 1958, p. 192). Brodnitz (1966) suggested breathing exercises when there is definite need to reduce the pressure of the breath against the vocal cords to teach adequate release of air during phonation. Wilson and Rice (1977, p. 26) suggested using breathiness as a means of reducing hard vocal attack. This can be demonstrated to a child by recording his voice after he has engaged in some sort of rigorous physical activity such as running up steps. The child's own breathy voice provides a model for him to follow. The child is told to use a breathy voice only in specified outside situations and at home. Wilson and Rice (1977, p. 28) also suggested teaching the child the concept of light contact of the vocal cords to establish easy vocal initiation.

Listening training is useful in teaching a child correct vocal attack to replace explosive or abrupt glottal attacks. The speech pathologist demonstrates abrupt and easy attacks for the child discussing the characteristics of each. The child identifies these attacks as they appear in the speech pathologist's demonstration. The child then is taught to use relaxed phonation (Moore, 1971a, p. 562). This can be done by using the three steps of teaching correct vocal practice. The first two steps, awareness and gross discrimination in his own voice, can be handled according to instructions in Chapter 7. The third step, fine discrimination of differences in his own voice, may require special handling for this type of problem. In learning a normal vocal attack have the child produce a breathy attack. This can be incorporated into the fine discrimina-

tion practice. The three productions for fine discrimination, then, are abrupt glottal attack (or explosive release), the desired normal attack, and breathy attack. In this way the child learns to identify and eliminate both forms of extreme attack and adopts the normal attack.

Laryngeal tension during abrupt glottal attacks should receive special attention. Have the child place the tip of his finger on the triangle of the thyroid cartilage as he uses an abrupt attack. The tension will be reflected in the elevation of the larynx. The child can then be shown that vocalizing in a relaxed easy manner results in little or no elevation of the larynx (West and Ansberry, 1968, p. 218). Brodnitz (1971a, p. 99) recommended the chewing method for reduction of abrupt glottal attack. This method will be described in connection with achieving balanced muscular tonus later in this chapter.

Negative-positive practice helps teach the child to modify his abrupt attacks to softer, easier initiations. A useful technique for this is the "clothespin-feather" game, using negative-positive practice techniques. A child emits an abrupt tone as he vigorously throws a clothespin into a large metal container. The clatter of the clothespin as it hits the bottom of the container is associated with his abrupt attacks. Then the child is asked to modify his abrupt attacks to easy initiations. Prolonging continuant consonants (Canfield, 1964) or beginning with an /h/ or breathy attack (Moore, 1971a, p. 563; Peacher, 1952, p. 11) helps prevent an abrupt attack. This time he drops a feather into the container as he uses an easy attack. The slow movement of the feather and its easy landing in the container are likened to the new easy tone initiation. Listening to tape recordings of this activity is useful in establishing the identification of easy tone initiation.

The child's notebook can be used as a visual aid in working on tone initiation. A page titled "Easy Voice" may contain three pictures of waves hitting a shore representing "easy," "hard," and "very hard" tone initiation. The size of the waves represents the three types of tone initiation. The child names each picture using the three types of initiation. Phrases and sentences for each picture can also be used. Prolonging initial sounds aids in developing a smoother less interrupted flow of tone.

We have used exercises similar to those

listed by Rubin and Lehrhoff (1962) to teach children correct attack on sounds. These can be copied and placed in their notebooks.

1. Make believe you are yawning and breathe out easily as you say the vowels /ɑ/, /o/, and /u/. Then say them easily without a yawn. Breathe in deeply and sigh as you let the air out and say a vowel sound as you gradually lower the pitch.

2. Remember to talk quietly with a good voice. Also talk clearly. Read a story or a poem in a quiet voice.

3. Whisper the vowels /ɑ/, /æ/, /i/, and /o/. As you do each one change the whisper to a good tone.

4. Say vowel sounds with an /h/ in front of each one. Be sure to say them easily with good tones. Get a list of words beginning with /h/ from your dictionary. Practice saying them easily. Then omit the /h/ in all words that still make a real word, such as hat/at or hold/old. Practice the new words easily with good tones.

Anderson (1977, pp. 117–120) presented exercises to establish quiet, effortless initiation of tone which are easily adapted to children. A person should produce voice easily, avoiding the use of muscles hindering optimal production. These exercises can be used not only for teaching easy initiation of tone but for eliminating excessive breathiness and introducing full resonant tones of good quality at the correct pitch and loudness.

1. Have the child yawn to relax and open the throat. Let him feel the air on the walls of the throat and become conscious of the rise of the soft palate by looking in a mirror.

2. Have the child take an easy breath, using abdominal breathing. Have him open the throat and quietly and carefully say *one,* then have him relax, take in another breath and say *two,* and then relax. Have him count to five at the rate of one count every 3 or 4 sec. Have him repeat the count with an upward pitch inflection on each number.

3. Have the child take an easy breath with open relaxed throat quietly whispering *no.* Then have him relax, take in a new breath and quietly vocalize the *no* without changing his mouth opening or his throat relaxation. Do the same thing on other words, such as see, boy, dog, girl, and rabbit.

4. Applying the same technique have the child read the following selection, pausing for a new breath indicated by the dashes.

Mike and Laura liked the snow.—They made snowmen—built forts—and had snowball battles.—They always hoped for snow—so they could stay home from school—and play outside.—Last year it snowed and snowed.

5. Starting from the yawn position have the child very lightly repeat *ho-ho-ho* holding each vowel 2 or 3 sec. Pay careful attention to the way the child initiates the tone. The child should avoid breathiness and harshness emphasizing easy tone initiation. Use this exercise with other vowels, such as /hu/ and /hɑ/.

6. Have the child begin /hu/ holding it for 2 or 3 sec and then very carefully and gradually merge into /o/, and /ɑ/ with continuous phonation, keeping the throat open as before, maintaining a constant pitch. This is done all on one breath at one pitch with a steady flow of tone so it will sound like /hu-u-u-o-o-o-ɑ-ɑ-ɑ/.

7. Next have the child sing /hu-ɑ/, merging the two vowels together. Do the same using /ho-ɑ/ and other vowels. Continue these drills until the vowels become clear and are easily initiated.

8. Now have the child practice initiating the vowel /ɑ/ several times, hitting it very lightly and easily, avoiding breathiness and abrupt attack.

9. Tell the child to take a comfortable breath and with open throat whisper the vowel /ɑ/ so quietly only he himself can hear it. Then after 2 or 3 sec have him very gradually begin to vocalize the /ɑ/ without disturbing the relaxed open condition of the throat. The vowel should be continued until it builds up to a full resonant tone with proper loudness.

10. Have the child count from one to six saying each number at 2 sec intervals. Have him begin very softly and gradually increase loudness with each count until he is speaking quite loudly when he reaches six. Do not allow him to raise the pitch level of his voice as loudness is increased, and check to make sure the muscles of the throat are not tensed. The voice quality throughout should remain full and resonant and not become tight and pinched.

Mueller (1972) suggested teaching easy tone initiation by having the child practice sustained breathy phonation of the vowels /ɑ/, /i/, and /u/ for two or three 5 min periods daily. Each vowel should be preceded by the sound /h/ or a sigh. Phonation should be synchronized with the onset of exhalation. Since there is considerable air escape during this type of phonation, the child will not be able to sustain the vowels for very long if he is doing the exercise correctly. Emphasis should be placed on giving the child the kinesthetic and auditory sensations of relaxed and effortless phonation. Next the child is asked to read with a breathy voice, avoiding strain and improper respiratory patterns. The vowel exercises and the breathy reading should be practiced about 5 min twice daily. Then easy tone initiation with a breathy voice is done in conversational speech, gradually resuming full phonation without breathiness, but always avoiding the abrupt attack.

Substitutions for Vocal Abuse

It is often necessary to help children find a substitute for vocal abuses or misuses which may be contributing factors in their vocal pathology. A notebook is useful here. A picture representing one type of vocal abuse can be put into the notebook and labelled. On the same page another picture is placed which shows an acceptable substitute to use in this situation. For example, a picture of a boy shouting "hello" to a friend from across the street illustrates an undesirable practice and a picture of a boy waving "hello" to his friend across the street illustrates the desired way (Wilson, 1961). Another page in his notebook can be titled "I don't have to shout to call my pets." A picture of a cat can carry the caption "I can click my tongue to call my cat" and a picture of a dog can have the caption "I can whistle to call my dog" (Fig. 32). Another page in the notebook can have a picture of a child with his mouth open (with NO written under it) and a child pursing his lips as if they were vibrating (with a YES written under this picture). The page can have pictures of cars, planes, boats, trains, and trucks with the couplet "I don't have to make sounds with my voice when I play with my toys, I can blow air through my lips and still make a lot of noise" (Fig. 33).

These pictures are used throughout the therapy program as an aid in listening training and in giving outside assignments for carryover. Other types of substitutes for voice activities should also be encouraged, blowing horns or whistles, clapping hands, and any other noises which do not require the use of the larynx. We have found a structured program of substituting vocally nonabusive ac-

tivities for abusive activities quite easy for children to use when motivation is high and rewards plentiful. Cooper (1973, p. 154) suggested role playing in which the child becomes voice conscious and assumes different voices as he tells stories or acts out plays. This can be useful in controlling vocal abuse.

Mime

Mime (pantomine) also can be used as a nonvocal substitute for some of the vocal abuses. Kipnis (1974, p. 15) stated that entering the world of mime requires a person to forget the talking world. Mime has considerable appeal to children; many of them have had experience at school participating in mime skits (Walker, 1969, p. 36). Children will readily recognize conventional mime gestures as part of their play and everyday living activities and as something they have often seen on television.

A look at conventional mime procedures will help the speech pathologist apply principles of mime to the clinic situation. Mime

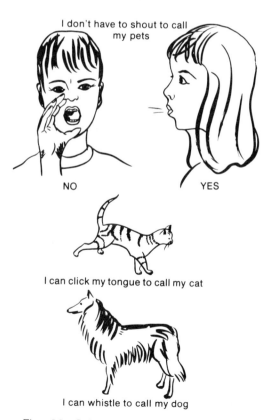

Fig. 32. Substituting nonlaryngeal sounds for vocal abuse. Illustration by Geraldine Balsam.

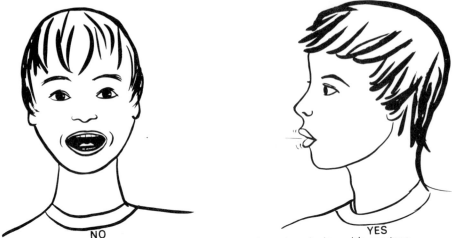

NO   YES

I don't have to make sounds with my voice when I play with my toys.
I can blow air through my lips and still make a lot of noise.

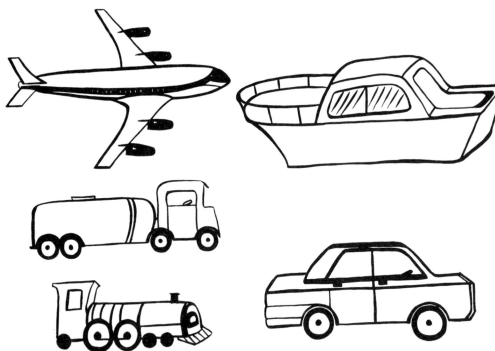

Fig. 33. Substituting nonvoiced for voiced sounds. Illustration by Geraldine Balsam.

communication techniques include facial expression, gestures, and body activities and postures, but no words and as few properties as possible. The mime uses his body and his skill to convey ideas and emotions to the audience (Hunt and Hunt, 1964, p. 10). There are four categories of mime (Walker, 1969, p. 161): (1) straight mimicry of action, (2) the use of specific gestures from a gesture vocabulary, (3) mimicry of action with objective reaction and thoughts added, and (4) expression of personal feelings and emotions. The first two will be most directly useful to the speech pathologist, though there are situations in which it is helpful to encourage expression of reactions and emotions. There are standard pantomimic gestures, many of which we use every day, such as placing the finger on the lips for quiet, or resting the forehead on the hand to express unhappiness (Hunt and Hunt, 1964, p. 102). Lawson (1957, pp. 83–114) presented a vocabulary of mimic gestures. Examining a few of these vocabulary items will give the pattern of how mime gestures can be developed. *To beckon*: Raise one arm. Fold all fingers except the index finger into the palm of the hand with the index finger upright. Make two circles inward with the index finger raised and toward yourself, and then move your arm through an arc towards yourself. *Listen*: Raise one arm with the palm facing the other person. Bend the forearm until the hand is cupped behind the ear.

Pantomime is regularly used in many situations as a substitute for unnecessary vocalization; for example, in outdoor sports where players are widely scattered and voice communication is impossible, pantomime activity is used to convey messages (Walker, 1969, p. 161). Walker also listed other situations where pantomime is useful: under water, in high level noise as in a factory, or in places where speech would be disturbing to others such as a concert, lecture, or study hall. Hunt and Hunt (1964, p. 9) gave the example of a traffic officer on a busy street holding up his hand to pantomime "Stop." The officer uses a pantomimic gesture because he could not be heard if he spoke. It is not even necessary for a driver to think of the word "stop" before applying his brakes.

In conventional mime the first step is to have a child analyze mime activities that are part of his everyday life (Walker, 1969, pp. 158–159); for example, how he mimes his likes and dislikes for food or uses mime to express his reluctance to follow orders. The second step is to have the child imagine he is in a foreign country and is unable to understand spoken language (Walker, 1969, p. 159). The child's task is to develop mime activities showing he is hungry, thirsty, sleepy, hot, or cold. Third, Hunt and Hunt (1964, pp. 101–102) suggested having the child pantomime pulling on a rope or digging with a shovel. Have him start by watching someone else perform the action and then he should do the actual digging or pulling. When he pantomimes he will need to exaggerate the motions a bit to insure accurate interpretation by others. He can try different degrees of effort, such as pulling on a rope easily, hard, and then very hard. Have him note differences in body positions which characterize the three degrees of effort. When he pulls easily his feet should be close together, as he increases his effort he should extend the leg

closer to the rope and he should bend his knee toward the direction he is pulling. Fourth, more involved situations are given the child to mime: "Imagine yourself... wading in a stream, coming in out of the snow, smelling fresh bread, tasting something bitter" (Walker, 1969, p. 123).

The speech pathologist need not go through all steps of pantomime training to use mime as a substitute for vocal abuse and misuse, but a discussion of pantomime activities in the child's everyday life is basic. Ask the child to describe nonvocal communication he has observed, and then give him an assignment to watch for pantomime situations and report them at the next session. Ask the child to suggest ways he can use pantomime as a substitute for his vocal abuse or misuse. He may be more comfortable using mime activities he has thought of, though the speech pathologist, of course, must be ready to guide him. A discussion of mime helps make each child critically aware of his own vocal abuses, and also helps him learn nonvocal activities which can be used as substitutes for undesirable vocal habits.

The speech pathologist should develop a list of typical mime gestures for use as substitutes for various vocal abuses and misuses. Figure 31 shows typical gestures or expressions for various vocal abuses. Substitutes are shown in Figures 32 and 33. Several useful mime gestures are the hand curved around the mouth to show shouting, the typical activity to show coughing, and the mime gestures for screaming and cheering. The listen gesture for louder voice can be used, or the arms may be positioned to indicate different pitch levels (Fig. 37). The child might point to his throat with an accompanying negative shake of the head to indicate he is not allowed to shout.

Mime requires very careful observation of others and their activities. A typical assignment for learning to mime shouting, for example, would be to have the child observe others in shouting situations. Then he can use this as a substitute for vocal shouting. Degrees of shouting can be paralleled to pulling on a rope or digging with a shovel easily, hard, and very hard.

Mime can work as a type of therapy for those who have psychological tensions or repressions by helping them move more easily, express feelings and emotions, and concentrate their attention on observing others (Walker, 1969, p. 36). This is especially true of the types of mime which convey reactions or thoughts and which express personal emotions and feelings. In these ways mime is especially useful in modifying behavior in children who are overaggressive, overtalkative, and vocally abusive, and whose voice problems appear to be related to these characteristics. For example, Balick, Spiegel, and Greene (1976) found training in mime decreased hyperactivity in a group of retarded children.

Mime can be used for nucleus situations during therapy and for carryover for children who need substitute activities for vocally abusive practices. It can also be used in programs to control pitch and loudness. Kipnis (1974) presented a definitive work on mime which is recommended for further study.

There are no suitable substitutes for some vocal abuses. Excessive talking, talking in noisy places, and screaming must be eliminated completely. Cheering must be avoided during the voice therapy period. Later, as we have seen, when children have been taught to use their vocal mechanisms easily and effortlessly, some are able to do moderate and limited cheering without trauma (Wilson, 1977, p. 265).

The following is an example of a child in whom reduction of excessive talking and eliminating other vocal abuses were the major goals of voice therapy (adapted from Wilson, 1962b):

> Terry's kindergarten teacher referred him to the speech clinic because he talked too fast and too loudly and had a hoarse voice. The medical report from the family physician described him as an essentially normal child in development and general physical condition. The child had always talked in a loud voice, and the parents had been unable to get him to talk with less intensity. They reported that he talked constantly at home and during play, although the mother denied excessive yelling or screaming. He occasionally became hoarse when he was fatigued, but never aphonic. Voice tests revealed a child with a hoarse, breathy voice with many pitch breaks and abrupt, hard initiation of tones. He talked loudly and excessively, using long sentences, and he was readily intelligible. Audiometric testing revealed normal hearing.

> The child was referred to a laryngologist for consultation because of the hoarseness. Examination of the vocal cords showed small vocal nodules at the junction of the anterior and middle thirds of each cord. It was felt that the nodules in all probability were due to improper use of the voice and also that the cords became more swollen as the day went on when he used his voice a great deal. The laryngologist noted that the child was very talkative and loud. He felt the nodules were too small for removal, and that voice training was indicated, especially if the child could be quieted down to a moderate degree. Psychological examinations revealed a child with adequate emotional maturity and with normal intelligence.

> During a period of 3 months the boy was seen for a series of 16 sessions with the speech pathologist. When voice therapy was initiated his voice was hoarse in a moderate degree rated 5 with much vocal abuse noted, such as excessive loud talking and forced high-pitched sounds made in play activities. The conversational voice was not abnormally high in pitch; therefore, voice therapy was designed only to reduce the amount of talking and to eliminate other vocal abuse. A laryngeal examination following voice therapy indicated the nodules were significantly reduced in size, and it was the impression that hoarseness had been practically eliminated. He was no longer abusing his vocal cords or talking as much. The laryngologist observed that the vocal cords did not seem to hit each other as abruptly and hard as they had prior to voice therapy. Subsequent voice evaluations over a period of a year following voice therapy revealed the voice to be clear and free from hoarseness.

MUSCULAR TONUS

Production of an adequate voice is based on a balance of muscular tonus. Balanced muscular tonus is present when proper tensions and timing in the musculature of the larynx and pharynx are present (Curtis, 1967, p. 218). Hyperfunction, which is overtense muscular tonus, and hypofunction, overly lax muscular tonus, are to be avoided. Most children with benign laryngeal pathology speak

1. I KNOW THE RULE ABOUT MUSCLE TENSION WHEN TALKING.   _____
2. I CAN TELL WHEN OTHER PEOPLE HAVE MUSCULAR IMBALANCE.   _____
3. I CAN TELL WHEN OTHER PEOPLE HAVE MUSCULAR BALANCE.   _____
4. I KNOW HOW MY VOICE *SOUNDS* AND *FEELS* WHEN I HAVE MUSCULAR IMBALANCE.   _____
5. I KNOW HOW MY VOICE *SOUNDS* AND *FEELS* WHEN I HAVE MUSCULAR BALANCE.   _____
6. I KNOW THE PLACES WHERE I HAVE MUSCULAR IMBALANCE.   _____
7. I KNOW THE PLACES WHERE I HAVE MUSCULAR BALANCE.   _____
8. I CAN TALK WITH MUSCULAR BALANCE *SOME* OF THE TIME.   _____
9. I CAN TALK WITH MUSCULAR BALANCE *MOST* OF THE TIME.   _____
10. I CAN TALK WITH MUSCULAR BALANCE *ALL* THE TIME.   _____

Fig. 34. Balanced muscular tonus.

in a hypertensive constricted manner characterized by tension in the lips, tongue, neck, throat, often in the shoulders, and sometimes in the whole body (Wilson, 1977, p. 269). It is necessary to modify or eliminate faulty vocal habits especially those producing excessive tensions (Murphy, 1964, p. 110). The 10 point therapy outline (Fig. 34) is followed in developing balanced muscular tonus.

For those with hyperfunctional and hypofunctional voice problems, Nichols (1977, p. 156) suggested the voice therapy goals should include control of muscular tonus and proper positioning of laryngeal, pharyngeal, and oral structures. Nichols added that the speech pathologist must teach modification of the force and duration of muscular contractions that underlie vocal functioning. We have found that the chewing method and progressive relaxation are useful in helping children reduce muscular tension, and that the pushing method is effective for increasing muscular tension. In cases of vocal nodules it is important to develop freedom from tension especially of chest, throat, and facial muscles. Freedom from tension in the extrinsic laryngeal and pharyngeal musculatures is a goal in therapy for harsh voices (Van Riper and Irwin, 1958, pp. 223–224). Boone (1973) stated the elimination of either excessive muscular force or inappropriate force in the wrong places will reduce hyperfunction and result in a better voice for a child. Hypofunction is the basis of nonorganic voice problems involving flaccid adjustments of the vocal mechanism. The voice typically sounds breathy and the voice therapy goal is to obtain firm closure of the vocal cords through increasing muscular tonus.

Our discussion of balanced muscular tonus is divided into two sections: (1) therapy for hyperfunction and (2) therapy for hypofunction. Normalizing muscular tonus helps to prevent vocal abuse and often results in adequate use of pitch (Brodnitz, 1966) and loudness without paying specific attention to pitch and loudness as such. Hyperfunction usually causes a higher pitch and hypofunction may cause an abnormally low pitch.

Hyperfunction

The correction of hyperfunction is one of the most important goals in vocal rehabilitation (Brodnitz, 1971a, p. 97). Perkins (1957, pp. 859–862) stated the person should be taught the kinesthetic sensations of an efficient voice and the feeling of getting the throat open and relaxed for efficient voice production: "The efficient voice . . . feels as cool and open and big as a sigh." In contrast he stated the inefficient voice is like an automobile being driven with the brakes on, with both the brakes and the motor straining during forward movement of the automobile. Instead, the person should feel as if his voice is coasting.

We feel it is important that the extrinsic muscles be kept as relaxed as possible and that the main work of the larynx should be done by the intrinsic muscles. Shipp (1975) found considerable variation in the amount of vertical laryngeal movement in six young adults as they phonated over a range of 2 octaves. In one subject the excursion of laryngeal movement was 6 mm and in another subject 14 mm before the mandible obscured the thyroid prominence. However, Shipp found the amount of upward laryngeal movement oftentimes was only 2 mm. Shipp and Izdebski (1975) reported that trained professional singers can produce their full frequency range with almost no vertical laryngeal movement. This means that apparently some professional singers use only intrinsic laryngeal adjustments to change pitch. However, subjects untrained in singing use a combination of both intrinsic and extrinsic muscle forces for pitch control. The untrained subjects tended to lower the larynx for low-pitched sounds and raise the larynx for high-pitched sounds (Shipp, 1975). Thus it appears that with the rise of the larynx there may be more extrinsic muscle activity accompanying the intrinsic muscle activity, producing increased hypertension or hyperfunction of the extrinsic laryngeal muscles. We think it would be best if individuals were taught to speak without any or with very little elevation of the larynx, especially during high pitches; this is the way trained speakers and singers use the larynx.

Procedures to Reduce Hyperfunction

The speech pathologist explains the need for avoiding muscular tension while speaking and demonstrates the difference between the child's hypertensive manner of speaking and the desired voice, which we often refer to as an *easy voice*. Achieving balanced muscular tonus is based on techniques to reduce generalized tension in the entire body and to reduce specific tension in the laryngeal area, neck, and shoulders. The basic procedures for reducing laryngeal hyperfunction are:

1. Posture instruction. Training in good posture is helpful in reducing hypertension of the extrinsic muscles of the larynx and pharynx of persons with vocal nodules (Van Riper and Irwin, 1958, p. 193).

2. Breathing exercises. Breathing exercises can sometimes be helpful in relieving tensions of muscles in throat and neck areas (Hauth, 1961).

3. Relaxation procedures. For problems of hoarse voice, relaxation to modify the upward displacement of the larynx is recommended (Van Riper and Irwin, 1958, p. 239). For problems of ventricular phonation of a non-organic nature the speech pathologist should obtain lowering of the larynx during phonation and relaxation of the suprahyoid muscles in order to get sustained tones without laryngeal tension (Van Riper and Irwin, 1958, p. 220). For young children rag doll games can be useful to teach the child the sensation of reduced tension while speaking. With older children and adolescents more formal relaxation procedures may be indicated.

4. Chewing exercises. Chewing exercises

are most useful in reducing hyperfunctional use of the vocal mechanism. They are an integral part of a program to improve voice through reducing hyperfunction.

Posture Instruction

The following suggestions for achieving proper posture are based on McClosky (1977, pp. 141–142):

1. Have the child stand erect and place one foot ahead and apart from the other, having him lightly curl his toes as if to grasp the floor.

2. Have the child place the small of the back against a wall with the feet several inches away from the baseboard. Have him slowly edge the heels up to the baseboard—but he must keep the small of the back against the wall. The posture is correct when the heels are against the baseboard and the small of the back is against the wall. Be sure the child keeps his knees relaxed.

3. Have the child sit in a straight chair with the front of his body facing the back of the chair. Have the child place his hands on the chair back and his toes on the floor on a line with the back of the chair. Have the child concentrate on his lower back, stretching the muscles upward. The results of this exercise are a stretching of the pelvic muscles and a feeling of expansion of the lower ribs. According to McClosky unconscious control of the breathing mechanism is a dividend of posture control.

Breathing Exercises

We currently are paying considerable attention to the breathing habits of children with voice problems. Often we find poorly coordinated breathing and speaking patterns even though silent breathing is normal. Many of these children, especially the ones with hypertensive voices with or without pathological changes, use upper chest (clavicular) breathing characterized by short shallow breaths. This type of breathing results in tension of the neck muscles and in diminished breath support especially at the ends of breath groups. Kelman, Gordon, Simpson, and Morton (1975) noted many dysphonic individuals show abnormalities in their breathing patterns even during quiet respiration, although other dysphonic individuals have quite normal breathing patterns. Lerman (1972, pp. 119–120) stated it should first be determined whether or not a person is breathing well enough to produce speech; for those who present improper breathing patterns such as clavicular breathing, exercises and training in breathing are necessary to establish proper breathing patterns. Eisenson and Ogilvie (1977, p. 317) stated a speaker must have an adequate supply of breath to be comfortable during speaking. They stated it is unusual for an individual not to have adequate breath for normal speech purposes; however, when improvement of breathing is necessary a child should be taught specific diaphragmatic-abdominal control. They stated that during inspiration if a person is lying down the abdominal area should move upward, and if he is sitting or standing the abdomen should move forward. On expiration the abdominal wall should pull in. Eisenson and Ogilvie advised eliminating upper chest and clavicular breathing because such breathing frequently results in a strained humping of the chest and shoulders and interferes with easy breath control. They stated it is often possible to modify and improve breathing used for vocalization without paying direct attention to breathing activity. Correct posture and speaking with easy tone initiation usually assure good breath control.

If improvement in posture and attention to proper vocalization result in a better voice, breathing exercises are not necessary. However, many children who demonstrate inadequate breath control during talking need special attention. The breathing exercises we use are based on those described by Connelly et al. (1970), Cooper (1977, p. 28), and McClosky (1977, pp. 142–143).

Breathing exercises for children with vocal nodules were described by Connelly et al. (1970). They suggested the following procedure to introduce correct breathing: (1) The child is asked to stand, place his hands on his stomach, and let all the air out of his lungs as if he were squeezing air out of a balloon. (2) With the hands still on the stomach, have the child imagine his waistline is a balloon filling up with air while he breathes in deeply. His hands should move outward. (3) After the child is able to breath systematically in this manner have him count on exhalation using correct breathing patterns.

According to Cooper (1977, p. 28) attention should be given to midsection or central breath support, avoiding upper chest breathing. He suggested the following procedure for this:

1. Have the child lie on his back, keeping the head and body flat. Have him place one hand on his chest and the other on his stomach.

2. Tell the child to inhale easily through the nose and exhale through the mouth. During this maneuver the midsection should gradually inflate and deflate with no movement of the chest.

3. Have the child repeat the exercise, but this time inhaling and exhaling through the mouth rather than through the nose. The midsection should inflate quickly and deflate gradually.

4. These exercises should be practiced next in a sitting position and then in a standing position. The new breathing patterns must be coordinated with optimum pitch level, tone focus, and comfortable loudness. The child practices the new midsection breath support beginning with mechanical exercises of *um-hum one, um-hum two*, etc.—followed by practice with isolated words, then phrases, sentences, and finally spontaneous speech.

The following exercises to develop and strengthen the muscles of breathing were suggested by McClosky (1977, pp. 142–143). The purpose of these exercises is to make the child feel strongly just which muscles he is dealing with when he exercises breath control. In breathing during singing and speaking, the child should avoid letting the rib cage fall during exhalation.

1. Have the child lean over, grasp his knees, and take a large deep breath which he holds until the end of this exercise. Then, with his head still down and his back arched, have him rise on tiptoes and draw in the abdominal muscles strongly. Now, still without releasing his breath, have him spring up from the knees and toes to an upright position, feeling a strong upward pressure in the back muscles. Now the child can release the air.

2. Have the child collapse his chest by exhaling as much air as he can. Then by sheer muscular effort without inhaling have him expand and contract the ribs three times, stretching them as wide as possible. Have him hold this position and tell him to take a deep breath, having him become aware of the strong outward action of the abdominal wall.

Relaxation Procedures

Children with hypertensive voice problems usually benefit from a structured program of relaxation procedures. A child who tenses the muscles of speaking and breathing while he talks benefits from relaxation training. This results in a lessening of tension and the production of an improved laryngeal tone. Relaxation procedures are especially beneficial for children with vigorous vocal abuses. The average relaxation period is about 15 min at the beginning of a voice therapy period.

Connelly et al. (1970) recommended relaxation procedures for relieving tension in children with vocal nodules. Lerman (1972, p. 119) stated improved habits of phonation can be taught if tension associated with a voice disorder can be reduced or controlled. Filter (1974) stated a child with a voice problem must be able to relax the laryngeal area before the speech pathologist begins to teach new voice patterns; unnecessary tensions during breathing as well as tensions of the arms, chest, neck, shoulders, and pharynx should receive attention to assure adequate relaxation.

Five exercises listed by Rubin and Lehrhoff (1962) are introduced to orient a child to laryngeal hyperfunction therapy. These aid in obtaining properly adjusted tonus of muscles.

1. Have the child sigh very gently to feel the openness of the throat. Have him yawn deeply with the mouth opened as wide as possible.

2. Ask the child to tense the large muscles of the body and then suddenly relax. Point out the different muscular sensations of contraction and relaxation.

3. Have the child relax the fingers first, then the hands, arms, body, and legs. Soft soothing background music may help the child relax.

4. Have the child roll his head forward and then around his shoulders in a slow circle as he says vowel sounds smoothly and easily.

5. Teach the child to tighten the muscles at the back of the neck. Have him move the head backward in a tense fashion. Then have him move the head from side to side, and then forward. Repeat the same exercise with relaxed easy movements, pointing out the difference in tension between the two.

Our relaxation procedures are based on those presented by Jacobson (1938; 1964; 1976), McClosky (1977), Moncur and Brackett (1974), and Phillips (1976).§ To obtain best results sessions should be individual in a quiet room where the child is not distracted by other children and noise. We will present

§ A 90 min audiocassette and manual *Relaxation* by E. Kass explaining and demonstrating Jacobson's methods is available from Ideas, P. O. Box 741, Tempe AZ 85281.

four relaxation programs in detail. Several techniques are common to all the programs, but they are presented individually in order to give the speech pathologist variety in selecting relaxation procedures.

Jacobson (1964, pp. 78–80; 1976, pp. 192–195) suggested the following program for specific relaxation in the speech region.

1. While the child is reclining grasp his chin and slowly move the lower jaw. Note the resistance.

2. Have the child stiffen the jaw a little and ask him to report where tension is noted. Usually he will report tension in the temporomandibular region and sometimes in the temple area.

3. Have the child relax his jaw by asking him to relax with the mouth open. It should now be possible to move the jaw shut and open with no resistance.

When the child can accomplish the above, Jacobson (1964, pp. 97–99; 1976, pp. 192–195) suggested the following procedures be used for each session until the child can be relaxed under all conditions. We have modified his procedures for use with children.

1. Close jaws firmly; open jaws; relax.

2. Show teeth as in smiling; pout; relax.

3. Push tongue forward against teeth; pull tongue backward as far as possible; relax.

4. Tense and round the lips saying /o/; relax.

5. Count to 10 with normal loudness; count again one-half as loud; relax.

6. Count to 10 very softly; count in a whisper; relax.

Imagination Exercises.

1. Keep speech musculature relaxed and imagine the following:

    a. Counting loudly.

    b. Counting softly.

    c. Saying the alphabet.

2. Still keeping the speech musculature relaxed imagine the following:

    a. Saying name three times loudly.

    b. Saying name three times softly.

    c. Saying address three times loudly.

    d. Saying address three times softly.

    e. Saying name of city three times loudly.

    f. Saying name of city three times softly.

3. Be sure the speech musculature is relaxed. Imagine the following:

    a. Loudly telling a waitress to bring your order.

    b. Softly telling a waitress to bring your order.

    c. Loudly telling the bus driver to stop at

the next corner.

    d. Softly telling the bus driver to stop at the next corner.

For each of the imagination exercises have the child describe where muscle tensions were felt. The exercises should be repeated until the child reports an absence of muscle tension during both the vocalized and the imaginary exercises and under both loud and soft conditions.

Now the child is ready to apply relaxation procedures to his specific vocal abuse. If, for example, his vocal abuse is cheering at sports events:

1. Have him do procedures 1 through 6 above.

2. Have the child imagine he is at an exciting football game.

3. Keeping the speech musculature relaxed imagine the following:

    a. Cheering loudly.

    b. Cheering softly.

    c. Shouting team's name.

    d. Softly saying team's name.

Phillips (1976) described a relaxation procedure at a seminar which we attended. This procedure is based on Jacobson's (1938) procedures. Children with hypertensive voice disorders respond nicely to this procedure with resulting improvement in laryngeal tone. For most children only a few minutes are necessary to obtain complete relaxation. (This is in contrast to adults where the minimum time is usually 20 to 30 min.) During the relaxation steps 1, 2, and 3 below, the speech pathologist carefully watches breathing patterns and the relaxation of the jaw, keeping a careful watch on the child's hands to make sure he is in a relaxed state before proceeding to step 4. Beginning with step 4, when the speech pathologist directs the child to tense specific muscle groups, the rest of the body should remain as relaxed as possible. At times throughout the relaxation procedure the child should be instructed to breathe fairly deeply two or three times, thinking "calm" with each breath. Be sure the child does not hyperventilate.

The following basic relaxation procedure should be used:

1. Get the child comfortable in an easy chair or recliner-type chair. A small child can curl up on a couch. A child can be told to feel like a wet noodle or to be as relaxed as hairs on a pussy cat. The use of a doll or a stuffed animal with the young child may be appropriate to help attain relaxation.

2. Have the child close his eyes. The eyes should remain relaxed and closed throughout the complete relaxation procedure.

3. The speech pathologist describes a relaxed imaginary scene to the child, for example a quiet beach. The description, usually lasting about a minute, should be done in a quiet, relaxed voice. The imaginary scene is presented again to the child if he becomes unduly tense at any time during the relaxation procedure.

4. Have the child clench his right fist tightly, feeling tension in the hand and arm and feeling the fingers bite into the palm. Then have the child very slowly relax the hand and arm. Do the same with the left hand and arm.

5. Have the child tighten the forehead by raising the eyebrows, not creasing between the eyes as in a frown, but raising the eyebrows as high as possible. Have him relax slowly until the forehead is smooth.

6. Have the child tighten his jaw, clenching the teeth tightly; the neck muscles should also be tensed. Have him relax slowly.

7. Have the child tense and raise the shoulders as high as possible tightening all the shoulder and upper back muscles, avoiding tensing the arms and hands. Have him relax slowly.

8. Have the child open his eyes, resuming a normal sitting position.

McClosky's (1977, pp. 139–141) procedure is as follows: He advised having the person sit in a comfortable position, thinking about peaceful untroubled scenes. Relaxation procedures should be done slowly and deliberately. We recommend that when the following procedures are used with children, the speech pathologist first demonstrate them so the child will be able to follow the directions and do the physical manipulations himself. This makes it possible for the child to do these procedures at home.

1. Have the child gently massage the muscles of the face and throat, beginning at his hair line and working down to the lower neck. While doing this have him keep his face as limp as possible, rubbing his fingers gently over his closed eyes, and allowing the jaw to hang slack.

2. Have the child let his tongue fall out over the lower teeth as if he were asleep. Tell him not to push it out. McClosky stated it is important the tongue should be as relaxed as possible, especially the back of the tongue.

3. Have the child relax the swallowing

muscles as follows: First, using the fingers of both hands, have him press gently on the soft part of the throat between the mandible and the larynx, starting under the hinge of the jaw. Second, have the child gently massage these muscles (mylohyoids) until he reports they are soft and pliable. Third, have the child move his fingers gradually until they are directly under the chin. Fourth, have him hold his fingers in this position and ask him to swallow and to feel the downward pressure in the throat. Emphasis should be placed on keeping this area relaxed during all talking.

4. Have the child hold his chin between his thumb and forefinger and move the chin up and down, first slowly and then rapidly. The jaw should be relaxed so it moves easily without resistance, with the tongue lying limply within the mouth.

5. Have the child make sure the lower neck muscles and sternocleidomastoid muscles are relaxed, allowing the head to nod up and down lazily while keeping all other muscles of the head and neck relaxed.

Moncur and Brackett (1974, p. 123) presented a series of procedures for throat relaxation.

1. Have the child do three types of yawning: gently, then more deeply, then vigorously. During the last yawn have the child close his eyes and stretch the muscles of his mouth and throat.

2. Have the child inhale, yawn gently, and then sigh a prolonged breathy /ɑ/.

3. Have the child inhale deeply, and sigh /ɑ/ in a relaxed, breathy manner (omitting the yawn used in No. 2).

4. Develop an awareness of the *feel* of throat relaxation as follows:
   a. Have the child inhale slowly and deeply and then vocalize /ɑ/ on a sigh. Have him concentrate on the kinesthetic sensation of both inhalation and exhalation.
   b. Have the child close his eyes and recall the kinesthetic sensations during slow and deep inhalation and the sensations felt as he sighs on a vocalized /ɑ/.

Relaxation procedures are of definite value for many children with hypertensive voice problems. Improvement in voice quality or resonance balance is often noted immediately following relaxation procedures. If a definite decrease in physical tension does not occur within about a half dozen sessions, other methods of tension reduction, such as chewing exercises, should be considered.

The Chewing Method

The chewing method is often effective for persons with hyperfunctional voice problems of various etiologies. Using this method it is possible to obtain good vocalizations free from voice deviations and at a pitch suitable for the child without paying direct attention to either voice quality or pitch. The child is made aware of the clear tones in his voice and then can contrast them to his old way of talking. Listening practice is based on recordings of these two qualities.

The chewing method has been used for some time in Europe and was described by Brodnitz and Froeschels (1954), Froeschels (1943), Froeschels and Jellinek (1941, pp. 179–180), Weiss (1971, pp. 17–20), and Wyatt (1951, pp. 70–99; 1977, pp. 281–286). Weiss (1971, p. 20) stated the chewing method is the main approach in the treatment of hyperfunction of the voice and can be applied to almost all aspects of voice therapy. Brodnitz (1971a, pp. 97–99) regarded Froeschels' method as the best way to correct hyperfunction and to reduce abrupt glottal attack. He felt an important by-product of the chewing method is the normalizing influence it has on pitch of the voice (Brodnitz, 1971a, p. 102). This method can also be used in voice mutational difficulties.

Froeschels (1943; 1952) recommended the use of his chewing method to improve the voices of hard of hearing and deaf children. He felt the use of this method, with special attention to the kinesthesia of chewing and of improved voice quality, helps to replace unusual voice patterns with more normal patterns for these children. Beebe (1951, pp. 58–69; 1976; 1977) also advocated the chewing method to enable hearing-impaired children to develop a natural voice quality. After practicing the movements of chewing as if chewing food, the child is taught to speak with the mental attitude of chewing, with the result that muscles function in a natural manner resulting in more adequate articulation. Beebe (1977) stated the strained high pitch and unnatural melodic pattern of the deaf can be changed into natural parameters by teaching vocalized chewing.

The chewing method has been used to normalize voice in children with other problems, such as myasthenia gravis, multiple sclerosis, scoliosis, and cerebral palsy. For example, Skelly et al. (1971) in working with children with scoliosis used the chewing method for reducing laryngeal tension and to determine adequate pitch range. Audiorecordings of the sounds emitted during chewing were also used for identifying hypernasality, the predominant voice problem in the scoliosis group. In the early stages of therapy these children were able to identify hypernasality more readily on the meaningless chewing sounds. It was believed this enabled them to make more reliable judgments in meaningful speech later on.

Weiss (1971, p. 17) stated, "The basic movement of the chewing procedure is a 'sonorous chewing'—a kind of generous munching, whereby vigorous but relaxed chewing movements are accompanied by a haphazardly emitted voice." The similarity between eating and speaking is explained (Wyatt, 1977, p. 281). Wyatt (1977, p. 283) stated patients' attitudes toward the chewing method vary. Uninhibited or extroverted persons, such as actors, singers, and most children, usually have little difficulty in doing simultaneous chewing and vocalizing. If a patient is uncomfortable doing chewing exercises with the speech pathologist, private practice at home usually overcomes this feeling.

Weiss (1971, p. 18) stressed it is important that the child not try to imitate the chewing of the speech pathologist in number of movements or extent of jaw movements. However, it is often useful for the speech pathologist to demonstrate chewing for a child (Wyatt, 1977, p. 281), but doing it in unison should be avoided. The child should be encouraged to develop his own method and kinesthesia of natural chewing (Weiss, 1971, p. 18).

The following is a description of the chewing method applied to a child. The speech pathologist demonstrates each step as the therapy progresses.

1. The child is told he can talk and chew at the same time using the same muscles for both functions. He is told he will learn how to chew his breath first and then later will chew while vocalizing. Ask the child to imagine he is chewing a piece of apple or a marshmallow (Weiss, 1971, p. 18). All chewing should be done pretending food is in the mouth and actual food or gum chewing is not advocated (Froeschels, 1952). Weiss (1971, p. 18) stated there are no advantages in using chewing gum or any other similar substance. The child must learn to adopt the purely psychological attitude of relaxed chewing independent of having anything in his mouth. Wyatt (1977, p. 281), on the other hand, stated it is helpful during introductory sessions to give a child a small piece of bread to chew; soon, however, actual chewing of food is not done.

2. The child is requested to chew either with the lips closed or slightly open and with energetic movements of the tongue and lips. During this activity the child is asked to be especially conscious of the movements of his tongue.

3. The child is told to chew "like a savage" (Froeschels, 1943) with an open mouth and with very vigorous movements of the lips and tongue. Special attention should be given to obtaining good tongue movement. It should not be cultured chewing with the mouth closed, but rather the sloppy chewing of a tired worker (Weiss, 1971, p. 18).

4. Now the child is asked to vocalize while chewing. Weiss (1971, p. 18) suggested asking the child to open his mouth and say a neutral sound without inflection or expression. Wyatt (1977, p. 281) recommended vocalizations not be initiated until a child feels no effort or tension while chewing silently. Then the child continues chewing while simultaneously producing a vocal tone. The child should chew vigorously and let himself go. A large variety of sounds should be produced and not a monotonous repetition of just a few sounds. Weiss (1971, p. 20) recommended the child be told to take a deep breath and to chew and vocalize as he maximally exhales. This is done five times during each of the first few sessions. The number of these exercises can be increased during later sessions. Weiss (1971, p. 18) stated the child can now be shown how to chew all kinds of vowels allowing the pitch of his voice to vary in an unorganized manner. Next Wyatt (1977, pp. 284–285) suggested asking the child to chew and slide into short phrases such as *I am in, I am out, I am alone*. During the exercises the child is asked to go from nonsense chewing and nonsense vocalization into chewing of short phrases and back again to chewing nonsense material. There must be no change in voice quality during these maneuvers and

vocal hyperfunction must be avoided. During the beginning sessions, transition from monotone to varying pitch and loudness may be difficult. A hypernasal quality may result from over-relaxation during chewing and should be avoided.

5. The child is asked to chew with vocalization about 20 times a day for a few seconds each time. It is helpful if he keeps in mind he is pretending he has food in his mouth. Wyatt (1977, p. 282) suggested the initial outside assignment should be to do the chewing exercise once an hour for only a few minutes each time. It can be done sitting, standing, or walking, keeping generally relaxed.

6. After several days of this chewing activity the child should begin to read aloud after each session of vocalized chewing. Weiss (1971, p. 19) suggested when the child is able to chew in a natural and relaxed manner, playing with his voice and vowels at the same time, a very potent instrument of therapy has been acquired. In spaced steps the child is asked to chew the numbers, then he is asked to answer questions by chewing the words of short answers, progressing to longer sentences, poems, and reading.

The child should now be ready to do the following exercises as suggested by Wyatt (1977, pp. 285–286):

1. Chewing while vocalizing.
2. Imaginary chewing while vocalizing.
3. Yawning, vocalized chewing—followed by phrases.
4. Imaginary chewing while saying phrases, concentrating on the feeling of chewing words.
5. Chewing phrases, then memorized short poems.

Next the following exercises are done emphasizing variations in pitch and loudness (Wyatt, 1977, pp. 286–287):

1. Have the child do vocalized chewing and then say the first three lines of a poem all on one breath.
2. Have the child yawn and say the whole poem on one breath.
3. Have the child yawn, take in a deep breath and repeat the poem as many times as he can on one breath.
4. Now have the child concentrate on pitch variation by having him begin the first line at a low pitch, raising the pitch a bit as he goes from line to line. Have him say the poem again, but this time starting at a high pitch shifting downward in pitch as he goes from line to line.

5. The child is now ready to approach variations in loudness. Using a short poem, have him begin in a soft voice increasing loudness as he goes from line to line. Next, have him do the reverse—beginning in a loud voice gradually decreasing loudness as he goes from line to line.

We have used the chewing method with children with hyperfunctional voice problems and have found it to be successful in reducing hyperfunction and in obtaining good clear tones. Its successful use in vocal tension reduction in children has been reported by Wilson and Rice (1977, p. 26). If the chewing method is done correctly laryngeal dysfunction is greatly diminished, and pitch is normalized (Wyatt, 1977, p. 284). In our opinion chewing exercises should be included in voice therapy programs when reducing vocal hyperfunction is a major goal. These exercises are useful also in normalizing pitch and establishing balanced oral-nasal resonance. We have found chewing exercises can be fun for the child but all efforts should be made to keep the activity of chewing free from silliness. The exercises can be terminated when optimal voice use is attained by the child.

The following is an example of a hypertensive voice problem for which tension reduction therapy was the chosen approach.

Kathy was 13 years old when she was referred to us by her laryngologist for consultation regarding a strident and breathy voice which had developed after a bout of bronchitis 1 year previously. The laryngeal examination by indirect laryngoscopy showed clear vocal cords that moved equally on phonation, but there was incomplete approximation of the cords posteriorly resulting in a posterior V-shaped glottal opening. The mother reported that Kathy did not seem to breathe properly, that when she talked she ran out of breath and her shoulders moved upward during inhalation. Kathy had a history of allergy affecting the upper respiratory system; this was considered a possible contributing cause but not the main cause of her voice problem. The major cause was attributed to carryover of a strained voice evoked by the bronchitis. The mother regarded Kathy's voice a severe problem often interfering with intelligibility; the teacher reported the same problem in the classroom. Kathy was a bright girl earning high grades at school. Both the mother and the teacher described her as quiet and shy. When we saw Kathy her voice was characterized by pitch breaks, stridency, breathiness, and low modal pitch level. She produced voice with extreme effort with tension manifested in her neck and face; clavicular breathing was characteristic. On the Buffalo Voice Profile she was rated 6 on laryngeal tone, 7 on laryngeal hypertension, 4 on too low modal pitch, and 3 on pitch breaks. On the Speech Anxiety Scale she was rated 6 on *rigidity* as manifested by hypertension noted in the shoulders, neck, and face, and 4 on *inhibition* shown by lack of facial expression and a monotonous voice of low intensity. Her maximum phonation time was 14 sec which was normal for her age. Her modal pitch level was 175 Hz, which was 85 Hz (7 semitones) below the average fundamental frequency for her age, 260 Hz (middle C). Her pitch was considered too low for a 13-year-old girl (premenarche). Voice therapy was begun with the following goals: (1) reduction of muscular hyperfunction to a state of balanced muscular tonus, (2) raising the modal pitch level to the average level for her age, (3) teaching the use of an "easy" voice free of hyperfunction, (4) improving the quality of the laryngeal tone, and (5) habituation of new vocal patterns.

Relaxation procedures, breathing and chewing exercises, and attention to posture resulted in eliminating clavicular breathing and reducing muscular tension associated with talking. Raising the modal pitch level to 260 Hz and increasing the loudness of her voice for efficient communication resulted in a clear laryngeal tone free of stridency and breathiness. After 23 one-hour therapy sessions over a period of 3 months Kathy was dismissed with a follow-up program planned to insure carryover and habituation of her new vocal patterns.

Hypofunction

Hypofunctional voice problems are characterized by excessive breath escape, weak laryngeal tones, low speech intensity, and low pitch levels. Inadequate glottal closure is also found in children with vocal palsy and laryngeal hypofunction due to trauma to the larynx as well as in problems of functional breathy voices. In some laryngeal problems such as chronic nonspecific laryngitis the voice is too breathy with a weak glottal attack and a voice of low intensity. With breathy voices it is necessary to reduce the amount of wasted air to achieve a better voice pattern (Van Riper and Irwin, 1958, p. 235). Exercises to overcome flaccid laryngeal muscle activity have been suggested in the treatment of hysterical aphonia (Bangs and Freidinger, 1949). Velopharyngeal insufficiency is often caused by hypofunctioning velar and pharyngeal muscles.

Procedures for Hypofunction

The 10 point therapy outline for balanced muscular tonus (Fig. 34) is used in eliminating hypofunction. The steps are carefully followed, from teaching the child the rule about balanced muscular tonus to carryover. Tension increase therapy is a basic approach in eliminating hypofunctional voice problems.

Tension increase therapy, according to Wilson and Rice (1977, p. 33), starts with obtaining full voice production, then getting full voice production on words and short phrases, and then using full voice within the child's peer group structure and at home. Their goals for increased tension therapy include: (1) Establish normal voicing by increasing muscular tension. (2) Teach the child differences between voice produced with tension and without it. (3) Teach the child to produce his improved voice with proper muscular force. (4) Improve the child's vital capacity so the vocal cords can operate with maximum efficiency.

Exercises to increase muscular tonus are necessary for problems of hypofunction. Pushing exercises are particularly helpful in eliminating hypofunction. Other exercises to innervate the speech mechanism for a more firm closure of the vocal cords are also useful. Van Riper and Irwin (1958, p. 237) suggested asking the person to initiate vocalization suddenly and strongly, perhaps initially employing abrupt tone initiation to do this. To obtain clear phonation they suggested having a person hold his breath against strong abdominal contraction and then suddenly explode the tone. We have found in working with a child with a breathy voice this technique is a good one. We ask the child to stand against a wall, and we have him place his hand flat against his stomach just under the rib cage and above the waistline. The speech pathologist places his hand on the child's hand pressing slightly inward. The child is asked to maintain steady abdominal pressure against his own hand as he says vowels, words, and sentences. This technique almost always results in good clear tones. The clear tones are tape recorded and contrasted to the breathy tones for listening training. Soon the abrupt initiations should be modified to easy initiations with full phonation.

In a breathy voice with excess waste of air during phonation Curtis (1967, p. 226) suggested asking the child to phonate in a louder tone thus increasing muscular tonicity resulting in elimination of breathiness. He stated when the child hears the difference between the breathy and clear tones, the loudness of his voice can be reduced to an appropriate level making sure the breathiness does not return. Another method of reducing breathiness is to note its occurrence on the plosive sounds /p/, /t/, and /k/. Canfield (1964) stated these sounds are apt to be more breathy than other sounds and this breathiness is carried over into the following sounds. He stated the speaker should be made aware of his breathiness on these sounds since more precise articulation of these particular plosives will often reduce a generalized breathiness of all sounds.

Pushing Method

Froeschels' pushing exercises are useful in increasing muscle tonus to eliminate hypofunction (Froeschels, Kastein, and Weiss, 1955). Brodnitz (1971a, pp. 100–101) discussed correction of hypofunction through the use of Froeschels' pushing exercises. He stated correction of hypofunction presents a particularly difficult problem for the speech pathologist. He recommended pushing exercises to get more muscular activity in cases of incomplete glottal closure during phonation. It is also used to obtain improved velopharyngeal closure especially in cases of velar paralysis (Froeschels et al. 1955). The objective of the pushing method is to get more activation and firmer closure of the vocal cords as well as improved velopharyngeal closure. When pushing exercises are used correctly, according to Weiss (1971, p. 21), they are the best and most expeditious way of remedying insufficiencies of the voice associated with hypofunction. He stated if they are used carefully, both as to how often and how long they are practiced, not only are the vocal muscles used with more force, but in

time they are actually strengthened. Pushing exercises consist of simultaneous phonation and movements of the arms (Froeschels et al. 1955). To do this a child stands and raises his fists to his chest and then pushes his arms down in one quick sweep with the hands opening just as the palms land on the front of the thighs. When this can be done without undue tension the child is requested to say consonant-vowel (CV) syllables. It is best to begin with CV syllables since the use of isolated vowels may lead to sharp and forceful closure of the glottis preceding phonation and in this way may be responsible for the undesirable habit of abrupt glottal attack. Weiss (1971, p. 22) suggested first using /pɔ, pα, pi, po, pu/ pronounced in a brief, sharp, explosive manner. Later isolated vowels such as /α/ can be used and then other vowels. Vocalization is initiated at the beginning of the downward movement of the arms and ends as the palms hit the thighs. Weiss (1971, pp. 21–22) stated it should be stressed that phonation must occur at exactly the same time as the sudden, energetic, and full-swinging downward motion of both arms. It is useful, therefore, to instruct the child to "Push your voice out with your arms!" When a good voice has been produced on the CV syllables and vowels, then other syllables and monosyllabic words are used. Five to ten pushes should be done every half hour on the 1st day and once an hour daily for.a week (Froeschels et al. 1955). The number is then reduced according to vocal progress. As laryngeal tone and loudness improve ask the child to say a sound, syllable, or word during the pushing movement and to follow this immediately with a repetition of the vocalization without pushing but matching the volume and tone of the pushed vocalization. When good phonation develops the actual movements can be stopped with the person only thinking of pushing while he is speaking or reading aloud. These exercises energize the whole body including the voice and speech producing mechanisms. In the beginning stages it may be necessary to initiate the vocalizations abruptly in order to get a clear tone free from breathiness. Very soon, however, these abrupt initiations should be modified to easy initiations to avoid possible trauma to the larynx. Weiss (1971, p. 21) cautioned that if pushing exercises are not used properly they can be harmful since they subject the vocal organ to sudden stress, and the speech pathologist must guard against overtaxing a weakened vocal organ.

Children with hypofunctional voice problems benefit from special exercises to increase muscular tonus to assure more firm vocal cord closure. Excessive breathiness is eliminated with a stronger more forceful voice the end result.

SUMMARY

Two major goals of voice therapy for laryngeal dysfunction are eliminating or modifying vocal abuse and developing balanced muscular tonus. The rules of voice hygiene must be strictly observed as a basis for the elimination of laryngeal dysfunction in the presence or absence of vocal pathology. Vocal abuse is approached directly; each abuse is identified and a careful listening training and charting program developed for its elimination. Substitute behaviors are used whenever possible. The majority of children with laryngeal dysfunction characteristically use hypertensive voice patterns as revealed by strident constricted voices. Reduction of tension is accomplished by attention to posture and assuring proper breathing technique during speaking. Specific relaxation procedures and chewing exercises help reduce vocal hyperfunction and promote adequate use of voice. Procedures for children with breathy weak voices due to muscular hypofunction call for muscle energizing procedures such as pushing exercises. Balanced muscular tonus will assure the correct use of a vocal mechanism free from undue tension or excessive flaccidity.

NINE

Voice Therapy for Laryngeal Dysfunction: II

Loudness, Pitch, Rate, Clear Voice, Special Problems

Children with laryngeal dysfunction usually need direction in controlling loudness, pitch, and rate. Attention may be needed for improving laryngeal tone to assure the production of a clear voice. Problems of incipient spastic dysphonia, hysterical dysphonia, and ventricular phonation require special attention.

APPROPRIATE LOUDNESS

Modifying loudness is necessary for many children. Loudness may be a problem by itself or it may be associated with other problems such as vocal cord thickening or polypoid degeneration. Most children with laryngeal dysfunction habitually talk too loud. A too-loud voice may be present in a child with vocal hyperfunction and a too-soft voice in a child with vocal hypofunction. Talking too loud is more common than talking too soft. We are referring to loud talking present on a habitual basis in contrast to the intermittent use of an extremely loud voice during shouting, which was discussed under vocal abuse. Loudness training should be coordinated with procedures to assure balanced muscular tonus (Wilson, 1977, p. 268). It is especially important to eliminate loud talking in children with vocal nodules (Wilson, 1961; 1962b; 1962c). Even in the absence of laryngeal pathology we are interested in reducing excessive loudness present on a habitual basis as a preventive measure to avoid possible pathological changes in the larynx.

Loudness control can be approached directly. The correct loudness level is reached when voice is produced without constriction (Perkins, 1971, p. 527). In some cases learning to talk more distinctly decreases the necessity to talk loudly (Van Riper and Irwin, 1958, p. 192).

Modifying Loudness

The pattern for loudness listening training is similar to that used for shouting and in some cases shouting and loudness training can be combined. It is necessary for the speech pathologist to develop awareness of excessive loudness or softness in speech intensity and then proceed to gross discrimination. For fine discrimination of loudness four loudness levels are selected: (1) a very high speech intensity approximating a shout, (2) high speech intensity termed very loud, (3) a level or range of loudness calculated to be most desirable or just right for the child to use under most circumstances, and (4) low speech intensity considered to be too soft. Pictures are placed in the notebook representing these four levels of loudness. These can be pictures of children using these loudness levels (Fig. 35). Another technique for loudness listening training is called the animal game (Wilson, 1961). The speech pathologist selects four pictures of animals ranging from very large to small in size to represent the four loudness levels. The child is asked to point to the correct picture as the speech pathologist uses various intensity levels.

After listening training has resulted in good discrimination of loudness the child is ready to demonstrate his own ability at controlling speech intensity. The loudness chart (Fig. 36) is used for loudness modification and control following the 10 steps of the voice therapy outline. As with similar charts, picture stickers or simply a written "O.K." may be used as rewards. The rule about loud talking is taught. The child is told a specific loudness level is to be observed in order to have a good voice (Step 1). The child identifies the undesirable and desirable loudness levels in others (Steps 2 and 3). He next learns the auditory characteristics of his own loud—or soft—talking (Step 4). He identifies situations where his loudness level is inappropriate and appropriate (Steps 6 and 7). Then habituation of the desired loudness pattern is programmed (Steps 8, 9, and 10).

The intensity of the speech pathologist's voice can be expected to influence the intensity of the child's responses (Atkinson, 1952; Black, 1949; 1950; Hanf and Corso, 1966). The greater the intensity of a speaker's voice the greater will be the intensity of the listener's vocal response. Therefore, when we are working to modify the intensity of a child's voice we can expect an increase in the loudness of his responses if we talk louder to

him; in contrast, softer talking by the speech pathologist will result in a decrease in the loudness of the child's voice.

Black (1961) found soft speech was accompanied by a slower rate while reading phrases. Some children may use an excessively slow rate at a low level of loudness. Increasing the rate of talking may help bring the loudness to a more normal level.

Various devices and instruments can be used to help the child monitor the loudness of his voice. An amplifier with earphones such as an auditory training unit can be used in teaching voice monitoring especially adequate control of loudness (Brodnitz, 1961; Van Riper and Irwin, 1958, p. 259). If we want a child to talk softer we turn the volume control up and he automatically decreases his loudness level. The reverse can be done in order to increase voice loudness. Feeding a masking noise into the child's ears through earphones also increases the loudness of his voice. The masking noise from an audiometer or a recorded white noise on a tape loop can be used. Careful listening training has to accompany these techniques for carryover from the auditory trainer or amplifier into conversational use. All these activities should be tape recorded for the child to listen to so he can learn to monitor his own voice. During the recording the child can watch the recorder's intensity meter or light, or a sound level meter, and listen to his own loudness levels when he is engaged in these activities with the speech pathologist (Wilson, 1962b). The pictures in Figure 35 can be used by the child for practice.

The "Voice-Lite I"* provides a visual feedback of voice loudness. It is a small instrument (8½ × 6¾ × 6¾ in) which can be placed

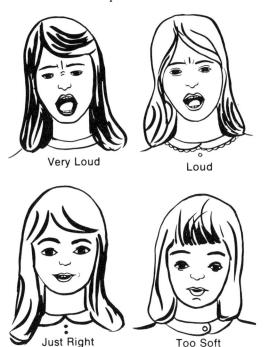

Very Loud   Loud

Just Right   Too Soft

Fig. 35. Loudness practice. Illustration by Geraldine Balsam.

* Behavioral Controls, Inc., P.O. Box 480, Milwaukee, WI 53201.

1. I KNOW THE RULE ABOUT HOW LOUD I SHOULD TALK.   _____
2. I CAN TELL WHEN OTHER PEOPLE USE INCORRECT LOUDNESS.   _____
3. I CAN TELL WHEN OTHER PEOPLE USE CORRECT LOUDNESS.   _____
4. I CAN TELL WHEN THE LOUDNESS OF MY VOICE IS INCORRECT.   _____
5. I CAN TELL WHEN THE LOUDNESS OF MY VOICE IS CORRECT.   _____
6. I KNOW THE PLACES WHERE I USE INCORRECT LOUDNESS.   _____
7. I KNOW THE PLACES WHERE I USE CORRECT LOUDNESS.   _____
8. I CAN TALK WITH CORRECT LOUDNESS *SOME* OF THE TIME.   _____
9. I CAN TALK WITH CORRECT LOUDNESS *MOST* OF THE TIME.   _____
10. I CAN TALK WITH CORRECT LOUDNESS *ALL* THE TIME.   _____

Fig. 36. Loudness.

in front of a child. The electronic circuitry changes sound energy into light patterns according to the intensity and duration of the sound—a short, soft sound makes a light come on briefly and dimly while a loud, long sound produces a bright light of longer duration. The Vocal Intensity Controller described earlier also can be used to control loudness through auditory feedback. Florida I, also described earlier, can be used for modifying loudness as well as for pitch control (Holbrook and Crawford, 1970; Holbrook and Meador, 1969). "Spright"† is an electronic instrument for demonstrating loudness. It has a row of 10 red lights which are consecutively lighted as loudness input increases. It operates on regular current; the size is $3 \times 4 \times 9$ in.

Instruments useful in teaching children appropriate loudness of the voice can be built in home or school workshops at minimal cost. Harper (1970) described a voice-activated battery operated instrument that can be assembled by an amateur. A microphone, preamplifier, and transistorized amplifier are housed in a clownlike figure. By using a stepped up transformer, voltage is provided for two tiny neon lamps in the clown's eyes. Any vocalization lights up the neon lamps. Aston (1973) reported the use of a large stuffed toy dog with a microphone in its nose and an amplifier inside the dog. Lights in the dog's eyes are activated when a child vocalizes. Special lights can be used to indicate two loudness levels. These lights have two concentric circles so when a soft sound is made only the center circle lights up, and with a louder sound both the center and the outside circles light up. One of our favorite instruments, which we built, resembles a miniature electric traffic signal light. It consists of a small box with three lights, red, yellow, and green. Connected to it with a 6 foot cord is a switch box with three manually operated on-off switches. The speech pathologist can hold the switch box under the table or out of the line of vision of the child and turn on the light that is indicative of a child's performance. For example, the green light can be used to indicate to the child he performed a certain task satisfactorily, the red light that his response was not the desired one, and the yellow light to indicate he approached or approximated the desired response. The elec-

† Electronics Inc., 4727 Fellow St., South Bend, IN 46614.

tric signal light can also be used for negative practice.

Singing

Improper singing can be a vocal misuse if pitch or loudness is misused during singing. Both boys and girls should avoid singing during voice change (Weiss, 1950). The singing of all children should be carefully supervised, but caution is particularly important if laryngeal pathology is present. Improper use of the voice in singing should be avoided, especially when a hoarse voice is purposely used and a breathy style combined with excessive exertion, strain, and loudness (Moses, 1959). The loud raucous rock style of singing, particularly when young men extensively use falsetto, can result in traumatic laryngitis and bilateral vocal cord nodules (Batza, 1971).

As a general rule if vocal pathology is present the child should be excused from singing until his voice has improved and the pathological condition has cleared up or significantly improved. Singing should be eliminated in cases with vocal nodules until the nodules are resolved and then it can be resumed but with different techniques (Baker, 1962; Holinger et al. 1952). If the youngster with vocal nodules is allowed to continue vocally unrestrained in singing class he will develop irreversible vocal changes (Holinger et al. 1952). Disturbances of the voice may not be apparent during speaking but become apparent during singing, for example subtle variations in vocal quality, the appearance of voice breaks, and the complaint of discomfort in the throat and neck during or following singing (Rubin, 1964). We suggest the speech pathologist and the singing teacher coordinate their efforts with children who have good speaking voices but have alterations in vocal quality during singing. The singing teacher may improve faulty singing techniques while the speech pathologist concentrates on the speaking voice. Many singers who have nodules or polypoid thickening of the cords make a good living and the pathology probably accounts for the distinctive character of their singing voice (Baker, 1962).

Recently we have been seeing teenage and young adult professional singers who have vocal cord pathology. With these young people the organic changes have made continuation of their style of singing impossible. Our approach has been to treat the speaking voice first and allow no singing during this time. Then as the speaking voice improves a coordinated program with a qualified vocal instructor is arranged. All attempts are made to direct the singer to use a singing technique that is appealing to him and one that is not organically traumatizing. See case example on pp. 43–44.

Loudness training, even though an uncomplicated procedure, requires careful application of the listening training program, followed by teaching the correct level of loudness through auditory cues reinforced by visual displays. Control of loudness is very important in maintaining good vocal hygiene and is an essential element in voice improvement.

DESIRABLE USE OF PITCH

The results of the pitch examination should be studied carefully before considering changes in pitch use. Recommendations for changing voice pitch level should not be made indiscriminately (Brodnitz, 1962) but are made only after careful evaluation. Children and adolescents exhibiting unsatisfactory use of pitch generally fall into one or more of the following five classifications: (1) pitch problems related to mutation, involving a high pitch level in the adolescent male or an unusually low pitch level in the adolescent female (appropriate changes in the voice pitch level are in order for these problems); (2) excessive pitch breaks usually associated with voice change (these should be eliminated); (3) frequent use of traumatizing high or low pitch levels under certain circumstances, such as in games and outdoor activities even though the voice pitch level and pitch range are adequate under normal speaking conditions. Also some children may use abnormally high pitch while speaking loudly under noisy conditions or talking under emotional strain (if these abnormal pitch levels are used enough to be considered damaging children should be taught to avoid even the intermittent use of unusually high or low pitch levels); (4) the habitual continuous use of too-high or too-low pitch levels considered to be traumatizing and contributing to the laryngeal dysfunctioning (changes in pitch level are indicated); (5) stereotyped and limited voice range (instruction for improved expression is indicated for these problems).

Pitch is not an isolated factor of the vocal characteristics of a person (Brodnitz, 1971a, p. 103). Teaching overall good use of voice in its various parameters of loudness, inflection, and quality often results in a suitable pitch level. For example, teaching a child to talk in an easier fashion rather than in a staccato, hard manner with abrupt attacks modifies his use of pitch to a more acceptable level without paying direct attention to the pitch of his voice.

Perkins (1971, pp. 508–509) stated any tone requiring strain to produce is undesirable whether it is high or low, but tension is less likely to be present when the voice is produced near the bottom of the range than when it is produced near the top of the range. He objected to the practice of mechanically analyzing the voice for the modal and optimum pitch levels and deciding to change pitch if there is an appreciable difference between the levels. He favored a more subjective approach in which the person is encouraged to use as low a pitch as is comfortable to get a voice production that is effortless and free from tension.

Laguaite and Waldrop (1964) stated as a general rule pitch should not be worked on directly but advocated therapy techniques for easy relaxed phonation. They stated the fundamental pitch of a person's voice should not be changed unless it is significantly different from the norm established for that particular age. They compared mean fundamental frequencies and acoustical analyses of subjects before and after therapy. They found the fundamental frequency did not change significantly but the acoustical analyses indicated more vocal energy in the higher frequencies and greater regularity in the harmonics. Therefore, they concluded that changes in voice as a result of therapy are due to factors other than changes in fundamental frequency.

Raising or lowering pitch level of the voice in cases of laryngeal pathology has been a subject of discussion and research. Connelly et al. (1970) reported children with vocal nodules tend to have a modal pitch level too low for adequate vocal efficiency. Fisher and Logemann (1970) analyzed high speed motion pictures and perceptual evaluations of a 19-year-old actress with bilateral vocal nodules at the junction of the anterior and middle thirds of the total glottal length. Analysis revealed her modal pitch was 190 Hz while her optimum pitch level should have been 250 Hz. After voice therapy for raising her pitch to the desired level she no longer experienced aphonia and vocal fatigue following a performance, nor did she have difficulty in vocal projection and expressiveness. Further, indirect laryngoscopy revealed a marked reduction in the size of the nodules. The actress resumed her career. Cooper (1971b) found all his subjects with papilloma needed their modal pitch levels raised from 1 to 3 tones in order to obtain optimal use of the laryngeal mechanism. Cooper (1974) reported on a spectrographic analysis of 155 patients aged 15 to 73 years with laryngeal dysfunction due to a variety of causes. Of the 155 patients, 150 were using too-low modal pitch levels before voice therapy. The rises in pitch for the latter group ranged from 4 Hz to 245 Hz. Thus Cooper concluded a major factor in dysphonia is the use of a pitch level which is below the optimal level. Mueller (1975), in disagreement with Cooper (1974), described 25 female patients with a variety of vocal cord conditions who had a mean fundamental frequency of 204 Hz. This level, Mueller stated, is considered within the normal range, and thus changing modal pitch for his patients was not indicated. In a reply to Mueller's remarks, Cooper (1975) stated that in his clinical experience he had found 90% of 2000 voice patients using a too-low modal pitch; the other 10% too high. We can see, therefore, that the question of changing pitch is an area of disagreement.

We emphasize *normalizing* pitch when it is inappropriate to a child's size, age, and sex and is thought to have a relationship to voice misuse or vocal pathology. We suggest a careful analysis of pitch should be made for each child. The study should include range, modal pitch level, and optimum pitch level. Optimum pitch level can be calculated by using Fairbanks' (1960, Ch. 11) method—one-fourth up from the basal pitch. We also suggest comparing the modal pitch level with the norms presented in Chapter 6, taking careful note of the acceptable ranges for each age level.

Changing Modal Pitch Level

Changes in modal pitch level can be achieved by administering a thorough program of listening training and then teaching correct pitch level and pitch variability. The listening training sharpens pitch discrimination ability and prepares the child for specific control of pitch. The basic outline for listening training can be used here. Awareness of

differences in pitch in the speech pathologist's voice and gross discrimination on two levels can be covered quickly. The speech pathologist can then concentrate on fine discrimination of three levels—high, middle, and low. These three pitch levels are based upon the child's pitch range and modal pitch level. If the child's pitch is too high, the speech pathologist selects a high level near the top of the range which often coincides with the too-high modal level. The middle pitch is carefully selected as the level to be established as the new modal level. The third level is a low level only slightly above his lowest pitch. The child is told the significance of each level: the high level is the old way to be avoided, the middle is the desired new way, and the low pitch is too low to use most of the time (Wilson, 1961).

Pictures for pitch practice can be placed in the notebook. For example the speech pathologist can use a picture of three children standing at different heights on rocks. These can be labeled "I can talk low," "I can talk in the middle," and "I can talk high" (Fig. 37). The speech pathologist demonstrates the three levels with words, phrases, and sentences for discrimination training with the child pointing to the appropriate figure.

Another technique for pitch training is called the space game (Wilson, 1961). The speech pathologist places three pictures of airplanes in the child's notebook, one at the

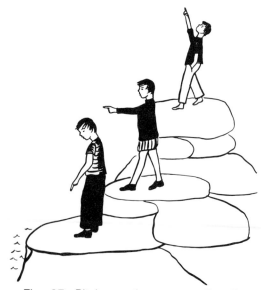

Fig. 37. Pitch practice representing three levels—too high, correct, too low. Illustration by Geraldine Balsam.

top of the page, one in the middle, and one at the bottom. These are captioned "high airplane," "middle airplane," and "low airplane," and the three pitch levels are repeatedly demonstrated by the speech pathologist and associated with each picture. When the child has begun to categorize pitch into the high, middle, and low levels the speech pathologist makes up stories about the three pictures and keeps changing pitch levels. Each time the level changes the child points to the appropriate picture. Pictures of birds, rockets, or balloons can also be used.

Practice by the child himself follows listening training when he has developed good pitch discrimination. The roles of the child and the speech pathologist are reversed with the child becoming the performer and the speech pathologist the listener and judge. The child knows from his listening training the significance and meaning of the three levels of pitch and can therefore strive to produce each pitch level. The pictures used to develop discrimination can be used for the child to practice the pitch levels. Other useful devices for identifying and establishing proper use of pitch level involve simple skits in which the child is encouraged to use the three pitch levels in impersonating characters. Puppets can be used as the basis for these skits.

The pitch chart (Fig. 38) following the ten step outline is to be used in a manner similar to other charts. The chart is placed in the child's notebook and each step rewarded appropriately as he progresses. The child is taught the rule about correct use of pitch (Step 1). He learns to recognize when other people use too-high and too-low pitched voices (Step 2) and when others use correct pitch (Step 3). The child knows when he uses incorrect pitch (Step 4) and when he uses correct pitch (Step 5). The places where he uses incorrect pitch are identified (Step 6) and where it is used correctly (Step 7). Carryover proceeds from partial to complete habituation of correct pitch use (Steps 8, 9, and 10).

Robby, a 6½-year-old boy, is an example of pitch misuse causing vocal nodules. Lowering the modal pitch level resulted in a normal laryngeal mechanism. He was referred to the speech pathologist by a laryngologist with the complaint of hoarseness and the diagnosis of "screamer's nodes" about 2 mm in size bilaterally at the junction of the anterior and middle thirds of the vocal cords. About 1 year prior to the referral the child had a series of colds and two attacks of bronchitis, and it was then that the parents began to notice the hoarseness. This hoarseness continued after recovery from the colds, however, and became increasingly worse. He was a very active boy with more hoarseness at the end of a day of hard playing and yelling. He habitually talked excessively in a loud voice with a high pitch level. He continually abused his vocal cords by using strained high-pitched sounds in play activities. The pediatrician felt that the boy was developing normally and was generally in good physical condition. The child was doing well in the first grade and was a leader among his peers.

Voice tests indicated the child's voice was hoarse in a severe degree (rated 6) with the conversational voice generally dysphonic and at times aphonic especially at the ends of breath groups. There was no hoarseness on sustained vowels when the voice was pitched 2 to 3 semitones below the modal level. A psycho-

1. I KNOW THE RULE ABOUT THE CORRECT PITCH FOR MY VOICE.   _____
2. I CAN TELL WHEN OTHER PEOPLE USE TOO-HIGH AND TOO-LOW
   PITCHED VOICES.   _____
3. I CAN TELL WHEN OTHER PEOPLE USE CORRECT PITCH.   _____
4. I CAN TELL WHEN I USE INCORRECT PITCH.   _____
5. I CAN TELL WHEN I USE CORRECT PITCH.   _____
6. I KNOW THE PLACES WHERE I USE INCORRECT PITCH.   _____
7. I KNOW THE PLACES WHERE I USE CORRECT PITCH.   _____
8. I CAN TALK WITH CORRECT PITCH *SOME* OF THE TIME.   _____
9. I CAN TALK WITH CORRECT PITCH *MOST* OF THE TIME.   _____
10. I CAN TALK WITH CORRECT PITCH *ALL* THE TIME.   _____

Fig. 38. Pitch.

logical evaluation revealed a child with adequate social adjustment and average intelligence.

The laryngologist and the speech pathologist conferred on the case, and it was decided to give the child voice training for a period of 3 months. Accordingly, the child was seen for 17 sessions. The objectives of voice therapy included: (1) lowering the modal pitch level of the voice, (2) reducing the amount of loud talking and yelling done in a high pitch, and (3) eliminating the hoarse voice quality. After 3 months of training by the speech pathologist the second laryngeal examination revealed a significant reduction of the nodules beyond that expected under normal procedures without voice therapy. Voice training was continued for an additional nine sessions over a period of 4 months. At the conclusion of these sessions vocal abuse was modified, the modal pitch level was lower, and the voice practically free from hoarseness. A third laryngeal examination at this time indicated the nodules were no larger than a pinhead. The child was placed on a bimonthly voice check with the speech pathologist. A fourth laryngeal examination 14 months after the initial one revealed that the nodules were no longer present. The voice was clear, the lower pitch level was being used, and subsequent rechecks by the speech pathologist over a period of 3 years indicated the child was free from any symptoms of hoarseness (adapted from Wilson (1962b)).

Disturbed Mutation of the Voice

The speech pathologist will find cases of delayed or partial mutation and mutational falsetto voice in teenage boys. Very infrequently boys have precocious vocal mutation, that is, sexual maturity with a low-pitched voice beginning before age 8 (Luchsinger, 1965, p. 197). Perverse mutation is also infrequent, that is, when the female voice changes into an abnormally low-pitched voice upon puberty. The speech pathologist should be prepared to handle all types of disturbed mutation. Phillips (1975, pp. 101–102) suggested that teachers should give special consideration to boys undergoing voice change. Teachers should be patient and sympathetic and should avoid placing them in embarrassing situations. Singing should be discouraged

and they should not be encouraged to maintain their little boy voices.

Treatment should be instituted for mutational falsetto when boys are in their teens or at the latest in their early twenties, because if the falsetto voice persists there may be some atrophy of the vocal muscles because of disuse (Weiss, 1950). Greene (1972, p. 227) stated treatment is most successful with teenage boys and also with men in their early twenties. However, Greene stated, it is less successful with older men, and most difficult in those with incomplete mutation. Aronson (1973, p. 61), in discussing psychogenic voice disorders‡ stated that not all high-pitched voices are mutational falsettos since a person may have a structurally small larynx. Mutational or structural causes cannot be distinguished by the sound of the voice. An effective test for mutational falsetto is to ask the person to breathe in deeply and say a vowel or cough with an abrupt glottal attack. In a mutational falsetto there will be an extensive downward break in pitch, but this does not occur in a person with a structurally small larynx. Anderson and Newby (1973, p. 277) also suggested having the adolescent clear his throat or sigh audibly. If these are done at a lower pitch, the sound produced can be held and merged into vowels such as /ɑ/ or /o/ and then immediately into isolated words on the new pitch level. We suggest recording this procedure so the adolescent can hear his use of lower pitch. Sometimes the boy can sing down the scale and reach a lower register with ease (Greene, 1972, p. 227). Anderson and Newby (1973, pp. 276–277) suggested a count-down technique. We use the rocket blast-off technique, having the boy start with 10 on a very high pitch, lowering the pitch on each count. Anderson and Newby suggested the counting should be vigorous. The speech pathologist reinforces the vocal and auditory aspects by counting with the boy while raising his hand on "ten" and lowering it downward with each count. Often a boy will reach the desired pitch level as he ends the count-down. This new level can be identified, practiced, and stabilized.

Greene (1972, p. 226) stated in boys who have not undergone the usual voice change to a lower pitch, the larynx is generally pulled up high and the throat musculature may be

‡ Audiotapes and manual on psychogenic voice disorders by A. E. Aronson are available from W. B. Saunders Co., W. Washington Square, Philadelphia, PA 19105.

noticeably tense. Some boys, Aronson (1973, p. 61) stated, who have shallow breathing and low infraglottal pressure have difficulty getting full vocal cord vibrations. Full vibrations can be obtained if the speech pathologist manually pulls the larynx down to a lower position in the neck.

We suggest the following sequence for determining if a lower larynx position results in a lower pitched voice. We teach the person relaxation concentrating on specific relaxation of the neck, laryngeal area, shoulders, and arms. We then firmly but gently do one or more of the following maneuvers as suggested by Aronson (1973, p. 61): (1) Tell the boy to extend his head backward and open his mouth widely. (2) The speech pathologist works the thumb and middle finger between the thyroid cartilage and hyoid bone and then exerts a firm pull downward on the body of the larynx. (3) While the larynx is held in a lowered position have the boy say a vowel or cough with an abrupt glottal attack.

The speech pathologist can begin a program to change the modal pitch level in a teenager if the laryngologist's examination reveals normal laryngeal structures and general normal functioning. Hoarseness and vocal strain and shallow breathing are frequent (Greene, 1972, pp. 226–227). Thus voice therapy is also indicated when laryngeal irritation is felt to be due to disturbed mutation. Psychotherapy should be synchronized with voice therapy when indicated. Aronson (1973, p. 63) described three main objectives of voice therapy for mutational falsetto. (1) Teach the boy to phonate at a low pitch by showing him how to use his phonatory and respiratory musculature to its full capacity. (2) Demonstrate that the new low-pitched voice is to be used and the old high voice is to be avoided. (3) The speech pathologist should see that the boy is comfortable with his newly acquired voice through encouragement and should help him use his new voice in nucleus situations.

Voice therapy for delayed or partial mutation or a persistent falsetto voice follows the general outline of voice therapy procedures. We first give the youth a structured program of listening training. This follows the three major steps of listening training, awareness of differences, gross discrimination, and fine discrimination of differences in others. When discrimination between the high pitch and the desired lower pitch has been established, the young man can be taught to produce the

lower pitch level voluntarily (Bryngelson, 1954). We make sure he is aware of his own incorrect pitch levels through tape recordings of his voice compared to recordings of the desired pitch levels.

Then we teach him to produce a correct pitch level. This usually can be done quite quickly in only a few sessions, sometimes in the first session. The adolescent can often be taught a new lower pitch by having him imitate the lower pitch of a male speech pathologist; it is sometimes useful to amplify the speech pathologist's voice by funneling it directly into the boy's ear (Bryngelson, 1954). Another method of obtaining normal pitch and quality of voice in cases of falsetto voice is to have the boy first produce a vocal fry in isolation and then in softly spoken speech (Anonymous, 1964b). Luchsinger (1965, p. 196) described a useful method. The boy is instructed to hum a sustained tone. The speech pathologist presses the thyroid cartilage inward and downward. The pressing inward relieves excessive contraction of the cricothyroid muscle. A low-pitched voice emerges almost automatically. Then the boy is taught to lower the pitch voluntarily without touching the larynx.

Cooper (1977, p. 27) stated a good way to find correct pitch level is to have the boy say *um-hum* in a spontaneous and sincere way with an upward inflection as if agreeing with someone. When done correctly a tingle or buzz about the lips or around the bridge of the nose should be felt by the boy. Also Cooper suggested having the person say *hello* several times in the same manner as *um-hum* in a slightly louder voice.

Greene (1972, pp. 229–230) suggested the following exercises to obtain lower pitch:

1. Have the person drop his head forward, keeping the neck and shoulders relaxed. Have him place his thumb and forefinger on either side of his thyroid alae to make sure the larynx does not elevate upon phonation of *hmm*.

2. Have the person hold his arms out sideways from the body in a horizontal position and then drop the arms to his sides as he vocalizes various vowels.

3. Have the person breathe in deeply two or three times and then have him vocalize on a deep sigh. He should keep as relaxed as possible.

4. Ask the person to sit with his knees apart and drop the upper part of his body forward between his knees as he says vowels.

5. Have the person stand with feet apart and bend over with the arms swinging loosely. Have him vocalize on a grunt as the speech pathologist pushes down on the shoulders.

Anderson and Newby (1973, p. 277) suggested having the person begin on a pitch level that is easy to produce, probably around middle C, and have him sustain various vowels such as /ɑ/ or /o/. Work gradually down the musical scale in sung vowel tones until the quality deteriorates. Start again at middle C and with repeated trials the range can be lowered to a point that represents the basal pitch level. From this level the optimum pitch can be calculated. We suggest using Fairbanks' (1960, Chapter 11) method and verifying the results according to pitch norms.

When the boy can produce the desired pitch we work to establish this pitch level. We introduce negative practice by having the boy produce his old high pitch and contrast it to the new low pitch. When he can do this we ask him to experiment with three levels of pitch, too high, correct, and too low. Bryngelson (1954) suggested the following steps in establishing the use of the desired pitch level in adolescents. Practice reading aloud under supervision with the speech pathologist restimulating the new lower pitch when necessary. Then proceed to nucleus situations where the new lower pitch is used for only a few sentences beginning with very short sentences. Then the boy is asked to use his new low pitch in social situations. Then he may be asked to do limited negative practice outside the clinic to gain voluntary control over the undesirable high pitch level. Soon he can be asked to tabulate the number of times the old high pitch level is used in outside situations. Anderson and Newby (1973, p. 278) advised carryover into speaking situations as each new gain is made. Special attention should be paid to the clearness or the quality of the sound at the new pitch level.

Frequently a boy is reluctant to use the new pitch level in outside situations. A marked change in voice can be traumatic to an individual because it may be a surprise both to the individual himself and to his associates (Van Riper and Irwin, 1958, p. 229). This type of patient, as well as his mother, first rejects the new low voice and persuasion may be necessary for permanent carryover (Luchsinger, 1965, pp. 196–197). If there is too much resistance psychotherapy should accompany voice therapy (Luchsinger, 1965, p. 197; Weiss, 1950). In some individuals abnormally high pitch and excessive loudness may be associated with emotional conflicts. Treatment may require psychological counseling as the speech pathologist directs conscious control of phonation (Aronson, 1973, p. 19).

Pitch Breaks

Both boys and girls are apt to go through a period during mutation characterized by many voice breaks. After this problem has been evaluated by the laryngologist and the speech pathologist a program of voice therapy is planned. An adolescent should not strain his voice during the period of voice change. He should follow good voice hygiene principles by avoiding vocal abuse and vocal misuse. Van Riper (1972, p. 151) stated control of pitch breaks can be taught fairly easily. He suggested the use of negative practice through deliberately practicing the pitch breaks. This helps make the youngster feel less self conscious about pitch breaks. The youth should be cautioned against developing tension in the laryngeal area in an attempt to avoid pitch breaks. If laryngeal tension is present the speech pathologist may need to follow some of the suggestions for achieving balanced muscular tonus (Ch. 8).

The principles we wish to emphasize regarding treatment of falsetto voice are best illustrated by the following case history.

Kevin was referred to us by his high school public speaking teacher during his junior year in high school. He was 17 years of age, a tall, slender, masculine-appearing young man, one of the top basketball players in high school. The basketball coach was preparing him for his senior year when he was expected to bring state honors to the high school basketball team. In a preliminary interview we found his modal pitch level was approximately 280 Hz when talking with normal loudness. During louder talking his pitch level went up to over 300 Hz. He reported he had not experienced any type of voice change during puberty and he was now becoming concerned about his voice. He stated he was occasionally teased about his high-pitched voice but since he was well known in the school it was generally accepted. He stated his most embarrassing times occurred when he answered the telephone and the caller thought he was a girl. He readily admitted one of the reasons he concentrated on athletics was in an effort to express his masculinity. Kevin reported he dated frequently, attending most of the social functions at the school with his steady girl friend. We requested a laryngological consultation. The laryngologist assured us all laryngeal structures were of normal size and function. The school physician assured us of Kevin's normal physical maturation and secondary sex characteristics. Psychological testing by the school psychologist included intelligence tests and various projective techniques. The test results were summarized by the school psychologist as follows: above average intelligence, a normal heterosexual adolescent without any deviant personality patterns. The psychologist noted strivings to prove himself to be masculine, probably mainly as compensation for his high-pitched voice. Following these tests the laryngologist, school physician, psychologist, and speech pathologist met to discuss the results of the tests and to formulate a treatment program for Kevin. The group felt if the modal pitch level of this adolescent could be lowered through voice therapy most of his problems would be solved. Voice therapy was recommended three times a week for half hour sessions. During the first voice therapy session through singing and experimenting with various pitch levels good vocal tones were isolated at approximately 135 Hz. During the next three sessions the new low pitch was used on nonsense syllables, words, phrases, and sentences. During the fifth session Kevin conversed with the speech pathologist in his new low pitch. Kevin was reluctant to try his new voice outside the clinic so we planned a gradual habituation program. We began carryover by having Kevin use his new low voice while making phone calls from the clinic room to stores and other places where he was not known. Kevin was particularly reluctant to use his new voice at home. With his permission we talked with his parents to arrange situations so he could use his new low voice without surprise from them or his

brother and sister. Kevin described his therapy experiences to them using his new voice. We devised a situation in Kevin's speech class where he could give a talk about his voice therapy program; this was appropriate because the general topic under discussion was personal improvement of speaking habits. As he began his speech he was to use his old high pitch level and as he explained the various techniques we had used he planned to demonstrate how he first lowered his pitch on an isolated vowel. He planned to increase his use of the new pitch level during his speech so that by the time he finished talking he was using his new low pitch continuously. Kevin came to the clinic after class to report on his speech and used his new low pitch to the clinic secretary before he came into our office. He had completely sold the class on his new voice. Fortunately several members of the basketball team were in the class so at basketball practice that afternoon he felt comfortable about using his new low pitch. We saw Kevin every other week for 3 months and then for an occasional check-up during the rest of his high school career. His new low voice became permanent.

CONTROLLED RATE OF SPEAKING

Many children with laryngeal dysfunction have problems in the rate of speaking. They may speak too rapidly or too slowly. Incorrect rate of speaking does not in itself constitute a problem in voice use, although a rapid rate may interfere with teaching correct use of pitch and loudness and usually makes control of vocal abuses difficult. Rate may be related to hypertensive or hypotensive manners of speaking, as children with vocal hyperfunction characteristically talk too rapidly while those with hypofunction usually talk too slowly. A rate problem also exists if there is lack of variation in rate or if staccato speech interferes with good voice production (West and Ansberry, 1968, p. 278). It is difficult to detect and change traumatic and damaging voice habits in a child who talks too fast; this is especially true if he uses abrupt glottal attacks along with a rapid, staccato style (Wilson, 1966). Often attention to problems of voice such as loudness and pitch will bring about normalization of rate of speaking.

However, it may be necessary to work directly on normalizing rate.

Therapy for Rate

When a child's rate has been judged to be too rapid he must first be made aware of his rapid rate by listening to tape recordings of his speech and comparing his recordings with pretaped samples of slow, average, and fast rates. Then his rate of speaking can be reduced to a desirable pace through oral reading and speaking exercises which stress suitable rate, correct use of pauses, and good vocal inflections (Wilson, 1966). Rate can be reduced by using correct duration of sounds in words (Strother, 1942, p. 225) and using adequate phrasing and smoothness (Pronovost and Kingman, 1959, p. 111). Rate may also be reduced by increasing pause time between words, phrases, and sentences (Strother, 1942, p. 225).

Inefficient breathing patterns may cause rate problems. Curtis (1967, pp. 217–218) noted that breathing exercises in themselves need not be used for most cases, but if there is insufficient breath for phrases of normal length, corrective drills and exercises can be used to lengthen phonation time in talking without the necessity of stopping to inhale frequently. This training makes certain a child has adequate breath reserve for good voice and gives a child the secure feeling of having sufficient air for talking (Hauth, 1961).

A study was made of the speaking rate of a group of children aged 5 to 7 (Salzinger, Salzinger, Portnoy, Eckman, Bacon, Deutsch, and Zubin, 1962). A clown head made of papier mâché with a red light for a nose was used as the reinforcing apparatus. The children were told to talk to the clown to make him happy and his nose would light up. This caused the rate of the children's speech to increase. If we wish to reduce a child's rapid rate of speaking we can reverse this process. That is, the clown would be unhappy with a rapid rate and would turn off the red light. A slower rate would be reinforced by turning on the light. A simple device like this could be used with the speech pathologist operating a hidden switch.

The speaking rate chart (Fig. 39) is used in a fashion similar to other voice charts using the 10 step outline. The child is taught the rule about proper rate (Step 1). He learns to identify too-slow or too-fast rate in others (Step 2) and when others use correct rate (Step 3). He knows when his rate is too slow or too fast (Step 4) and he knows the correct rate for himself (Step 5). He knows the places where his rate is incorrect (Step 6) and where it is correct (Step 7). Carryover from partial to complete habituation follows (Steps 8, 9, and 10). Action pictures are placed in the child's notebook. He is asked to tell stories about them as he practices slow, fast, and correct rate of talking. For example, he can tell a story about the dog (Fig. 40) varying his rate according to the picture being described.

Practice in talking rapidly and slowly is useful in obtaining rate control. Hanley and Thurman (1970, Ch. 7) suggested using the symbol ⊢⊣ before a sentence or phrase that should be read quickly and ⊢——⊣ to indicate a slower rate. The speech pathologist can choose sentences and stories and use these symbols to teach children rate control:

⊢⊣ Give me a cookie.
⊢————⊣ Thank you for the candy.
⊢————⊣ I like soup and sandwiches.
⊢⊣ I want a dime.

Paragraphs can be marked the same way.

⊢————⊣ On the way home ⊢⊣ Bob slipped and fell. ⊢————⊣ He spilled grape

1. I KNOW THE RULE ABOUT MY RATE OF TALKING. _____
2. I CAN TELL WHEN OTHER PEOPLE'S SPEECH IS TOO SLOW OR TOO FAST. _____
3. I CAN TELL WHEN OTHER PEOPLE USE A CORRECT RATE. _____
4. I CAN TELL WHEN MY SPEECH IS TOO SLOW OR TOO FAST. _____
5. I KNOW WHEN THE RATE OF MY SPEECH IS CORRECT. _____
6. I KNOW THE PLACES WHERE MY SPEECH IS TOO SLOW OR TOO FAST. _____
7. I KNOW THE PLACES WHERE THE RATE OF MY SPEECH IS CORRECT. _____
8. I CAN TALK WITH THE CORRECT RATE *SOME* OF THE TIME. _____
9. I CAN TALK WITH THE CORRECT RATE *MOST* OF THE TIME. _____
10. I CAN TALK WITH THE CORRECT RATE *ALL* THE TIME. _____

Fig. 39. Speaking rate.

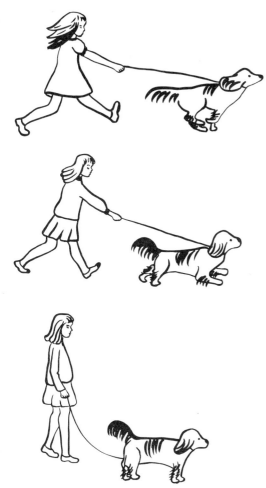

Fig. 40. Rate practice representing three levels—too fast, correct, too slow. Illustration by Geraldine Balsam.

soda ⊢—⊣ all over his shirt. ⊢———⊣ Mary laughed and laughed. ⊢———⊣ Bob said ⊢—⊣ "I couldn't help it. ⊢———⊣ I think you pushed me."

Eisenson and Ogilvie (1977, p. 68) stated children often can learn correct rate of speaking if they let the pitch and loudness reflect their feelings. For example, through puppetry or creative dramatics children can play characters representing slow, moderate, and fast speech. The three rate levels can be represented by a sauntering bear, a parading elephant, and a racing horse. Three levels of pitch and loudness can be worked into a skit using pictures to represent the three rates.

The following rate exercises, all based on suggestions by Eisenson and Eisenson (1974, pp. 112–115), are given as samples for the

speech pathologist to use with children needing work on rate control.

1. Read these sentences slowly; read each italicized word even more slowly.

I *like* to drink *soda pop* when I *eat* pizza. *All* the *children* were *very* quiet *during* the *movie*.

2. Read these sentences at a moderate rate; read each italicized word more slowly for emphasis.

The *horse* jumped *over* the *fence* and the *rider* fell *off* and *hurt* his *arm*.
The *boys* and *girls* were playing *hide* and *seek* and *three* came *in* home *free*.

3. Find a short story. Place slash marks (//) where pauses should be made for meaning and correct rate.

Paul and Susan who // lived in Texas // went to visit their uncle. // He lived in Florida // which was a long drive // but they didn't mind // because they had a new car.

Attention to rate is necessary when a child with a voice problem has an inappropriate rate of speaking that interferes with good voice production. Successful control of rate is accomplished following the 10 step voice therapy outline.

PRODUCTION OF A CLEAR VOICE

Obtaining a clear and resonant voice is a major goal in voice therapy for laryngeal dysfunction (Peacher, 1963). Teaching adequate vocal patterns usually begins with the first session and is done concurrently with the elimination of inadequate vocal patterns. That is, as an inadequate pattern is being eliminated it is replaced by an adequate pattern. This rule applies to all vocal rehabilitation procedures except those vocal abuses which must be eliminated when there are no suitable modifications or substitutes.

Eliminating vocal abuses, teaching the proper use of pitch and loudness, establishing balanced muscular tonus, and controlling rate of speaking often result in a clear laryngeal tone with balanced oral and nasal resonance. With some children, however, additional procedures may be necessary to develop a voice free from the undesirable laryngeal characteristics. A clear voice chart (Fig. 41) can be placed in the child's notebook to keep track of his progress in improving quality. This chart is used in the same manner as the charts previously presented following the 10 steps of the voice therapy outline.

The rules about a clear voice are explained and demonstrated. The speech pathologist describes the characteristics of a clear laryngeal tone and presents audiorecordings of clear voices (Step 1). The child is told he must learn to recognize deviant and clear voices in others (Steps 2 and 3). He is next taught the auditory features of his voice so he can *hear* his own deviant voice (Step 4). He is then shown how to produce a clear voice and learns the auditory features of his improved voice (Step 5). Now he is ready to learn the kinesthetic features of his deviant voice (Step 6) and of his clear voice (Step 7). Lastly, he is guided through the habituation steps of using a clear voice some, most, and all the time (Steps 8, 9, 10). A concentrated program of listening training is necessary before direct methods to improve voice are approached.

Listening Training for Improved Laryngeal Tone

To begin listening training, awareness of laryngeal tone deviations in others is approached. The child indicates when the speech pathologist produces sounds with excessive breathiness, harshness, or hoarseness. Next comes gross discrimination of differences. A principal technique for this is the cloudy-clear game. The top half of a page of the child's notebook is designated the "cloudy" part and the bottom half the "clear" part. Related pictures are pasted on the two halves. For example, a picture of a cloudy sky is placed on the top half and described by the speech pathologist in a voice that is an imitation of the child's deviant voice, and a picture of a sunny day on the clear half is described in a voice free from deviancy. The child is asked to point to the picture indicated by the quality being used by the speech pathologist. When the child can identify the presence of both clear and deviant laryngeal tones produced by the speech pathologist he is ready for fine discrimination of differences. Pictures of the three palm trees (Fig. 42) can be used for this training. The pictures are labelled "clear," "rough," and "very rough." The child designates the quality being used by the speech pathologist by pointing to the correct picture. He is rewarded by having stickers placed on Steps 2 and 3 of the Clear Voice Chart.

An important adjunct in the listening training of children is to have them listen and judge their own performance from recordings. Samples obtained during the examination can be used. The child listens to these recordings which contain samples of sounds or words, some of which have clear laryngeal tones and some defective laryngeal tones. The child points to the picture of the palm tree represented by each of his own taped samples. Tabulations in the notebook on a 3 point scale are used for older children and teen-

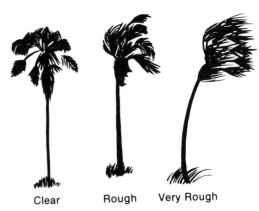

Clear   Rough   Very Rough

Fig. 42. Clear voice practice. Illustration by Geraldine Balsam.

---

1. I KNOW THE RULE ABOUT USING A CLEAR VOICE.
2. I CAN TELL WHEN OTHER PEOPLE HAVE BREATHY/TIGHT VOICES.
3. I CAN TELL WHEN OTHER PEOPLE USE A CLEAR VOICE.
4. I CAN *HEAR* BREATHINESS/TIGHTNESS IN MY VOICE.
5. I CAN *HEAR* WHEN I USE A CLEAR VOICE.
6. I CAN *FEEL* BREATHINESS/TIGHTNESS IN MY VOICE.
7. I KNOW HOW IT *FEELS* WHEN I TALK WITH A CLEAR VOICE.
8. I CAN TALK WITH A CLEAR VOICE *SOME* OF THE TIME.
9. I CAN TALK WITH A CLEAR VOICE *MOST* OF THE TIME.
10. I CAN TALK WITH A CLEAR VOICE *ALL* THE TIME.

Fig. 41. Clear voice.

agers as they listen to their own recordings, with *1* representing clear voice, *2* rough voice, and *3* very rough voice. When the child correctly identifies the occurrence of deviant and clear quality he is rewarded for Steps 4 and 5 on the chart. When listening training is well under way the child is ready to be taught to produce a better voice.

In teaching correct voice use the basic steps of listening training are used. Here, however, the child is the performer and the speech pathologist the listener and judge. Production of correct voice follows three steps. (1) Awareness of the deviation in his own voice: The child is taught to recognize his own incorrect use of a specific voice parameter. (2) Gross discrimination of differences in his own voice: He is asked to produce two levels of the voice characteristic, the correct and incorrect. (3) Fine discrimination of differences in his own voice: He produces three levels of the specific voice parameter.

The problem of hoarseness is used to illustrate these three steps. (1) To develop awareness of the deviation in his own voice the child listens to tape recordings of his own production of vowels. The speech pathologist uses a random arrangement of hoarse and clear vowels selected from the diagnostic tests. The child signals each time he hears a hoarse vowel and is rewarded appropriately. (2) The child then progresses to the next step, gross discrimination of differences. Here he produces vowels or words containing the old hoarse quality and contrasts them with his best approximation to the desired quality. The speech pathologist selects vowels on which the child can achieve some success for initial practice. These productions can be tape recorded on language master cards and the child can stack the cards into the piles representing his two types of production. (3) The child next proceeds to fine discrimination in his own voice using three degrees of hoarseness, his old faulty hoarse voice, an intermediate amount of hoarseness, and his closest approximation to clear voice. These, too, may be recorded on tape or language master cards. If the child experiences difficulty producing intermediate stages of this defective quality, the speech pathologist may prefer not to have the child spend much time on discrimination of fine differences in his own voice. It may be more productive to spend time teaching the child correct production rather than an intermediate stage. However, using several

levels of quality in his own voice may serve a useful purpose when it does not present difficulties.

Locating a Satisfactory Tone

Special techniques are necessary to discover good tones in some children. Voice scanning techniques described by Van Riper and Irwin (1958, p. 286) are useful as a basis for teaching improvement of voice. They suggested finding the child's new voice by having him go through the whole repertoire of possible phonations to locate the desired tones. Good vocalization can usually be found by varying loudness or pitch levels on vowels or words. Van Riper (1972, pp. 163–164) stated when a person can identify his deviant voice and vary it, the speech pathologist helps him locate and stabilize a new vocal tone. Van Riper compared this procedure with learning target shooting, in that the child may miss the new vocal tone more than hitting it. A child must be shown new patterns of muscular contractions and laryngeal and pharyngeal functions. The speech pathologist constantly informs the child about the accuracy of his efforts.

After the child has found an acceptable voice he then is taught the auditory and kinesthetic images of this voice. When he has learned the kinesthetic sensations of deviant and clear voice production he continues through Steps 6 and 7 of the Clear Voice Chart. It is usually necessary to use progressive approximations to obtain a better voice with the person being encouraged as he more closely approximates the desired voice (Van Riper, 1972, p. 164). Cooper (1973, p. 74) suggested that clear tones can be obtained and at the appropriate pitch level through the use of his *um-hum* technique. Have the child repeat *um-hum* easily and effortlessly as though agreeing with someone and a good voice emerges. Cooper (1977, p. 27) stated proper tone focus is thus obtained and the child should feel a tingle or buzz about the lips or around the bridge of the nose. Cooper also suggested having a person say *hello* spontaneously several times to obtain the same result.

In some cases a good tone or quality is not found in the repertoire of a child's productions, so special techniques are used to locate a satisfactory tone. A method we use for finding a good tone is as follows:

1. Have the child assume a good standing

posture where he is at ease, perhaps against a wall where he has some support.

2. Have the child breathe through his nose, the speech pathologist places a finger above the larynx.

3. Have the child sustain a good /m/. The tone should come through the nose with good resonance and with the throat open and relaxed. The larynx should not move upward; the neck muscles in particular should be relaxed.

4. The child initiates a good /m/ in this manner at various pitch levels.

5. Have the child phonate a good /m/ as in No. 3 above with his throat open, being sure there is no upward movement of the larynx and that the neck muscles are relaxed. Without interrupting phonation have the child open his mouth to produce the sound /ɑ/. The sound should be soft at first and then gradually increased in loudness with repeated production. Practice all the vowels in this manner. When a satisfactory tone is isolated, it is tape recorded immediately so the child can identify its desirable characteristics.

6. The acceptable vowels are combined with other initial consonants for syllable drill and then practiced in nonsense syllables where consonants both precede and follow the vowel. Exercises using words, phrases, and sentences follow. During these exercises emphasis should be placed on clarity of sounds, correct pitch placement, adequate loudness, and good resonance.

McClosky (1977, pp. 143–144) suggested four exercises for locating good tone. (1) Have the child assume proper posture. Be sure his throat and jaw muscles are relaxed. Have him take in a short breath, starting out on a high-pitched, breathy sound (e.g. /ɑ/) inflecting downward as on a sigh. (2) Have him do the same on a downward inflection and when he reaches his optimum pitch level have him bring his lips together easily to produce /m/ then /ɑ/, and repeat /mɑ/ at this pitch level—/mɑ, mɑ/. (3) Do the same exercise but change the vowel so it sounds like /mɑ/, /mi/, /mo/, /mu/. (4) Have the child start with a high pitch and descend to his optimum pitch level and at this level have him prolong vowels. We feel this should be a good exercise for locating tones by placing emphasis on good posture, proper breathing, and relaxation. With all these things working for a child the likelihood of producing good

clear tones free from laryngeal disturbance should be possible. These exercises should be recorded so the clear tones can be identified by the child.

Breathiness may present a special problem in modification. Eisenson and Ogilvie (1977, p. 321) suggested having the child become aware of the difference between a breathy and a normal voice quality by having him place his hand in front of his mouth while saying sentences with all voiced sounds, such as "My bunny's name is Lanny." There should be only a minimum of breath felt on the hand. For contrast have the child say sentences with stops and fricatives, such as "Polly likes to eat thin crackers" with the hand placed where it will be struck by the breath. Eisenson and Ogilvie also suggested having the child say a vowel such as /i/, which is a relatively tense and high pitched vowel and likely to have little breathiness.

Production of improved quality by the child can be based on imitation if it is done under expert guidance and a good voice is selected as the ideal (Perkins, 1957, p. 874). For example, a binaural amplifier can be used with the child's voice fed into one of his ears and the speech pathologist's voice into the other ear or both voices into the same ear.§ Van Riper (1959) stated the speech pathologist can begin blending his voice to match that of the child, speaking in unison, repeating words or sentences several times. The speech pathologist then gradually modifies the stimulation, introducing variations toward the desired pitch or voice quality. When this is done correctly the child follows the slight gradations until a more normal voice results. As a result of using these techniques some children are able to produce good tones free from laryngeal deviations. With other children we are able to obtain improved tones which need additional attention.

Teaching adequate stress on words, Scholl (1961) suggested, improves voice quality and eliminates forced tones. He suggested having the child sing to obtain a continuous flow of phonation being sure he uses an appropriate pitch level and firm articulation. Also he recommended attention be paid to lengthening and strengthening voiced continuant consonants such as /z/, /v/, and /l/; sometimes prolonging or giving due phonation time to

§ Binaural Speech Trainer, HC Electronics, Inc., Mill Valley, CA 94941.

these types of consonant sounds eliminates breathiness and harshness. Canfield (1964) suggested these sounds should be sustained for two rhythmic beats or counts as a person talks to obtain better and stronger phonation. Also, he stated, when this added time is given to the voiced continuant consonant sounds the articulators develop more tonicity and sounds become clearer as well as more accurate. Emphasis should be placed on obtaining an easy voice production that is free from strain and excessive loudness. This can be aided by having the child take an easy breath and use an easy voice, making sure that an adequate breath supply is maintained while talking (Baynes, 1967).

In some instances negative practice helps a child produce an improved voice. For example, in the case of hoarseness the child listens as the speech pathologist demonstrates both desirable quality and hoarseness on vowels, words, and phrases. The hoarseness does not necessarily have to be an exact imitation of the child's hoarseness but should approximate it. The child is then asked to repeat the same vocalizations alternating his usual hoarse quality with as clear a voice as possible. This is recorded and played back on a tape recorder and the child is requested to evaluate the success of his attempts at producing a clear voice.

We should pay attention to the excessive dropping of the mandible in speaking. In a radiographic study Shelton and Bosma (1962) found when their subjects had a wide opening of the mouth the tongue was quite consistently humped and the pharyngeal airway was reduced in some subjects. In studying the pharyngeal airway with various head positions they found a wide opening of the mouth produced the greatest airway reduction. In contrast they found while a lax opening of the mouth resulted in some reduction of the pharyngeal diameter this was less extensive than during the wide mouth opening. With a lax opening tongue humping was not observed. They found the dorsal portion of the tongue is apparently the " . . . key mobile pharyngeal element in airway regulation. Its strategic role is indicated by the multiplicity of its function. It regulates the airway in the mesiopharynx and in the laryngeal vestibule, and it rises to approximate the soft palate."

Canfield (1964) stated that excessive or wide excursions of the jaw add to reduced tongue tip activity which results in poor voice

quality. To increase tongue tip activity for improved voice quality he recommended the person be told to hold his upper and lower teeth lightly together during practice periods, thus forcing the tongue to move more. He stated attention to precision of articulation during this type of practice will result in better oral, nasal, and pharyngeal resonance. Thus if we say to a person, "Open your mouth more" or "Move your jaw more" we may be promoting inadequate tongue tip activity and a reduction of the pharyngeal airway. This may result in poor articulation and poor voice quality. We should be very cautious in giving these commands unless the child actually has an inadequate mouth opening and little jaw movement.

Carryover is sometimes difficult in establishing permanent use of good voice habits. A child may have difficulty making use of new voice patterns because he is accustomed to his old way of talking and the new voice sounds and feels strange to him. However, practice in using new vocal patterns gradually adjusts him to his new voice. Steps 8, 9, and 10 on the voice chart are used as the child progresses from partial to complete use of his new voice.

SPECIAL PROBLEMS

Incipient Spastic Dysphonia

Incipient, beginning spastic dysphonia affects the voice in subtle ways and is a mild form of advanced spastic dysphonia. It will be easier to describe incipient spastic dysphonia if we first describe advanced spastic dysphonia.

Aronson (1973, pp. 42–51) classified spastic dysphonia as a conversion phenomenon of two main types, adductor and abductor. He stated (1973, p. 44) in a severe form of adductor spastic dysphonia both the true cords and the ventricular bands hyperadduct, but in the milder form only the true cords hyperadduct. Inappropriate vocal cord movements and adductor spasms may be noted during laryngeal examinations, with the spasms being intermittent and nonregular (Rabuzzi and McCall, 1972). In the abductor type of conversion spastic dysphonia a sudden widening of the glottis occurs as a person phonates, resulting in a stoppage of vocal cord vibration (Aronson, 1973, p. 50). Both types of spastic dysphonia, adductor and abductor, may be present in any one person

(Aronson, 1973, p. 50). The laryngeal examination is negative, revealing essentially normal laryngeal structures (Aronson, 1973, p. 44; Rabuzzi and McCall, 1972). Dedo (1976) stated advanced spastic dysphonia usually begins after age 40, but in his series one of his patients was in her twenties.

The main voice feature of advanced adductor spastic dysphonia, according to Aronson (1973, p. 44), is a choppiness of phonation caused by the intermittent hyperadduction of the cords. The abductor type is characterized by moments of sudden aphonia or excess breathiness (Aronson, 1973, p. 50). According to Rabuzzi and McCall (1972) the features are harshness, a low modal pitch level, monotonous use of pitch, noticeable tremors, and intermittent strain and voice stoppages.

Incipient spastic dysphonia characteristics are similar to those found in advanced spastic dysphonia, except the symptoms are present in a mild or moderate degree. Over the years we have seen teenagers with symptoms of early spastic dysphonia. The symptoms characteristically include moderate stridency, harshness, breathiness, and a slight vocal tremor. Usually there are no instances of sudden aphonia. The laryngoscopic examination is usually negative, but vocal cord spasms may be observed. Aronson (1973, p. 44) noted that in its beginning stages spastic dysphonia often first appears as a nonspecific hoarseness. Cooper (1973, p. 172) stated the symptoms of incipient spastic dysphonia are less severe, occur less frequently, and disturb the person less than the advanced stage. The characteristics of incipient spastic dysphonia depend on whether it is the adductor or abductor type. Stridency and constriction are symptomatic of the adductor type, and breathiness of the abductor type. In some adolescents with incipient spastic dysphonia we have observed muscle tightening in the neck and elevation of the larynx during phonation. Cooper (1973, p. 173) stated incipient spastic dysphonia may be present in a person for a number of years. Spastic dysphonia may often be misdiagnosed when in an incipient, beginning stage. Brodnitz (1976) stated that no doubt mild cases of spastic dysphonia are not properly labeled. Cooper (1973, pp. 173–174) noted incipient spastic dysphonia is frequently overlooked and misdiagnosed.

Although spastic dysphonia is usually considered a voice problem of adulthood, it has been diagnosed in teenagers. Aronson (1973, p. 50) presented a case of a 16-year-old girl with abductor type spastic dysphonia. Hall and Jerger (1976) described a 15-year-old boy diagnosed as having spastic dysphonia. Our youngest patient with diagnosed incipient spastic dysphonia was a 16-year-old boy. Indirect laryngoscopy on him revealed the typical intermittent and nonregular spasms described by Rabuzzi and McCall (1972). These could be observed first-hand without the aid of stroboscopy. He is our case presentation for this section.

In our experience we have found voice therapy successful if the spastic dysphonia remains in the incipient stage. Therefore, we feel it is important for the speech pathologist to recognize the identifying features of beginning spastic dysphonia. As stated by Cooper (1973, p. 177), prognosis for incipient spastic dysphonia is good to excellent. This is in contrast to the unfavorable prognosis for advanced spastic dysphonia. Dedo (1976) reported voice therapy is usually not successful if advanced spastic dysphonia has been present 3 months or more.

Goals of voice therapy for incipient spastic dysphonia include relaxation procedures, breathing exercises, and procedures designed to promote easy initiation of tone and establish vocal patterns free from tremor. With some adolescents it may be necessary to change their modal pitch level, usually to a somewhat higher level. A new modal pitch level combined with a decrease in loudness often makes easy nontremorous phonation possible. The use of psychotherapy by reciprocal inhibition often counteracts anxiety evoking situations which may contribute to vocal instability.

The following is an example of incipient spastic dysphonia in which early intervention prevented the development of an advanced problem:

> Paul was a 16-year-old boy active in high school theater. He was also in a city theater program for the preparation of professional actors and singers. Long hours of play rehearsal and singing lessons continued week after week. Six weeks before we saw him he began to have periods of hoarseness, especially after long rehearsals. The family physician referred Paul for a head and neck examination. The laryngologist reported the vocal cords moved equally upon

phonation, but spasms were observed which were localized in the area of the junction of the anterior and middle thirds of both cords. A mild inflammatory condition of the vocal cords suggested vocal strain. The diagnosis was incipient spastic dysphonia, adductor type. Paul was referred to us for consultation. Paul's speaking voice was rated essentially normal in laryngeal tone; however, a tremulous characteristic reflected small fluctuations in laryngeal tension. His modal pitch level of 150 Hz indicated voice change was almost complete. Paul reported frequent bouts of hoarseness associated with much talking, play rehearsals, and singing. We analyzed his voice during one of his periods of dysphonia. His laryngeal tone was rated *4*, being characteristically harsh. Laryngeal tension was rated *5*, manifested by increased muscular effort during talking as revealed in his neck and shoulders. Maximum phonation time was essentially normal at 20 sec, but during this task increased vocal tremor was heard. We placed him on a program to reduce the amount of talking for two purposes, first, to reduce the vocal cord inflammation, and second, to restructure his own vocal-auditory feedback. When we saw him it was late spring with the theater season near its end, so it was easy to place him on a restricted talking regimen with a complete "vacation" from singing. He reduced the amount of talking about 50% and after 2 weeks he reported no recurrences of his hoarseness, that his voice sounded clearer to him, and though the voice tremors remained they were less severe. We saw Paul weekly during the summer. Our immediate objective in voice therapy included relaxation procedures, breathing exercises, listening training for voice tremors, and production of voice free from tremor. As soon as clear tones were produced at will, negative practice was used to dramatize the differences between the two productions. Soon Paul had voluntary control of his voice so carryover was started. He reported difficulty in controlling his voice in certain situations, while having no difficulty in others. Following procedures of behavior therapy by reciprocal inhibition, sit-

uations were listed in order of their anxiety evoking character from near 0 on his *suds* scale to those evoking a *sud* level near 100. Paul was soon desensitized to the low anxiety evoking situations so we gradually worked up the *suds* scale until the high anxiety evoking situations were no longer affecting his voice. At the end of the summer Paul was placed on a long-term follow-up schedule. At this point Paul realized the demands of acting and singing on his voice made a career in this field uncertain. He reassessed his vocational goals with his school counselor and took several aptitude tests. He changed his goal to dentistry, a profession in which he had interest and aptitude. We have followed Paul over the years, most recently during his first year of dentistry school. He reported his voice had remained free from hoarseness and tremor. This we could easily verify as he talked with us in an easy relaxed manner with clear laryngeal tone free from tremors.

Hysterical Dysphonia

Hysterical dysphonia, although not common in children and adolescents, occurs frequently enough especially in adolescents so that a section about it is appropriate. Hysterical dysphonia characteristically has a sudden onset where the individual's voice is characterized by excessive breathiness because of inadequate adduction of the vocal cords. In addition to the breathiness, several adolescents we have seen exhibited excessive muscular tension as they attempted to gain fuller phonation. In some a normal voice returned as quickly as it had disappeared. In others, with help from a clinical psychologist or counselor, we have seen a gradual lessening of the dysphonia and a gradual return of full voice.

Goals for the adolescent with hysterical dysphonia include the following: (1) The speech pathologist and the clinical psychologist or counselor help the person resolve emotional problems, especially those problems related to the onset of the dysphonia. Psychotherapy by reciprocal inhibition often is useful in decreasing the anxiety evoking situations related to voice instability. (2) Relaxation procedures and breathing exercises are used to reduce the effort used in speaking and to establish balanced muscular tonus. (3)

Adequate phonation may be regained through chewing exercises when there is hypertension; pushing exercises are appropriate when there is hypotension.

Brodnitz (1969) stated treatment of hysterical aphonia is often difficult but success is possible. His approach to the treatment of hysterical aphonia is as follows: The speech pathologist should aim to obtain a clear phonatory voice in one session. He suggested a slight digital pressure on the larynx to 'steady' the vocal cords may help the person produce a clear tone. The use of pushing exercises often results in clear phonation. With some a slight cough can be prolonged and changed to a lower-pitched /o/ sound. Once samples of clear voice have been obtained negative practice is started immediately. Brodnitz suggested telling the person that everyone has two voices which can be used alternately at will, a tuneless whisper and true phonation. The person is asked to read, constantly switching from a whispered sentence to one in his rediscovered new voice (Brodnitz, 1969).

Here is an example of the effectiveness of voice therapy in hysterical dysphonia, conducted in coordination with psychological counseling:

> Sandy was 17 when she was referred to us by her high school counselor. About 10 days previously, following a quarrel with her parents about coming home late from dates, she had suddenly developed dysphonia. Her voice was constricted (rated 6 on laryngeal tension) and breathy (rated 5 on laryngeal tone). She was dysphonic, but not aphonic, speaking with great effort and tension in her face, neck, and shoulders. She could not understand why she had "lost her voice," but she did wonder if the screaming and crying during the quarrel with her parents had precipitated the problem. A head and neck examination was negative with good vocal cord closure on a high-pitched /i/. Psychological examination revealed a normal girl but one overly sensitive to others' opinion of her. She was especially tense about her relationships with her parents, specifically her father. She felt insecure because her 12-year-old sister obviously was the father's favorite. A program of voice therapy was initiated with Sandy in conjunc-

tion with psychological counseling involving Sandy with the family group: mother, father, and sister. During the first voice therapy session following a 15 min relaxation period clear tones were isolated and audiotaped. Clear voice was produced on isolated vowels, which were then combined with consonants for consonant-vowel (CV) drill. By the end of the session she could say several common phrases without dysphonia. During six 1 hour sessions her dysphonia gradually diminished until her voice was free from tension and breathiness. Counseling was resulting in improved relationships with her family. Just before our seventh appointment the school counselor called to tell us Sandy had not been in school that day; her parents were keeping her home because she had returned from a date at 4 a.m. instead of the agreed 11:30 p.m. It was reported that her voice at breakfast that morning was again dysphonic. Appointments were continued with weekly family counseling and voice therapy sessions resulting both in resolving family problems and improving voice. Within 2 months the major family problems were resolved. Sandy's voice was again normal. We followed Sandy over a period of 2 years. Her voice remained stable and her family relationships were satisfactory.

Ventricular Phonation

Ventricular phonation presents a special problem requiring special techniques. In a very few instances the true cords may be absent or deformed. For these cases ventricular phonation must be continued and this substitute voice should be trained to function as well as possible (Brodnitz, 1971a, pp. 81–82). In cases where the true cords are present with the possibility of normal functioning, the goal of voice therapy is to eliminate the ventricular phonation and transfer this phonatory effort to the true cords. The person should be taught to speak at an optimum pitch and learn to control the laryngeal muscles so true vocal cord vibration can be encouraged and the vibration of the false vocal cords decreased and eliminated (Fred, 1962). Van Riper and Irwin (1958, p. 221) felt that if the speech pathologist regards the problem of ventricular phonation as a respiratory abnormality more success is assured. Sometimes voiced inhalation prior to regular phonation brings the true vocal cords into use. They (1958, p. 221) also have found that initiating tones using a glottal fry helps mobilize the true vocal cords. Children with ventricular dysphonia present on a psychogenic basis respond well to voice therapy especially when it is combined with encouragement and discussions regarding the basis of the disturbance. Progress in this type of problem is slow and it may be necessary to have a period of prolonged supervision in order to prevent recurrences; in severe cases psychiatric consultation should be sought (Brodnitz, 1971a, p. 82).

We have found all these techniques useful in working with cases of ventricular phonation, but one approach we have found most useful is a program of listening training combined with direct teaching of an improved voice. This is illustrated by the following case example (Wilson, 1968):

A physician noticed during a routine physical examination that Susan, 14 years old, had an extremely hoarse voice. This hoarseness had been present consistently since infancy. She was very self conscious and often refused to talk because she was teased about her low hoarse voice quality. The physician referred her to a laryngologist who diagnosed the disorder as dysphonia plicae ventricularis neonatorum—a congenital anomaly in which phonation is accomplished by the ventricular bands instead of the vocal cords (Jackson, 1967, p. 31). A voice evaluation by the speech pathologist revealed the girl could use the vocal cords in phonating several vowel sounds of good quality. These vowels and several hoarse vowels were recorded so the girl could contrast the two qualities. Beginning with this listening training she was taught to use the true vocal cords more and more and to eliminate ventricular phonation. She received voice therapy for 4 months. A laryngeal examination 8 months after the original one revealed adequate action of the vocal cords and elimination of the phonatory movement of the ventricular bands. This child was fortunate in that the true vocal cords were present. When the true cords are absent on a congenital basis a low-pitched and hoarse voice using the false vocal cords may be the maximum that can be obtained.

SUMMARY

Correct use of loudness and pitch is necessary for optimal voice use. Children often have deviations in these parameters which contribute to laryngeal dysfunction and a poor voice. Proper rate of speaking is necessary to avoid voice misuse and to help the child use his voice correctly. Directing a child toward a clear voice free from stridency and breathiness requires the application of a structured listening training program and the use of special procedures to locate and stabilize a clear voice. Problems of incipient spastic dysphonia, hysterical dysphonia, and ventricular phonation, although not common, need special attention when they occur in children and teenagers.

TEN

Voice Therapy for Resonance Problems

This chapter contains a discussion of voice therapy for hypernasality and hyponasality when voice therapy has been recommended as the treatment of choice. Hypernasality may be due to velopharyngeal insufficiency caused by either cleft palate or some other structural, muscular, or nerve disability in the velopharyngeal area; or the problem may be present on a functional basis with a normal velopharyngeal mechanism inefficiently used. Major emphasis will be placed on voice therapy procedures for children with a physical velopharyngeal insufficiency in the presence or absence of an overt cleft palate. These procedures can also be applied to resonance problems with other etiology. Therapy for hyponasality is also presented.

Nasal sounds have been found to constitute approximately 11% of the phonemes in speech, /n/ 6.43%, /m/ 3.16%, and /ŋ/ 1.27% (French, Carter, and Koenig, 1930; Tobias, 1959). We can expect nasal consonants to be present in normal connected speech at an average rate of more than one a second, assuming phonemes are produced at the rate of 10/ sec (Glenn and Kleiner, 1968). Mader (1954) found /n/ was the most frequently occurring consonant sound in the speech of children in Grades 1, 2, and 3. Thus if a child nasalizes some of the oral sounds in addition to the normally nasalized consonants, the impression of hypernasality is indeed marked. Therefore it is important to correct undue hypernasality on non-nasal sounds.

Children respond negatively to severe hypernasality in other children as early as kindergarten age. Blood and Hyman (1977) had kindergarten, first, and second grade children respond to the following five questions after listening to audiotapes of young girls with hypernasality: "1. Did you like the person telling the story? 2. Did you like the way the person talked? 3. Do you think she had trouble talking? 4. Would you like to talk like that person? 5. Do you think she needs some help with her talking?" Negative reactions were shown by the children, such as "She sounds funny" and "She needs speech."

Voice therapy for hypernasality is highly individualized. The speech pathologist must know the specific cause of the hypernasal voice to plan appropriate voice therapy procedures. In many cases therapy is designed to teach the child to compensate for a velopharyngeal insufficiency or other structural anomaly. Shelton, Hahn, and Morris (1968, p. 258) stated that only when physical management is impractical should compensatory therapy be considered. They said, "The decision to initiate voice training when the voice problem is the result, at least in part, of inadequate oral structures, is made according to the same criteria as the decision to provide speech training for an articulation disorder when the deviations are the result of inadequate oral structures." They stated further that if a decision is made to attempt compensatory therapy the goals will be limited in nature and this should be explained to the patient and other involved professional workers. The authors stated the speech pathologist must be alert to any signs of defeatism or frustration on the part of the child, and if these reactions occur the speech pathologist must decide whether to terminate or modify the therapy program. Morris (1972, p. 155) stated trial therapy may be in order for patients with marginal velopharyngeal sufficiency to determine if voice therapy produces positive results.

Greene (1972, p. 270) stated the major emphasis in therapy for a child with cleft palate should be on improving articulation and decreasing hypernasality; also, the speech pathologist should not become obsessed with the idea of treating a disorder of nasal escape.

Throughout the therapy program careful monitoring should be made of oral-nasal resonance balance and nasal emission. Several instruments are available for the speech pathologist to use.*

Improvement of hypernasality is based on structured voice and speech procedures and selected physical exercises. Voice and speech procedures include improving articulation and speech intelligibility and establishing correct oral-nasal resonance balance through a listening training program and special techniques to reduce or eliminate hypernasality. Also, attention is given to loudness, pitch, and rate. Vocal abuse is controlled and facial grimaces and nares constriction eliminated. Physical exercises are designed to develop adequate oral breath pressure and oral air flow. Specific attention is given to muscle exercises, developing correct breath direction, assuring correct breath pressure and muscular tension, and activating lips, tongue, and mandible. Improved velopharyngeal closure may be obtained through observing velar activity, and exercises involving swallowing, sucking, whistling, and blowing.

VOICE AND SPEECH PROCEDURES

Articulation and Speech Intelligibility

According to Van Hattum (1974, p. 330) the greatest improvement in communication in cleft palate individuals comes from improved precision of articulation; this results in improved intelligibility and less perceived hypernasality. Arnold (1965, p. 673) stated the correction of articulation errors reduces nasal emission of sounds and decreases hypernasality. Eisenson and Ogilvie (1977, p. 325) suggested that more precise and energetic articulatory activity results in a lessening of hypernasality. Van Demark (1974a) demonstrated a close relationship between good articulation and satisfactory resonance. He found that children with cleft palate who achieved velopharyngeal closure made greater gains in articulation therapy in fewer sessions than did children who had marginal or inadequate velopharyngeal closure. McWilliams (1954) in studying adults with cleft palate speech found a correlation of 0.720 between intelligibility scores and nasal-

* Florida II, Saber, Inc., Cocoa Beach, FL 32931; Nasal Indicator, Special Instrument, Stockholm, Sweden. United States Distributor: SI America, 255 South 17th Street, Philadelphia, PA 19103; Vega-Speech-O-Meter, Vega Electronics Corporation, Santa Clara, CA 95050; R-D Nasal Manometer, Stell-Will Products, P.O. Box 151, Grand Island, NY 14072.

ity ratings. A correlation of 0.821 was found between consonant articulation errors and nasality ratings.

Activating tongue tip, lip, and mandible movements (Van Riper, 1972, p. 370) and assuring an adequate mouth opening (Moore, 1971a, p. 568) are necessary to improve articulation. Specific exercises and procedures for this are to be found in other sections of this chapter.

All defective sounds should be approached through a well organized program of articulation remediation. The speech pathologist should review the child's performance on the general articulation test, the Iowa Pressure Articulation Test, and the stimulability test. Attention should be given to eliminating hypernasality and nasal emission of consonants, especially /s/, /k/, / ʃ /, /z/, and /g/. Philips (1972, p. 235) stated in improving articulation skills in children with cleft palate the child should be encouraged to use the speech sounds he can produce correctly. Play situations can be built around words containing these sounds and this can give the child a feeling of accomplishment.

Jacobs et al. (1970) stated emphasis in improving articulation in a cleft palate child should be on correct articulatory placement. Focusing on the perceived characteristics of sounds may interfere with improvement of articulation in the child with cleft palate who does not have adequate velopharyngeal valving since he cannot control nasal emission even with correct placement. Philips (1972, p. 235) stated in using placement methods to develop articulation skills, imitation based on both visual and tactile stimulation should be used. After correct placement is achieved a correct production often results. Van Hattum (1974, p. 330) stated tactile and visual approaches to improving articulation in cleft palate speakers are superior to using the auditory channel.

The /k/ and /g/ are especially difficult for a child with velopharyngeal insufficiency; as a result he substitutes a glottal stop. To produce /k/ and /g/ Greene (1972, p. 269) suggested the speech pathologist hold the front of the child's tongue down firmly with a tongue depressor and have the child attempt to say /t/. As he does this the back of the tongue comes up and a good /k/ emerges. Using the same tongue depressor technique, ask the child to attempt to say /d/ and the result will be a good /g/. Shelton et al. (1968,

p. 252) suggested teaching forward placement of the tongue and forward palatal-tongue contact practicing vowel-consonant-vowel (VCV) syllables such as /iki/ and /igi/. Specific attention is necessary to be sure the child is raising the level of tongue carriage. The child can be helped by having him hold the tongue tip lightly against the back of the lower incisors and pressing the body of the tongue upward against the palate. Holding the chin down aids in maintaining a higher level of tongue carriage. With a tongue depressor the speech pathologist can tap the posterior portion of the tongue and the correct spot on the palate to show a child where the physical contacts should be made for good /k/ and /g/ productions. All movements should be made without excessive effort and with light contact.

Fricatives usually need special attention. Shelton et al. (1968, pp. 252–253) suggested a fricative can be taught by emphasizing light, quick constriction of the breath stream with a small and brief amount of oral breath pressure. It should be noted, the authors stated, prolongation of a fricative often only increases nasal emission. Special attention should be paid to the /s/ and /z/. A child can be shown that a light closure of the teeth with a short oral airflow time is sufficient to make the /s/ and /z/ intelligible. Stress should be placed on forward placement for these sounds, avoiding retracting the tongue.

Improving articulation and speech intelligibility hopefully has had a positive effect on decreasing hypernasality. In many children, however, there is enough hypernasality remaining to warrant a direct approach to its elimination. Our program for this is in the following section.

Oral-Nasal Resonance Balance

Improvement in oral-nasal balance is primarily based on an auditory approach using listening training techniques. Visual placement cues as well as tactile and kinesthetic aspects of adequate oral-nasal resonance balance are used. The basic 10 step voice therapy outline applied to resonance (Fig. 43) is followed for eliminating excessive hypernasality in order to establish the proper emphasis or balance of oral-nasal resonance. Applied to resonance, a typical 10 step procedure is as follows: (Step 1) The speech pathologist explains how balanced resonance depends upon an adequate velopharyngeal seal except during production of the nasals /m/, /n/, /ŋ/, with the rule being to use correct resonance balance. Then listening training begins with the child learning to discriminate (Step 2) resonance imbalance in others and (Step 3) resonance balance in others. Then he turns his attention to himself, learning (Step 4) how resonance imbalance *sounds* and *feels* in himself and then learning resonance control by (Step 5) how his voice *sounds* and *feels* when he has resonance balance. The child next discovers (Step 6) the places where he uses resonance imbalance and (Step 7) the places where he uses resonance balance. Carryover then progresses to using adequate resonance balance (Steps 8, 9, and 10) *some, most,* and *all* the time.

Listening Training in Hypernasality

Listening training teaches a child the differences between hypernasal resonance and normal resonance. Fisher (1975, p. 104) stated where structures are normal but do not function efficiently in cases of hypernasality, improvement in resonance can be accomplished

---

1. I KNOW THE RULE ABOUT RESONANCE BALANCE.   _____
2. I CAN TELL WHEN OTHER PEOPLE HAVE RESONANCE IMBALANCE.   _____
3. I CAN TELL WHEN OTHER PEOPLE HAVE RESONANCE BALANCE.   _____
4. I KNOW HOW MY VOICE *SOUNDS* AND *FEELS* WHEN I HAVE   _____
   RESONANCE IMBALANCE.
5. I KNOW HOW MY VOICE *SOUNDS* AND *FEELS* WHEN I HAVE   _____
   RESONANCE BALANCE.
6. I KNOW THE PLACES WHERE I HAVE RESONANCE IMBALANCE.   _____
7. I KNOW THE PLACES WHERE I HAVE RESONANCE BALANCE.   _____
8. I CAN TALK WITH RESONANCE BALANCE *SOME* OF THE TIME.   _____
9. I CAN TALK WITH RESONANCE BALANCE *MOST* OF THE TIME.   _____
10. I CAN TALK WITH RESONANCE BALANCE *ALL* THE TIME.   _____

Fig. 43. Resonance balance.

by improving auditory discrimination between hypernasal and non-nasal resonance. Williamson (1944) found that in 84 cases with few exceptions velopharyngeal closure exercises are not necessary if a person with hypernasality is given a remedial program stressing the auditory aspects of good voice. Many children with hypernasality interpret their own voices as not being different from others. Therefore, they must be taught to hear the difference between a non-nasal and a hypernasal voice (Mysak, 1966, p. 173; Porterfield, Trabue, Terry, and Stimpert, 1966). It is necessary in cases of velar paralysis to develop the ability to listen carefully to voice and speech in order to produce the most intelligible communication possible (Moore, 1971a, p. 568).

We have found improvement of resonance is based upon thorough listening training following the general outline in Chapter 7. Listening training is designed to decrease hypernasality as well as reduce the emission of sounds through the nose. Listening training follows the three major steps: (1) awareness of the difference in others, (2) gross discrimination of differences in others, and (3) fine discrimination of differences in others. In all steps the speech pathologist is the performer while the child is the listener and judge. The speech pathologist uses the child's most hypernasal phonemes for listening training. These procedures teach the child to listen and to make judgments about voice quality in the speech pathologist's speech.

The listening training program for hypernasal resonance begins with awareness of the difference. For example, the speech pathologist uses pairs of sounds or words, saying one of the pair with hypernasal resonance and the other with normal resonance. The child signals the presence of the defective aspect by raising his hand or dropping a bead in a box when he hears hypernasality. Many similar techniques of interest to the child can be devised to teach awareness of defective resonance as the speech pathologist speaks sounds, syllables, words, or sentences using undesirable resonance on some of the items. In gross discrimination two levels, excessive hypernasality and normal resonance, are presented for the child to judge differences. Pairs of sounds using the two vocal parameters are spoken by the speech pathologist while the child judges which is which.

During the diagnostic examination the vowels and consonants were rated as to presence and degree of hypernasality. We suggest the speech pathologist select from these lists the phonemes which are excessively hypernasalized and those which are non-nasal. Van Riper (1972, pp. 160–161) stressed the importance of having a child recognize hypernasality when it occurs in his speech. Van Riper suggested the speech pathologist select the vowels least defective in the child's speech. Then have the child say them as he self monitors his resonance. Immediately after the child says each vowel the speech pathologist says it using excess hypernasality. In this way the child readily recognizes the differences. Fine discrimination of differences calls for even more careful listening and judging by the child. He is required to make judgments of the extent of defectiveness of resonance in the speech pathologist's speech. Usually three levels are selected representing excessive hypernasality, moderate hypernasality, and normal resonance. For example, the speech pathologist produces a series of three /ɑ/ sounds with the three degrees of voice resonance. The child can indicate his judgment by placing a bead or block in one of three designated boxes or by simply giving verbal indication of recognition of variations. The differences at first can be quite great but as listening training proceeds the differences are decreased until expert listening by the child is required.

As a result of the listening training program the child has now progressed through Steps 2 and 3 on the resonance balance chart. He is now ready to work directly on improving resonance in his own voice.

Negative practice is an integral part of a program for improving oral-nasal balance. As soon as a child can produce hypernasal and non-nasal vowels (Steps 4 and 5) negative practice is started and used throughout the resonance program. Negative practice can be used to reinforce and strengthen the use of improved resonance. For example, to reduce nasal emission the child is asked to produce a sound with nasal emission immediately followed by production of the sound without nasal emission. Fisher (1975, p. 105) suggested using negative practice by having the child deliberately produce /ɑ/ with hypernasality, then have him produce the vowel as free of hypernasality as he possibly can. Negative practice usually begins by using isolated sounds and progresses to syllables, words, and finally sentences. A child with velopharyngeal insufficiency especially needs negative practice during all aspects of his program. This type of practice allows the child to gain control over new habits and leads to eventual habituation.

Reduction or Elimination of Hypernasality

Van Riper and Irwin (1958, pp. 248–251) stated reducing the assimilation effect of nasal sounds and increasing the amount of nonnasal phonation in general is essential. They recommended selecting a phoneme that is excessively hypernasal and reducing the hypernasality on that one phoneme. This greatly increases the amount of non-nasal phonation in general. They reported that their most successful cases have been those who were taught normal production of one or two of the most hypernasalized vowels and then fixing and stabilizing these phonemes.

Cooper (1973, pp. 181–182) described procedures for the elimination of hypernasality. He suggested beginning with vowels which stress oral resonance such as /o/ and /u/. Here is the sequence of therapy for hypernasality based on Cooper applied to a child:

1. Have the child repeatedly say /o/, using his lowest level of the optimal pitch range until the resonance is acceptable. The speech pathologist acts as a model. Audiorecordings are made and evaluated.

2. The /u/ is introduced next and the process repeated. Careful tabulations are made of the child's progress.

3. Next, numbers follow the vowels, such as "/o/ one," "/o/ two," and "/u/ one," and "/u/ two," counting to 10 in this manner. Emphasis is placed on good oral resonance on the vowels and oral consonants.

4. Now the child can advance to combining vowels such as "/o/, /u/, one," "/o/, /u/, two" counting to 10 in this way. The child should monitor resonance very carefully, making sure to produce a sound free from hypernasality.

5. Next, single words are added to the stimuli, such as "/o/, /u/, one hello," "/o/, /u/, one house." More words are added such as "/o/, /u/, one hello there," "/o/, /u/, two only tomorrow."

6. Sentences follow the production of the

/o/, /u/ combination, such as "/o/, /u/, one, the sun is setting tomorrow."

7. Appropriate and balanced oral-nasal resonance is now approached in spontaneous speech. Samples of spontaneous speech are audiotaped with the child monitoring his speech so that hypernasality is under control.

Eisenson and Eisenson (1974, pp. 80–81) suggested having the child pinch his nostrils closed as he says sentences that have no /m/, /n/, or /ŋ/ sounds in them. The child can practice saying these sentences alternately pinching his nostrils in a nasal flutter style. There should be no noticeable difference in resonance when the nostrils are open and closed. For this type of practice we use these sentences:

> He saw the boy.
> The baby is cute.
> I like big red apples.
> Jack likes to play ball.

Hanley and Thurman (1970, pp. 214–220) suggested that when a child can produce hypernasal and non-nasal vowels at will, he combine them with non-nasal consonants, first in VC syllables such as /at/, /ap/, /af/ and then reverse the syllables into CV syllables such as /ta/, /pa/, /fa/. Then CVC syllables are practiced, such as /tak/, /bas/. The syllable drills should be audiotaped for evaluation of success in eliminating hypernasality. Next, one syllable words with nonnasal consonants are introduced being certain the child has wide mouth openings and active articulation to help him say the words without hypernasality. Then two syllable words and multisyllable words are practiced. Mirror work helps stimulate more active articulation. When hypernasality is controlled or eliminated on non-nasal sounds, Hanley and Thurman recommended having the child say one syllable words containing nasal consonants. The purpose is to keep normal nasality on the nasal consonants and to prevent this nasality from influencing the adjoining vowels. First start with /am/, /an/, /aŋ/ and then combine nasal consonants in syllable drill such as /ma/, /na/, /mɔ/, /nɔ/. Next one syllable words are approached with nasal consonants before each vowel, such as *map, nap*. Then have the child say two syllable words with a nasal consonant between two vowels, such as *Annie, tuna,* and combine nasal consonants with vowels in initial, medial, and final positions such as *meet, Amy, ream.* Next consonant and nasal-consonant word pairs are practiced, such as *hot-not, sit-knit, see-me.* Hanley and Thurman further suggested having the child practice sentences loaded with /m/, /n/, and /ŋ/ being certain nasality on these consonants does not spill over into the vowels. We use these and other similar sentences: *In rainy times, Nan phones Tom. Ring me when Mama comes home.*

An exercise suggested by Fisher (1975, pp. 105–106) which we like to use is called the pull-out exercise. A child is asked to repeat a word such as *house* 10 times, gradually pulling out of an initial hypernasal quality. He begins with a hypernasal quality on the first few productions, gradually reducing the hypernasality until the last few productions are free from hypernasality. A record is kept of his success; audiotapes are useful here for evaluation of his attempts. Next Fisher suggested using voiceless stop consonants such as /p/ and /t/ at the beginning of a word in which air pressure must be increased in the oral cavity with the resulting tight velopharyngeal port closure. Word pairs are also used in this pull-out exercise, such as *pie-my, peat-meat, pet-met, tea-knee, tip-nip, tail-nail.*

At this point the child should recognize the places where he has resonance imbalance (Step 6 on the resonance balance chart). These places can be listed and the number of times he hears imbalance can be charted. The same procedure can be followed for Step 7 with the child counting and charting his use of resonance balance. Steps 8, 9, and 10 for carryover can now be approached. Programs for carryover are given in Chapter 12.

Loudness, Pitch, and Rate

Often attention to loudness, pitch, and rate is necessary to assure good use of resonance. During the examination by the speech pathologist, evaluations of a child's use of loudness, pitch, and speaking rate were made. Any significant deviations from normal should receive attention. Specific problems with loudness, pitch, and rate of speaking often occur in children with hypernasal speech. For example, it may be noted that a child's loudness drops below the optimal level on specific phrases or at the ends of breath groups. Also, pitch inflections may go higher and lower than is usual and occur more often

than is desirable. Then, too, rate of talking may be too rapid for optimal communication. The speech pathologist can compare these voice parameters in a particular child with norms or standards and plan a program for making the appropriate changes. If the voice is too loud or too soft the loudness training program described in Chapter 9 can be followed. Children with pitch and rate deviations can receive programs described in the same chapter for appropriate modifications. Changes in loudness, pitch, or rate should not be made unless they deviate from normal.

Loudness

Fisher (1975, p. 104) stated increasing vocal intensity may help reduce hypernasality especially for those who habitually talk softly. An increase in loudness requires a person to make more efficient use of the pharyngeal and oral cavities; this also tends to offset cul-de-sac resonance. Further, increasing loudness tends to increase the activity of the velar-lifting muscles and results in a general increase in muscle tone. Fisher suggested that even for those who use adequate loudness it may be profitable to experiment with a louder voice to determine the effect on perceived hypernasality. If improved resonance results, this can be pointed out to the child and audiotaped for listening practice. Therapy then proceeds to maintaining good resonance at a reduced loudness level.

Particular attention, according to Zimmerman and Canfield (1968, pp. 254–255), is indicated when the voice fades out at the ends of sentences. For example, a child may say, "I would like a sandwich with peanut butter," with *peanut butter* hypernasalized and too soft. The child is told *peanut butter* is an important part of the sentence and should be stressed and said at appropriate loudness. Maintaining adequate loudness levels throughout a sentence may be improved by breaking up sentences into phrases, words, or even syllables. For example, instruct a child to say a sentence pausing and taking a breath at the // marks, "I would like // a sandwich // with peanut butter." A sentence can be broken down further for loudness practice, "I would // like a // sand // wich // with // pea // nut // bu // tter." When loudness control is demonstrated the sentences are then practiced without the pauses.

Moncur and Brackett (1974, pp. 169–170)

suggested special procedures if a child has the tendency to diminish loudness between syllables or words. The end effect is a perception of "choppy" delivery because phonation is not adequately sustained. They suggested using any instrument with a volume unit (VU) meter, such as a sound level meter. The objective is to have the child keep the VU meter needle in a steady position as much as possible as he says words, phrases, and sentences. At first have him use spondee words, attempting to peak the needle of the VU meter equally on both syllables. Typical spondee words to use are *railroad, toothbrush, barnyard, cowboy, moonlight, hotdog.* Then as soon as a child can maintain adequate loudness on each syllable of the words with good resonance, negative practice should be introduced saying spondee words first choppy and then maintaining a smooth delivery on both parts of each word, not letting the needle fall back to 0. Moncur and Brackett suggested following the same procedures with phrases and sentences.

Pitch

Fisher (1975, pp. 103–104) stated if the optimum pitch is lower than the modal pitch, lowering the pitch of a person's voice may result in an automatic shift in resonance characteristics and in this way reduce or eliminate hypernasality. Starting sentences at too high a pitch level and then raising the pitch level even higher on stressed words is frequently a characteristic of a person with hypernasality (Zimmerman and Canfield, 1968, p. 254). Audiotapes of samples of these pitch variations can be made. The child can be taught to start sentences at a lower pitch level within his optimum range. The pitch level on stressed words also must be kept within the optimum range. This type of pitch control results in decreasing perceived hypernasality.

Tarlow and Saxman (1970) reported on the speaking modal frequency level of children with cleft palate. The group consisted of 12 children between the ages of 7 years and 8 years 11 months compared to a similar group with normal oral structures. The modal frequency levels for both groups did not vary dramatically from those reported in other studies. The modal level for the cleft group was 251.7 Hz and for the noncleft group was 241.5 Hz. No statistically significant differences were found between the groups on measures of modal frequency level. The cleft group, however, had a significantly greater number of upward and downward inflections while the noncleft group had a greater extent of inflection. Thus the speech pathologist may want to work on more normal upward and downward inflections in children with velopharyngeal insufficiency.

Thurman (1977, p. 252) stated there may be less perceived hypernasality at certain voice pitch levels than at others. Saying vowels at various pitch levels may isolate vowels which are free from hypernasality. We have found scanning techniques asking a child to say vowels at various pitch levels often helps locate non-nasal sounds which can be used as target models for improved resonance even though the pitch temporarily may not be appropriate. From these non-nasal target sounds we can then work toward normal resonance in the optimum pitch range.

Rate

We have found varying the rate of speaking in some cases reduces the amount of perceived hypernasality, both in organic and nonorganic hypernasality. Greene (1972, p. 266) suggested that the person with hypernasality should use slow speech. Colton and Cooker (1968) reported a study which showed that normal speakers are perceived as more nasal when speaking at a reduced rate compared with their normal rate. Lass and Noll (1970) compared rate characteristics of a group of 20 male cleft palate speakers 18 to 26 years of age with those of a similar group of noncleft speakers. The results indicated the cleft palate group exhibited slower reading and speaking rates than the noncleft group, though both were within normal limits. We recommend trying faster and slower rates to determine the effect on amount of hypernasality. It is possible a change in one direction or the other, keeping within normal rate limits, may improve oral-nasal resonance balance. If not, attention to rate is not recommended unless it is abnormally slow or fast.

The following teenager represents our approach where the major therapy goals were improving oral-nasal resonance balance and making the necessary modifications in loudness, pitch, and rate. This is an illustration of voice therapy for functional hypernasality.

Carol was 16 years old when we first saw her. She had come to the Clinic voluntarily after she listened to an audiotape made during her story-telling period in a nursery school where she worked as a volunteer. Carol said she had been concerned about her voice for about 2 years and hearing the tape motivated her to seek help. Hypernasality was her chief complaint and she also felt the pitch of her voice was too high and that her voice sounded "whiny." One year previously after a deviated septum had been corrected, the physician told her the hypernasality had no organic basis. Our ratings on the Buffalo Voice Profile included the following deviations: 5 for hypernasality, 3 for lack of adequate loudness, 3 for too high pitch, 2 for too slow rate, with an overall voice efficiency of 4. The combination of hypernasality and too-high pitch did indeed give the impression of a "whiny" voice. We checked her on several instruments. The Nasal Indicator revealed hypernasality present on vowels especially /æ/ and /ɔ/ and voiced consonants. Her oral manometer ratio was 0.98. Loudness analysis showed an average of 65 dB at 18 in from a sound level meter, about 5 to 10 dB too soft. Pitch analysis using the F_0 Indicator revealed her modal frequency level was 255 Hz, which was at the extreme upper end of acceptable limits for her age, about 3 semitones above the norm of 215 Hz. We audiotaped a sample of her spontaneous speech which we judged as representative of her rate of speaking. Her rate averaged 125 words per min, which was judged to be about 25 to 35 words too slow. Stimulability testing revealed she could produce non-nasal phonemes including the /æ/ and /ɔ/ and could lower her voice pitch level to the target of about 215 Hz. Her overall vocal efficiency potential was rated excellent when she was stimulated to monitor her resonance balance as she used lower pitch, faster rate, and increased loudness. The results of the voice examinations demonstrated quite clearly the necessity for the following therapy goals:

1. Establishing appropriate oral-nasal resonance balance through a concentrated program of listening training, also emphasizing tactile and kinesthetic aspects of good resonance use.

2. Increasing modal loudness about 5 to 10 dB to 70 to 75 dB 18 in from the measuring source.

3. Lowering the modal pitch approximately 3 semitones—about 40 Hz—from 255 to 215 Hz.

4. Increasing the rate of speaking from 125 to about 150 to 160 words per min.

Carol was seen for 20 one hour sessions over a 3 month period. The overall plan followed the 10 step resonance balance chart. Initially work was done using non-nasal words and progressing rapidly to non-nasal sentences and paragraphs. Work was concentrated on the /æ/ and /ɔ/, the two most hypernasalized vowels. Carol then proceeded to work with /m/, /n/, /ŋ/ in words, phrases, and sentences. Initially she experienced difficulty with assimilative hypernasality but soon little difficulty was encountered. Negative practice on the major aspects of resonance, loudness, pitch, and rate was begun as soon as Carol was able to produce the correct and incorrect form of each parameter. Negative practice was used throughout the program. At the end of the program normal oral-nasal resonance balance had been established and stabilized and loudness, pitch, and rate were within normal limits. Carryover of the new speaking parameters proceeded from nucleus situations and was soon generalized to all speaking situations.

Vocal Abuse

The speech pathologist should listen for hoarseness or any other signs of laryngeal dysfunction since children with velopharyngeal insufficiency may have vocal cord abnormalities. Bernthal and Beukelman (1977) stated vocal abuse should be checked in speakers with inadequate velopharyngeal valving who are attempting to increase modal loudness levels. McDonald and Baker (1951) stated vocal cord hyperemia and hyperplasia are characteristic of many persons with cleft palate. McWilliams et al. (1969) found 84% of a group of 32 children with cleft palates and hoarse voices had vocal nodules or vocal cord changes. Follow-up examinations about 4.7 years later showed vocal cord problems in 70% of the original 27 children who were reexamined (McWilliams et al. 1973). These studies were presented in detail in Chapter 2.

Luse, Heisse, and Foley (1964) reported on three patients with repaired cleft palates whose speech had marked cleft palate resonance. Two of them had vocal cord pathology, one, aged 10 years, had vocal nodules and the other, aged 21, had contact ulcers. The vocal cord pathologies and the hypernasality were felt to be due to pharyngeal and laryngeal tension. Initial x-ray lateral head plates showed a retracted tongue and a constricted pharyngeal wall. Following therapy procedures which emphasized release of tension in the laryngeal and pharyngeal areas, the vocal pathologies were no longer present and resonance was reported to be close to normal in all three patients. At this point x-ray lateral head plates showed the ball of the tongue tended to move away from the pharyngeal wall and the pharyngeal airway assumed a more normal appearance for phonation.

We recently saw a 15-year-old boy with a repaired cleft of the soft palate. He spoke with excessive muscular tension in his face, neck, and shoulders. He complained of chronic hoarseness and loss of voice after much talking, yelling, or singing. Indirect laryngoscopic examination revealed bilateral vocal nodules at the junction of the anterior and middle thirds of each cord. Voice therapy over a 4 month period concentrated on easy phonation and having the boy observe the rules of voice hygiene. A second laryngoscopic examination showed the vocal nodules were no longer present. The boy's laryngeal tone was clear reflecting normal vocal cord function.

The speech pathologist should note any vocal abuse, analyze it carefully, and proceed with a program for its elimination or modification. Our program for eliminating or modifying vocal abuse described in Chapter 8 can be used for children with velopharyngeal insufficiency.

Facial Grimaces and Nares Constriction

A child with velopharyngeal insufficiency may unconsciously constrict or flare his nares in an effort to prevent nasal emission of sound. He may also have associated facial grimaces. Improving velopharyngeal closure and articulation may eliminate nares constriction and facial grimaces since they are no longer necessary. However, it may be necessary to work directly on eliminating these

habits if they have become a firmly fixed part of the speaking pattern.

We have had success in eliminating facial grimaces and nares constriction using a direct approach through mirror work, negative practice, and teaching light quick articulation contacts (Greene, 1972, p. 267; Shelton et al. 1968, p. 251: Van Riper, 1972, p. 379). Moller, Starr, and Martin (1969), using operant conditioning procedures, had limited success in reducing facial grimaces in an adult with velopharyngeal insufficiency. Van Riper (1972, p. 379) suggested bringing these habits to the conscious level by using negative practice and eventually eliminating them through mirror work. Each child's pattern of facial grimaces should be carefully analyzed. For example, Moller et al. (1969) analyzed grimaces by describing the sequence of facial movements and the frequency of occurrence. Based on their description, the sequence most frequently seen in children is (1) an upward movement of the cheeks, (2) a slight squinting of the eyes, and (3) a downward pull of the nose with compression or flaring of the wings of the nose. Facial grimaces may be present in varying degrees of severity from a slight compression of the wings of the nose to the vigorous use of the full grimace sequence. Greene (1972, p. 267) stated emphasis should be placed on the fact that air will be coming through the nose, but that it should not be audible; practicing in front of a mirror to watch and inhibit any excess facial muscle tension may be indicated.

Shelton et al. (1968, pp. 251–252) stated teaching light, quick, and appropriate articulation contacts for the plosive sounds results in eliminating undesirable facial grimaces. For example, the /p/ and /b/ may be practiced as clicking sounds, making sure the child is relaxed and that he brings his lips together lightly for these sounds. At first the sounds may be whispered and the child encouraged to reduce the facial grimace; watching in the mirror may be helpful. Then words and short phrases loaded with /p/ and /b/ are used having the child concentrate on the tactile sensation of easy lip closure making sure the plosives are not distorted. The /t/ and /d/ are attacked similarly paying special attention to the mandible which should be held in a depressed position when the tongue tip taps the gum ridge. The /k/ and /g/ are similarly approached emphasizing light quick contact of the back of the tongue with the palate. Sometimes a more forward tongue contact is necessary to eliminate a glottal stop substitution for these plosives. Facial grimaces are reduced as the pressure behind the closure is reduced. Shelton et al. emphasized that requesting a "harder try" for improved articulation may only increase grimaces; an "easy try" for improved articulation on plosives decreases or eliminates grimaces.

PHYSICAL EXERCISES

Children with velopharyngeal insufficiency need adequate oral breath pressure and oral air flow. Oral breath pressure should be increased until the proper amount is attained to produce any misarticulated sound correctly. High pressure should be reduced if it is causing misarticulation and hypernasality. When improved velar and pharyngeal contractions result in better velopharyngeal closure the oral air flow is increased since air is not lost through nasal emission. Audible nasal emission of air during speaking should be eliminated (Van Riper, 1972, p. 370).

Some children improve valving and articulation as a result of vocal motor exercises and pressure building activities. In cases of short palate, exercises can be given to train the palatal and pharyngeal muscles to function more efficiently in making the sphincter-like closure needed for normal speech (West and Ansberry, 1968, p. 381). This is true also in cases of hypernasality following removal of adenoid. Westlake and Rutherford (1966, p. 113) stated some persons can as a result of exercises involving tactile stimulation improve valving so it becomes functional. They stated exercises are " . . . worth a *good* try."

In this section we are presenting a series of physical exercises for the speech pathologist who wishes to use exercises designed to develop adequate oral breath pressure and oral air flow. The exercises are based on the assumption that some children, especially those with marginal insufficiency, can benefit from a program of exercises. It is further assumed that these exercises will increase action in the velopharyngeal area, resulting in a decrease in the size of the opening. A reduction of nasal emission of sounds and hypernasality would be the dividend.

Muscle Exercises

Various types of muscle exercises may help increase muscle strength and improve muscle tonus in the velopharyngeal area. These exercises include maintaining adequate breath pressure and tension, developing correct breath direction, obtaining more oral activity, observing velar activity, swallowing and sucking exercises, and whistling and blowing activities.

Before initiating a program of muscle exercises for a child he should be evaluated carefully to see if he meets certain criteria. Van Riper (1972, pp. 372–373) stated evidence must be presented that shows closure is possible but not being done habitually. Van Riper also stated if velopharyngeal muscles are weak they can be strengthened through special exercises if physical management has made closure possible. If the person with velopharyngeal insufficiency can blow a balloon or whistle or if tests have shown good occlusion in the nasopharynx, the speech pathologist should be able to help the child make use of this closure in speech. Van Riper also said if in phonation, yawning, or other activities the velum can be seen to lift or the side walls of the pharynx contract or the rear wall come forward slightly, it can be presumed that improvement of the velopharyngeal function should be possible. Shelton (1963) stated individuals who are inconsistent in closure during speech are usually capable of learning normal speech. He also stated careful study should be made of the effectiveness of exercise in increasing the range of motion of the closure mechanism. Yules and Chase (1969) stated some patients with minimal velopharyngeal dysfunction may benefit from special exercises if cinefluorography demonstrates good "knee action" of the soft palate, if there is at least 2 mm posterior pharyngeal wall movement, and when nasal air escape is less than 200 cc/12 sec.

If a child meets the criteria suggested by Pannbacker (1973) chances for maximal benefit are high. Based upon the Pannbacker criteria velopharyngeal therapy may be indicated as a procedure of choice if the answers to the following questions about a child are in the affirmative:

1. Does the child have inconsistent hypernasality and nasal emission?

2. Can he produce defective sounds correctly with visual and auditory stimulation?

3. Is there evidence of normal velopharyngeal function during gagging, swallowing, and blowing?

4. Does he have a manometric ratio near 1.00?

Pannbacker stated if improvement at the end of a 3 month period of muscle training is not noted, consultation regarding physical management is indicated.

The following is a case history of Steve, who exemplifies the success of a combined program of physical exercise and speech and voice therapy:

Steve was born with a bilateral cleft lip and palate. When we saw him at 5 years of age he had had four operations on the lip, hard and soft palate, and nose. The results of the physical management were excellent. The hard palate had been closed without scarring and the soft palate had considerable motility with apparent adequate closure upon visual inspection. The lip appeared somewhat stiff and immobile. Steve could blow up a balloon and had a good gag reflex. Steve's oral manometer ratio was 0.93. Lateral head plates showed he could achieve adequate velopharyngeal closure on /s/, /ɑ/, and /i/. However, ratings on the Buffalo Resonance Profile showed he did not habitually achieve closure. Inconsistent nasal emission on plosives and fricatives was rated 3, inconsistent hypernasality was rated 5, and his speech intelligibility was rated 6, almost unintelligible. Stimulability was rated excellent for phonemes and resonance. Steve fulfilled Pannbacker's (1973) criteria as a candidate for velopharyngeal therapy using physical exercises. He had inconsistent hypernasality and nasal emission, high stimulability for correct phoneme production, evidence of normal velopharyngeal function on blowing a balloon, gagging, and on lateral x-rays, and a high manometric ratio. Speech and voice therapy goals for Steve were formulated as follows:

1. Improve articulation ability and speech intelligibility using the listening training approach.

2. Develop adequate oral breath pressure and oral air flow through physical exercises designed to develop orality of breath direction through observing velar action and getting increased oral activity.

3. Increase lip mobility through physical exercise.

4. Reduce nasal emission and hypernasality through listening training with tactile and kinesthetic reinforcement.

Steve was scheduled for an initial concentrated period of therapy of three 1 hour sessions/week. After 12 sessions six phonemes had been approached /m/, /p/, /b/, /w/, /θ/, /ð/ with satisfactory production in isolation and words, with about 50% carryover. A key to correct articulation was emphasis on placement and light contact of the articulators. Intelligibility had increased to about 60%. Oral breath pressure had increased and Steve had more orality of speech direction. Listening training for resonance following the 10 step outline had progressed through Step 5 so Steve was aware of the auditory and kinesthetic aspects of resonance imbalance and balance in his own voice. After this we saw Steve weekly over a period of 8 months. He soon progressed through the remaining steps of the voice therapy outline for resonance training. At the end of therapy his articulation was acceptable with difficulty remaining only on the fricatives, especially the /s/ and /z/. Speech intelligibility was rated as near 100% with strangers. Hypernasality had decreased to a rating of 2 and nasal emission had been eliminated chiefly through stressing light articulatory contacts specifically on the plosives /p/, /b/, /t/, /d/, /k/, /g/. We followed Steve over a three year period through phone calls with the parents. His articulation and resonance remained stable with only a trace of hypernasality appearing when he was fatigued.

Breath Pressure and Tension

Children with velopharyngeal insufficiency often distort articulatory movements and have nasal emission because they characteristically build up too much pressure on stop consonants or fricatives. Also they are likely to develop abnormal muscular tensions when they attempt to speak clearly. Zimmerman and Canfield (1968, p. 257) stated a person with a cleft palate may tend to speak with undue tension resulting in an emission of excess air. This leads to the development of vocal strain, which in turn results in a husky quality, nasal snorting, resonance imbalance, and excess breathiness.

Zimmerman and Canfield (1968, p. 257) stated cleft palate patients need a minimal amount of air passing through the vocal cords to produce clear phonation and a strong tone;

emphasis should be placed on developing proper control of the muscles involved in phonation. Greene (1972, p. 266) suggested that a quiet voice and slow speech without undue tension or stridency should be encouraged, with emphasis being placed on effortless but understandable speech. Reduced nasal emission can be obtained through reducing pressure and tension during speaking (Morris, 1972, p. 151; Van Hattum, 1974, p. 350; Van Riper, 1972, p. 370). Some children do not build up enough breath pressure or they have too lax muscle tension for good speech and resonance. When any unusual tensions are present in children with velopharyngeal insufficiences our procedures for achieving balanced muscular tonus described in Chapter 8 can be incorporated into the program. The speech pathologist may need to make particular use of the exercises for reducing hyperfunction in laryngeal and pharyngeal areas. All efforts should be made to prevent the development of excess muscular tensions as the child strives to improve articulation and to establish adequate oral breath pressure.

Van Riper (1972, p. 370) suggested air pressure controls should be carefully evaluated in the person with velopharyngeal insufficiency. In order to provide the best speech a person with cleft palate is capable of producing, Morris (1972, p. 151) suggested the use of very light contacts on pressure consonants so they are articulated only enough to be perceived and with not so much force that nasal emission ensues. Van Riper (1972, p. 370) also stated that less air pressure should be applied whenever possible, and that more oral direction rather than nasal direction of the air should be emphasized. Moore (1971a, p. 568) stated that developing gentle stop consonants reduces the apparent hypernasality and air noises in velar paralysis. Teaching children to use less air pressure on stop consonants or fricatives by loose contacts of the articulators allows more oral air flow; at the same time the use of larger jaw movements may facilitate better articulation and resonance (Anonymous, 1964a). For example, a technique using a repetitive /bɑ/, /bɑ/, /bɑ/, or /tu/, /tu/, /tu/ emphasizing easy pressure buildup and a gentle release of the /ɑ/ and /u/ sounds may be useful.

Warren, Wood, and Bradley (1969) found that in the presence of palatal incompetency the use of larger volumes of air for consonant production results in increased nasal emis-sion. They studied respiratory volume in 16 normal speaking and 18 cleft palate speakers over 16 years of age to determine how velopharyngeal incompetency influences respiratory effort. The volume of air released from the lungs during phonation was used as the measure of respiratory effort. Each subject was asked to produce "bat," "pat," "zat," "sat," "dat," "tat," "vat," and "fat" in the phrase "Say ____ again." Subjects with inadequate closure had air volumes approximately twice those of normals. The authors suggested that oral-nasal resonance and intelligibility may be modified by reducing respiratory effort.

Changing the location of tension may be necessary for some children. For example, some children with velopharyngeal insufficiency may substitute a glottal stop for various pressure sounds; what they do is substitute a buildup of pressure at the level of the glottis for a buildup of pressure within the oral cavity. The speech pathologist can have the child listen through a stethoscope with the bell of the stethoscope near the speech pathologist's larynx; the speech pathologist then demonstrates the difference between a glottal stop and the correct production of the sound. Then the child listens in a similar fashion to his own production of glottal stops. He continues to listen as the gottal stops are eliminated and he learns good production of pressure sounds (Anonymous, 1964a).

In the correction of excessive hypernasality on vowel sounds the teeth should be well separated; the back of the tongue, pillars of fauces, and pharynx should be relaxed (Greene, 1972, pp. 266–267). Negative practice can be used by contrasting the hypernasality present where more and then less force is used (Massengill and Phillips, 1975, p. 70).

Moncur and Brackett (1974, pp. 167–168) suggested the following guidelines in preparing a child for syllable exercises to develop oral and pharyngeal resonance. We have found these useful as a child works toward establishing proper air pressure and muscle tension in the oral and velopharyngeal areas. (1) Have the child relax his mandible and tongue. (2) Tell him to get maximum downward movements of the mandible and tongue for vowels. (3) Have him concentrate on keeping the pharyngo-oral tract relaxed and open. (4) Be sure he uses good breath support. (5) Tell him to pause between syllables in the exercises that follow, pausing for a normal unhurried inhalation at the slash // marks.

(6) Have him briefly prolong the vowel in each syllable. (7) Instruct him to use a downward inflection on each syllable. The syllable chains to which the above directions apply are exemplified by the following (Moncur and Brackett, 1974, p. 167): *rah, rah, rah // rah, rah, rah; yaw, yaw, yaw, yaw // yaw, yaw, yaw, yaw.* They also suggested starting syllables with vowels that are open such as /ɑ/ and /o/: *ahm, ahm, ahm // ahm, ahm, ahm; ohm, ohm, ohm // ohm, ohm, ohm.* Sentences are approached next concentrating on keeping the throat open and relaxed. For example, Moncur and Brackett (1974, p. 168) used the following sentences: "'Where are you?' she cried, aiming her flashlight down the road." "Bonnie's bouncing baby boy scowled and howled at Papa's Siamese cat."

Sometimes children have difficulty building up and maintaining appropriate breath pressure. In some children muscle fatigue may be a factor; others may have inadequate breathing patterns. Shelton et al. (1968, pp. 258–259) recommended evaluating the effect of fatigue on amount of hypernasality in the person with borderline or marginal velopharyngeal competence. In these patients it has been observed that the degree of hypernasality increases with fatigue. Therefore, if the patient learns to predict the situations where he will have hypernasality due to fatigue, he can make a concerted effort to achieve nonnasal speech.

Van Riper (1972, p. 372) suggested cleft palate clients be given training in control of breath if their breathing records show many instances of air wastage, speaking on tail ends of breath groups, opposition, and shortness of breath. Training in breathing through the use of exercises may pay dividends in improving speech and decreasing nasal emission and hypernasality. A child should inhale a normal amount of air and start his uttterances gradually rather than suddenly and he should monitor the amount of air used. Van Riper stressed that children must learn to monitor their phrasing and breathing patterns. Breathing exercises are presented in Chapter 8.

Breath Direction

Emphasis should be placed on directing air and sound through the mouth rather than through the nose (Wells, 1971, p. 238). Increasing the size of the mouth opening may

be helpful assuming that with a wider mouth opening the oropharynx will be larger and hypernasal resonance will be reduced (Morris, 1972, p. 151). Greene (1972, p. 267) stressed the importance of correct articulatory placement to get the air stream directed through the mouth instead of through the nose. Van Riper (1972, p. 371) stated this emphasis on the mouth as a major channel for speech and airflow is among the major objectives of speech therapy for those with velopharyngeal insufficiency. Van Hattum (1974, p. 329) stated directional exercises are useful for those with cleft palate—directional exercises being defined as those with the goal of stressing orality of breath and voice, and deemphasizing nasal direction.

Van Riper (1972, pp. 371–372) suggested concentrating on wider mouth openings to improve oral airflow as this tends to produce looser contacts of the lips and tongue and directs attention to the mouth rather than the nose. Van Riper also suggested lip exercises to help children become more mouth conscious. He suggested having children talk through fringed holes in a sheet of paper, through various sizes of slits and blowing tubes, or through fringed paper mustaches, anything to get children more mouth conscious. Shelton et al. (1968, p. 258) stated instruction to increase the size of the mouth opening and to lower the elevation of the tongue carriage is in order for a person with a small oral port. They suggested speech drill during which the child is asked to observe the articulation of /ɑ/ in contrast to that of /i/ and /u/ noting the difference in oral port opening on these vowels.

Massengill and Phillips (1975, p. 70) suggested whistling, playing wind instruments, playing suction games, humming, and yawning to help develop correct breath direction. A child can practice holding air under pressure in the mouth by blowing out the cheeks, holding the nostrils if necessary, and alternating oral and nasal emission of air. Thurman (1977, pp. 250–251) stated emphasis in therapy should be on wide mouth openings; in this way oral resonance will be increased in proportion to nasal resonance. Thurman suggested drills should begain with the open vowels such as /ɑ/. At first vowels should be practiced with non-nasal consonants in VC, CV, and VCV combinations. Then to overcome the assimilation effect of nasal consonants, the CV combinations can be made up of /m/, /n/, and /ŋ/ sounds.

For orality of speech and resonance we have found two of Fisher's (1975, pp. 104–105) exercises useful. The first one is to place a cold mirror underneath the nostrils during the following exercise: Tell the child to open his mouth wide and inhale and exhale through the mouth. This should require the velum to be raised in order to close off the nasal port. However, if any breath leaks through the velopharyngeal port, it will cloud the mirror as it strikes it. The second exercise suggested by Fisher is the /ŋ–ɑ/ drill. Have the child say /ŋ/, having him feel the velum lying relaxed against the humped back part of the tongue. Then have him say /ɑ/, noting the feel of muscle pull as the soft palate is lifted and retracted, and at the same time listening for hypernasality in the vowel. The /ŋ/ and /ɑ/ should at first be alternated very slowly and deliberately, then faster as the child gains increased auditory and kinesthetic awareness. Wells (1971, p. 235) suggested having the child imitate a person who talks using a very active mouth, or a howling wolf or dog (emphasize mouth postures; minimize loudness).

The following are exercises from Anderson and Newby (1973, pp. 254–255) for attaining the goal of openness and relaxation of the pharynx and oral direction:

1. Have the child yawn and note the kinesthesia of having the tongue at the bottom of the mouth.

2. Have the child use a small mirror to look in his mouth and throat during yawning. Have him note the position of the tongue, the soft palate, and how the throat opens.

3. Have the child look in the mirror and prolong /ɑ/ with the throat open.

4. Have the child make believe he is yawning and singing /o/, keeping the throat as open as possible.

5. Tell the child to get into the open throat position and sing /u/. Then go from /u/ to /ɑ/, keeping the feeling of the open relaxed throat. Moving from one vowel to the other should be gradual and continuous with no break in phonation.

6. Tell the child to do the same on the vowels /u/, /o/, and /ɑ/, beginning with /u/, changing to /o/, and then to /ɑ/. Keep phonation continuous.

To attain a wider mouth opening and re-laxation of the jaw, Anderson and Newby (1975, p. 255) suggested the following sequence:

1. Have the child relax the jaw, allowing his mouth to fall open.

2. Instruct the child to keep his jaw relaxed and passive; see if he can move it around while grasping it.

3. Tell the child to repeat *ouch* a number of times opening the mouth wide for each production.

4. Have him say the following words with an exaggerated mouth opening for the initial vowels: *open, almond, army, oddly, habit, action, offer, outfit.*

5. Tell the child to repeat rapidly the vowels /u/ and /ɑ/, merging them together until he can hear a /w/ between them.

6. Now have the child repeat the vowels /i/, /ɑ/, and /u/ with exaggerated lip and jaw action: lips wide for /i/, mouth open for /ɑ/, lips pursed and rounded for /u/.

Greene (1972, p. 268) suggested the following exercises for breath direction:

1. Have the child blow softly through his lips a few times and then interrupt the breath stream by gently closing the lips with a soft easy contact on /p/, then on /b/.

2. Have the child place the upper teeth on the lower lip, blow air, interrupting it with the /f/ and /v/ sounds.

3. Have the child sigh a breath over the tongue held between the teeth and obtain a /θ/ followed by a /ð/.

4. Show the child he can control nasal air escape on the /t/ by prefacing it with a /b/ sound /b–t/.

5. Emphasize the need for air to flow over the tongue tip as a child produces /s/ and /θ/.

6. To improve the /tʃ/ sound have the child sign a prolonged /ʃ/ interrupting it with /t/. Repeat several times until they merge.

We suggest doing the exercises in this section using negative practice procedures. First have the child use a narrow oral port and then an open oral port. Have him listen to the differences in oral-nasal resonance balance between the two productions.

Oral Activity

Attention to activity of the mouth, tongue, and mandible is helpful in obtaining improved resonance. If abnormal mandible and tongue movements are present, the child should be taught correct mandible movements and tongue positioning. For some children lip, tongue, and back of tongue exercises are suggested (Buck and Harrington, 1949). When indicated, attention should be given to lowering the dorsum of the tongue especially if it is high riding (Adler, 1960). The exercises should be accompanied by vowels, words, and connected speech. Vigorous speech mechanism exercises and practice on nonsense syllables, words, and sentences using voiceless fricative consonants (/s/, /ʃ/, /f/, and /θ/) and stop-plosive consonants (/p/, /b/, /t/, /d/, /k/, and /g/) are suggested in order to improve the action of the velopharyngeal mechanism (Curtis, 1967, pp. 224–225).

Anderson and Newby (1973, pp. 253–254) stated if a child speaks with sluggish tongue movements and immobile lips he may also have a sluggish and slow-moving velopharyngeal mechanism. They suggested the basic procedures in overcoming hypernasality should include: (1) vocal gymnastics for the speech organs to make them more active; (2) exercises for wider mouth openings to get full emission of tones; and (3) clear, precise formation of phonemes, emphasizing the role of the mouth in achieving orality of production.

To obtain increased oral activity Wells (1971, p. 236) suggested having the child talk in a highly exaggerated articulatory manner with some increase in loudness, and having the child imitate and exaggerate without tension activities depicted in pictures that show chewing, yawning, puffing, and swallowing. With small children Wells recommended pantomiming an imaginary dinner party where food is chewed vigorously, but this also should be done without tension.

Massengill and Phillips (1975, pp. 68–70) suggested exercises to increase tongue and lip mobility in patients with cleft palate. For example, to create awareness of tongue position and place of contact the speech pathologist, using a swab stick, touches spots on the child's tongue, lips, and in the mouth and pharynx, and the child touches the same points. To increase tongue mobiity, the speech pathologist can have the child follow movements of objects with his tongue, such as an airplane, car, flag, or bird. To innervate a tight and inert upper lip "Simon Says" can be played, with the speech pathologist making exaggerated faces while smiling, frowning, using wide mouth openings, and pouting.

Massengill and Phillips suggested the following exercises to reduce hypernasality, stressing oral activity: (1) Have the child relax the tongue on the floor of his mouth. (2) Have him say /ɑ/, /u/, /i/ keeping the tongue flat and relaxed. Be sure he does not close his teeth together and tell him to keep his tongue within his mouth behind his teeth as he says vowels. (3) Have him prolong /m/ gradually opening his mouth as he adds vowels.

A palatal stimulator may help some children with velopharyngeal insufficiency. Massengill, Quinn, and Pickrell (1971) reported on the use of a palatal stimulator to decrease velopharyngeal gap. A palatal stimulator is made of acrylic covering the hard palate and has an acrylic extension which fits against the soft palate. It is similar to a palatal lift but differs in that the stimulator extends only to the velum and fits against it in a rest position. The purpose is to stimulate movement away from the device. A person whose soft palate appears to have adequate potential for movement is a suitable candidate for a stimulator. Massengill et al. (1971) reported on five children ranging in age from 4 to 9 years who were fitted with palatal stimulators. Two of them had experienced excessive hypernasality after undergoing tonsillectomy and adenoidectomy, two had submucous cleft palates with short palates, and the fifth child had a short palate. These five children had velopharyngeal gaps ranging from 3 to 13 mm at the onset of the study. Massengill et al. reported after 1 year the gaps were 0 to 7 mm showing that velopharyngeal gaps were decreased considerably during the period of time of the study.

Velar Activity

Froeschels' pushing exercises may be useful in improving velopharyngeal closure and helping speed up the ascent rate of the soft palate (Arnold, 1965, p. 673). Pushing exercises are described in Chapter 8. Rochmis and Doob (1970, pp. 69–71) stated there are several forms of nonorganic hypernasality where observing velar action may help gain conscious control during speaking. The cause may be lax inefficient organs of speech or a tight strained muscular condition.

The child should observe the speech pathologist's palatal movement in a mirror (Van Riper, 1972, p. 373). Moore (1971a, p. 568) suggested having a patient observe his oral structures in a mirror as he protrudes the tongue and says vowels, such as /ɑ/; thrusting the tongue out strengthens and stimulates the palatal elevators and tensors. Wells (1971, p. 235) suggested having the child voluntarily yawn, stretching with lifted head, breathing in through the mouth, and phonating on exhalation; this stretches the muscles of the soft palate briefly in a nonspeech activity.

Yules and Chase (1969) suggested exercises for teaching voluntary contraction of the pharyngeal wall and elevation of the soft palate. Yules and Chase prefer the use of electrical stimulation to teach voluntary contraction although other types of stimulation are effective. These include visual observation in a mirror of attempts to control velar movement and pharyngeal wall contraction. Then the child can be taught the kinesthetic sensations of pharyngeal wall contraction. These exercises should be accompanied by speech. Fisher (1975, pp. 104–105) suggested having a child learn to feel where the velum is when the velopharyngeal port is closed by visually inspecting the action of the soft palate in a mirror as various vowels are produced. The child should open his mouth fairly widely but not in a strained manner. He then takes a deep breath through the nose and exhales through the mouth. Fisher stated that as this is repeated attention should be given to the kinesthesia of velar movements. Wells (1971, p. 237) suggested for better awareness and to encourage muscular control of the velopharyngeal sphincter, have the child sustain a tone and shift from oral to nasal emission of the tone; this will help him sense the velar movement that occurs.

For functional laxness of the soft palate Rochmis and Doob (1970, pp. 69–71) suggested teaching the raising of the soft palate by exercises using the /ŋ/ phoneme. Applying some of their procedures to children we would use the following sequence with mirror work:

1. Tell the child to pant vigorously while looking in a mirror. Have him watch the soft palate rise and fall and then practice raising the soft palate without panting or vocalizing.

2. Ask the child to yawn slowly and easily and watch the palate rise. Now see if he can raise the palate without yawning.

3. Have the child look in the mirror, raise the palate, prolong the vowel /ɑ/ and then, keeping the palate raised, have him say words beginning with /ɑ/ such as *are, art, army.*

4. Have the child say a word ending in /ŋ/ such as *bang.* Have him prolong the /ŋ/

and note how the back of the tongue humps up against the palate. Next have him say /ŋ/ and blend it into /ɑ/, keeping the soft palate raised.

5. Ask the child to say other words ending in /ŋ/ adding /ɑ/ such as *bringah,* keeping the palate raised.

Swallowing Exercises

Practicing swallowing is often suggested to strengthen muscles in the velopharyngeal port. Reseach studies do not agree regarding the effectiveness of swallowing exercises in improving velopharyngeal closure. For example, Flowers and Morris (1973) found no evidence to support a program of swallowing exercises. They studied cinefluorographically the swallowing patterns of four 8-year-old children, two with surgically repaired cleft palates and two with normal oral structures. They found that for some speech activities velopharyngeal competence is maintained for a longer period of time than during swallowing. Further, for some speech activities the rate of velar elevation and descent must be faster during a specific period of time than is necessary during swallowing. The authors concluded the differences between velar functioning during speech and during swallowing and other nonspeech activities are great enough that using nonspeech activitities is of questionable validity in evaluating as well as exercising the velopharyngeal mechanism. Powers and Starr (1974) administered a program of exercises to study the effects of blowing, sucking, swallowing, and gagging on palatal functioning and speech in four children aged 8 to 11 years with surgically repaired cleft palates. The results did not support the use of voluntary muscle exercises to improve velopharyngeal closure or decrease hypernasality.

On the other hand, Massengill, Quinn, Pickrell, and Levinson (1968) found swallowing exercises useful. They studied 13 cleft palate subjects aged 8 to 18 years. None of them demonstrated velopharyngeal closure when studied by cinefluorography. They investigated the effect of blowing, sucking, and swallowing exercises upon velopharyngeal closure. The subjects were divided into three groups with one group practicing blowing exercises on a manometer or with a blowing device. A second group practiced sucking exercises such as sucking through a straw or with a meter to indicate amount of pressure. The third group practiced swallowing exercises which consisted of placing the index finger on the neck in the area of the thyroid cartilage to feel neck movement during swallowing. The subjects were instructed to stop momentarily as they began to swallow and then to continue swallowing. In this way the length of the swallow was gradually increased in time. All subjects performed their specific exercises for a 20 min period each morning and each afternoon for 27 consecutive days. All subjects received intensive articulation therapy. Analysis of cinefluorographic films before and after this regimen for the three groups were made on /i/ and /u/. Significantly smaller velopharyngeal closures were shown only for the group which had swallowing exercises.

The speech pathologist may find some children benefit from swallowing therapy. Moore (1971a, p. 568) considered swallowing one of the best exercises for improving velopharyngeal closure. He suggested having the person swallow many small sips of liquid, being sure to carry out each swallowing act completely. Moore suggested swallowing exercises should be practiced regularly and frequently. We feel swallowing exercises may well be an appropriate part of a program for patients with velopharyngeal insufficiency, especially in the absence of cleft palate such as functional hypernasality and resonance imbalance associated with submucous cleft or palatal paralysis.

Sucking Exercises

Sucking exercises have been used for many years to stimulate and exercise muscles in order to provide better velopharyngeal closure. Wells (1971, p. 237) suggested alternation of sucking and ejecting movements can provide stimulation to muscle action. This can be performed simply by having the child pretend to move liquid from one imaginary container to another sucking it up from one and then ejecting it into another imaginary container. We have a child use a straw to help stimulate the activity. This also makes it a good lip exercise.

The Hunter Oral Manometer (bleed valve open) can be used for sucking and blowing tasks. The force of each effort is measured in ounces per square inch of pressure and a record is made of the time in seconds for each effort.

Massengill and Quinn (1974) reported on an 18-year-old male with repaired cleft palate who began experiencing an unusual amount of air pressure coming through his nose when he played the bassoon or saxophone. Radiograms of him at age 10 years revealed marked hypertrophy of adenoid tissue. In contast radiograms at 18 years of age showed atrophy of adenoid tissue. The patient was placed on a program of exercise as follows: The exercise was to hold a small piece of paper over the bottom of a straw by sucking on the straw. He was instructed to practice this exercise for approximately 10 min per day. After 6 months he reported no air escape during the playing of wind instruments. The patient was followed for approximately $2^1/_2$ years with no further difficulty reported. The authors stated the use of a sucking exercise to aid better velopharyngeal competence may seem a bit old fashioned. However, they stated with this patient sucking exercise appeared to be a successful method of solving the problem of excessive nasal emission of air.

Whistling and Blowing Activities

There is controversy concerning the use of blowing exercises in cases of velopharyngeal insufficiency. We are presenting both points of view since we feel the speech pathologist should select remedial procedures according to the apparent needs of a child. The arguments against the use of routine blowing exercises are (McDonald and Baker, 1951): (1) attention should be centered on correct mandible and tongue positions instead of velopharyngeal closure; (2) movements used in blowing are different from those used in speaking; (3) undesirable accessory movements, such as constriction of the nares and other facial grimaces, sometimes come about as a result of blowing exercises; (4) blowing exercises result in a misuse of breath pressure; (5) blowing exercises may result in failure and frustration. Calnan and Renfrew (1961) found practice in blowing brings into play mechanisms that are useless in speech, and they concluded success in blowing activities may lead both the patient and clinician into a false hope that speech will vicariously improve. McWilliams and Bradley (1965) felt the act of blowing involves a different pattern of physiological responses than those required in connected speech. Shelton et al. (1968, p. 257) stated we have no specific evidence to indicate motor exercises are valuable in increasing velopharyngeal competence or that exercise of palatal structures helps accomplish good and automatic articulation.

On the other hand, blowing exercises may be indicated in the treatment of hypernasality for the following reasons (McDonald and Baker, 1951): (1) they are sometimes considered to be useful in increasing mobility of the velopharyngeal structures; (2) a nonspeech activity such as blowing exercises may motivate a person who is emotionally disturbed about his speech and resists training. Blowing exercises can improve muscle function if used with reason and for a specific purpose. Indiscriminate use of blowing exercises should be avoided (Van Hattum, 1974, pp. 329–330). Stimulating velopharyngeal closure by modified blowing exercises should be approached early in therapy. Sustained exhalation of a narrow stream of air with rounded lips may not at first result in a tight velopharyngeal seal, but may help with this after practice (Wells, 1971, p. 236).

Anderson and Newby (1973, pp. 251–252) stated where there is some structural or physiological deficiency associated with velar control, blowing exercises have considerable value. Whistles, toy boats, pinwheels, balloons, and soap-bubble pipes can be used. They caution that blowing exercises have certain limitations in a program of reducing hypernasality; blowing and speaking are two quite different activities and there may not be automatic carryover from blowing to speech. Shprintzen, McCall, and Skolnick (1975) stated some individuals who have incompetent speech do not achieve closure because of an error in learning. Therefore, under the proper circumstances they should be able to learn competent closure. In these cases whistling or blowing exercises may make it possible for a child to achieve competent closure during speech. Shprintzen, Lencione, McCall, and Skolnick (1974) studied front and lateral cinefluorographic projections of velopharyngeal closure during various activities. Their study indicated that normal subjects utilize the same observable patterns of closure for speech as for whistling and blowing. The authors hypothesized that persons with cleft palate who have adequate closure during whistling or blowing but have incomplete closure during speech may benefit from approaching speech through the blowing or whistling mechanism. Sprintzen et al. (1975) applied this hypothesis in a study using operant therapeutic techniques for the treatment of velopharyngeal incompetence in four subjects. All had been examined videofluoroscopically and had shown normal-like velopharyngeal closure during blowing and whistling but abnormal closure for speech. Previous speech therapy had been ineffective. The subjects were a 19-year-old male with a repaired complete bilateral cleft of the lip and palate with an inferiorly based pharyngeal flap. The second subject was a 4-year-old boy with a repaired complete unilateral cleft on the left side. The third subject was a 6-year-old boy who had a submucous cleft of the palate with a superiorly based pharyngeal flap. The fourth subject was a 10-year-old girl with postadenoidectomy velopharyngeal incompetence, who also had a severe hearing loss with no hearing in the right ear and a 60 dB speech reception threshold in the left ear. The results of their study showed that some persons can be taught to obtain closure during speech through blowing and whistling exercises. Their procedure was as follows: Teach the child to blow and phonate or to whistle and phonate simultaneously. Then eliminate the blowing or whistling and obtain non-nasal phonation. To do this ask the child to blow or whistle as he phonates and then to cease whistling or blowing but maintain continuous voice. When blowing and whistling are faded the subject is instructed to phonate the /i/ vowel because the tongue position for /i/ is similar to that of whistling. When nonnasal vowel phonation is stabilized instruct the child to produce the /i/ vowel preceded and followed by non-nasal consonants, such as in /pit/, /sit/, /dip/. When monosyllabic words are produced without hypernasality ask him to say short non-nasal sentences such as "Popeye plays baseball" and "Susie sees Sally." Then have him use longer sentences, eventually going into spontaneous speech. Careful monitoring and the use of operant procedures are followed throughout the exercise.

Whistling and blowing exercises may help speed up palatal ascent rate. Yules and Chase (1968) measured the ascent rate of the soft palate in 94 cleft palate patients, 25 velopharyngeal incompetent patients, and 36 normal subjects by the cineradiographic method.

Most of the subjects were under 19 years of age. The rate of ascent in good velopharyngeal closure for the normal group was 65 mm/sec. In contrast the velopharyngeal incompetent group had an ascent rate of 38 mm/sec, while the cleft palate group was the slowest with 26 mm/sec ascent rate. We feel it may be possible to speed up the rate of palatal ascent in a child with velopharyngeal incompetence through vocal motor exercises and pressure-building activities. Many of the exercises for whistling and blowing are applicable here. In this way we may obtain better closure for speech and thus decrease hypernasality and nasal emission. Improved articulation and resonance should result.

We leave this section on physical exercise with certain reservations. First, there is conflicting evidence regarding the usefulness of such exercises. Second, we feel exercises are worth a thorough trial to determine any carryover into speech. Third, we feel all exercises should be communication oriented and should have accompanying phonation or speech. Fourth, we wish to reconfirm our belief that physical exercise can be effective in improving velopharyngeal closure if the speech pathologist carefully follows Pannbacker's (1973) criteria.

The following is an example where physical exercise resulted in consistent velopharyngeal closure for speech. These exercises combined with articulation and resonance therapy made a successful outcome possible:

At 5 years of age during a physical examination prior to entering kindergarten, the examining physician noted Pat had indistinct speech and a hypernasal quality. Pat was referred to us for speech and voice examinations. His parents reported that his speech development had been slow and that he had always "talked through his nose." Physical milestones and intelligence were normal. Our evaluation revealed that Pat had normal language development in general, but that his speech was only about 10% intelligible—knowing the subject of his conversation improved perceived intelligibility to about 25%. He presented mild to moderate hypernasality rated *4* on a *7* point scale. Pat could produce non-nasal vowels with minimal stimulation. There was no nasal emission of sounds. Lateral x-rays revealed essentially normal structures except that the soft palate was short. The distance between the soft palate and pharyngeal wall was 2.5 mm when Pat produced an /s/ at low intensity. However, upon phonating at a comfortable loudness level the velopharyngeal seal was tight with no measurable opening. Therapy goals were set as follows: (1) Therapy to improve articulation and speech intelligibility. (2) Vocal motor exercises designed to obtain consistent velopharyngeal closure during speech. These included pressure building exercises. (3) Exercises designed to direct the air stream orally. (4) Voice therapy designed to improve the oral-nasal resonance balance to eliminate hypernasality.

Over the next 8 months Pat was seen twice weekly, a 1 hour individual session and a 1 hour session with two other children with similar problems. At the end of this time his articulation errors had been eliminated and his speech intelligibility was almost 100%. Hypernasality was reduced to acceptable limits, rated *1* on a *7* point scale. Behavioral management had been successful.

IMPROVING RESONANCE IN HYPONASALITY

Voice therapy is essential when hyponasality is present on a functional basis. It may also be indicated following operations for removal of nasal obstructions. In some cases the person's auditory feedback is such that he continues to use hyponasal speech even though the nasal passage is open. The basic procedures for improving resonance in hypernasality can be modified to apply to children with hyponasal resonance. The 10 step resonance balance chart (Fig. 43) is followed. The listening training procedures are the same with the speech pathologist using a hyponasal voice. The speech pathologist must teach the child how to produce nasal sounds and when they should be used. A child can be taught to hum a prolonged /m/ and then taught to produce the /n/ and /ŋ/; after these have been learned in isolation the child is ready to practice them in syllables, words, and then sentences in free conversation (Arnold, 1965, p. 686). Increasing the phonation time on /m/, /n/, and /ŋ/ in connected speech decreases the impression of hyponasality (Scholl, 1961).

An unusual combination of hypernasality

and hyponasality sometimes occurs (Arnold, 1965, p. 687; Murphy, 1964, p. 59; West and Ansberry, 1968, p. 389). Some persons may have a partial obstruction in the nasal passages interfering with production of normal nasal sounds /m/, /n/, and /ŋ/, but strangely they may nasalize some vowels or consonants. The program for this problem, according to West and Ansberry (1968, p. 389), includes the following: (1) explain the causes of both types of resonance problems, (2) administer a thorough program of listening training, (3) practice control of velopharyngeal closure, (4) teach adequate nasalization on /m/, /n/, and /ŋ/, and (5) improve articulation ability especially in connected speech.

Another special problem of resonance is present in a person with chronically open eustachian tubes. This condition alters auditory feedback resulting in hyponasality and autophony—the latter a phenomenon in which a person's voice reaches both sides of the eardrum simultaneously causing him to perceive his own voice as having hollow rain-barrel resonance. In persons with this condition Batza and Parker (1971) suggested that occasionally occluding the external auditory canals provides temporary relief from autophony. Another technique is to have a person monitor his own amplified voice through earphones to provide a cancelling effect on sounds reaching the middle ear from both sides of the ear drum. Batza and Parker stated a person must have high motivation to learn to tolerate the autophony and benefit from remedial help by the speech pathologist.

The following are sets of practice materials to use for children with hyponasality to develop full nasal resonance. We have selected three sets, from Eisenson and Ogilvie (1977), Anderson and Newby (1973), and Fisher (1975), which we feel are representative of the type of material useful for improving nasal resonance.

Eisenson and Ogilvie (1977, p. 326) suggested exercises loaded with words, phrases, and sentences that have the nasal sounds /m/, /n/, and /ŋ/ in them for improving hyponasality as follows: first, have the child gently hum the three nasal sounds; second, have him begin a hum on one of these sounds and then blend it with a vowel; third, have the child prolong one of the nasal sounds and blend it with a vowel such as *mmm-ah* and *nnn-oh*; and fourth, have the child begin with a lengthened nasal sound, blending it with a vowel, and ending with a lengthened nasal sound, for example, *mmm-ah-nnn.*

Anderson and Newby (1973, p. 244) presented exercises to develop nasal resonance:

1. Have the child hum /m/ at various pitch levels up and down the scale, paying particular attention to the tingling on the lips and the resonance in the nasal passages.

2. Tell the child to hum /n/ in the same manner he used with /m/; although the lip sensation is not present he should get vibratory sensations in the nasal cavity.

3. Instruct the child to repeat rapidly /mi/ six times. Do the same with /meɪ/, /maɪ/, /mo/, /mu/. Next do the same exercise using /n/. Be sure the child uses full nasal resonance.

4. Give the child words and short phrases which have the /ŋ/ sound such as: *running, coming, going, ting-a-ling, ding-dong.* Have the child prolong /ŋ/ in each word with full nasal resonance.

The following exercises for hyponasality are based on Fisher (1975, pp. 110, 113–114). First, have the child practice humming exercises, placing his fingers on both sides of the bridge of the nose to feel the vibrations transmitted from the nasal cavity. Next, sprinkle confetti on a piece of cardboard. Have the child hold it under the nares as he gently and steadily prolongs /m/ to make the confetti move slowly across the cardboard. Have him do the same exercise using /n/ and /ŋ/. Bits of facial tissue or cotton balls can be used to vary the procedure. Tell the child to make the materials move slowly across the cardboard. Finally, have the child say word pairs that are the same except the second word of each pair contains a nasal sound. Using the cardboard have the child stress nasal resonance on the second word, moving the material on the cardboard. Word pairs suggested are *be-me, bet-met, by-my, cub-come, rib-rim, wig-wing, tug-tongue.*

SUMMARY

Children with resonance problems need carefully programmed voice therapy. Correctly balanced oral and nasal resonance is based upon improving articulation and speech intelligibility. Special attention should be given to listening training in the programs to reduce or eliminate hypernasality and hyponasality. Eliminating facial grimaces and nares constriction results in cosmetic improvement. Modifying or eliminating vocal abuse and establishing balanced muscular tonus are necessary for improving the quality of the laryngeal tone. Adequate use of loudness, appropriate pitch, and suitable rate of speaking are basic to improved resonance. Using proper oral breath pressure and oral air flow improves both resonance and articulation. Special therapeutic exercises may improve resonance in selected children. A comprehensive voice therapy program enables a child to use good resonance with adequate speech intelligibility.

ELEVEN

Voice Problems of Children with Hearing Losses

The program of voice therapy presented in this chapter is designed for use by the speech pathologist in handling voice problems of hearing-impaired children in a variety of settings including schools, college and university speech and hearing centers, and community and hospital clinics.

Voice problems may be associated with all types and extent of hearing loss. A child with a mild to moderate loss may only have difficulty with oral-nasal resonance balance while a child with a more extensive hearing loss may not only have resonance problems but other problems involving pitch, loudness, laryngeal tone, and rate and rhythm of talking.

Levitt and Nye (1971, p. 20) reported the most noticeable features of the speech of the severely hearing impaired are that intonation is frequently flat and monotonous, rhythm is either lacking or incorrect, and phrasing is inaccurate. Sounds may be produced inefficiently and the person may have to pause for breath frequently. There is also a tendency to speak more slowly with short breath groups of only a few words. Other typical problems are a too-high or too-low modal pitch level, breathiness, harshness, and resonance problems. An important observation of Levitt and Nye is that although voice use may have a secondary effect on meaning, an unpleasant or abnormal voice may nevertheless be an important psychological impediment to communication. Ling (1976, p. 211) stated deviant voice patterns in the hearing impaired are likely to occur when too much and too early emphasis is placed on articulation skills and not enough attention paid to controlling breath and voice production.

It has been observed that infants with severe hearing losses babble and vocalize spontaneously until they are about 9 months of age (Pronovost, 1977, p. 196). After these first months hearing-impaired infants are unable to produce the normal transitions between sounds (Jones, 1967). Teachers and parents are advised to listen carefully for the natural quality and pitch of a very young hearing-impaired child's voice as he babbles and vocalizes during play; the child should be helped to maintain this pleasant voice quality, avoiding the development of a nasal or strained voice (Miller, 1960). Magner (1971, p. 246) advised using an informal approach to speech development starting as early as possible. She noted the child's spontaneous vocalizations and speech attempts should be promoted and encouraged and more formal analytical methods in speech begun when the child is ready for them.

VOICE THERAPY

Vorce (1974, pp. 49–50) stated attention to the voice of the hearing-impaired child should begin very early. He must be given every encouragement to use his voice for communication. Vorce suggested the parent and teacher should consistently respond to a young child's use of voice, though it may be only an approximation of speech or a random vocalization. The adult should respond by giving the child a strong auditory signal and encouraging the child to reply, preferably by repeating. In this way a child establishes the idea of conscious vocalization and he can be expected to use his voice for communication. The early use of amplification provides the child with the stimulation of feedback of his own vocalizing; parents and other adults should reinforce this feedback by imitating the child's vocal patterns (Pronovost, 1977, p. 196). General voice training as a part of a child's regular program helps prevent the development of voice problems and insures a more adequate voice for effective speech communication (Wilson, 1972, p. 497). Then if voice problems arise they should be approached through therapy.

With appropriate modifications our general programs of voice therapy for children with normal hearing can be used for hearing-impaired children. The modifications depend mainly upon the child's aided hearing. We will suggest some of the appropriate modifications and will include supplementary exercises from programs for deaf children. We recommend the following general principles for voice therapy in the presence of a hearing loss: (1) full use should be made of the auditory pathway; (2) the voice therapy program must always be coordinated closely with the child's overall program, including auditory training, lip reading, improvement of articulation, vocabulary building, and speech; (3) the auditory approach should be supplemented by visual stimuli and training in the use of kinesthetic and tactile cues.

Our program of voice therapy for hearing-impaired children makes full use of the auditory pathway through the use of our listening training program. This program should be based on the child's previous auditory training and combined with his current auditory training program. According to Sanders (1971, p. 205), "Auditory training constitutes a systematic procedure designed to increase the amount of information that a person's hearing contributes to his total perception." Auditory training is an integral part of the program for a child with a hearing loss, and it ranges all the way from gross discrimination of noises to fine discrimination of speech sounds.

Although we place primary emphasis on an auditory approach, we recommend supplementing it with visual stimulation and with kinesthetic and tactile cues. Pollack (1970, p. 19) advocated a primarily auditory approach to teaching very young children; then when the listening function has been established she recommended supplementing auditory cues with visual cues. According to Berg (1970, p. 305) supplementation of auditory stimulation with visual and tactile aids should occur when the child is between 3 and 5 years of age. The use of tactile and kinesthetic cues, according to New (1945), helps the child develop an "inner feeling," specifically in the region of the throat and neck, as to what is desirable and undesirable; this helps him control quality and pitch. The speech pathologist signals to the child when he is producing the desired pitch, loudness, or quality. With training the child can develop the ability to supplement his auditory cues with the tactile and kinesthetic sensations of the desired voice productions. Froeschels (1943; 1952) and Beebe (1977) recommended the use of the chewing method, described in Chapter 8 to improve the voices of hard of hearing and deaf children. They felt the use of this method, with special attention to the kinesthesia of chewing and of improved voice quality, helps to replace unusual voice patterns with more normal patterns for these children. Full use should be made of a child's individual hearing aid. He may need to be encouraged to wear it and instructed to take care of it carefully. The speech pathologist should have information about the specifications for the aid a child is wearing. The audiologist, parents, and hearing aid dispenser are all good sources for this. The information is necessary as the speech pathologist makes a daily check of each child's hearing aid. Ling (1976, p. 157) recommended making a brief check of the child's aid at the beginning of each session to see how well the child hears speech. He suggested speaking the sounds /u/, /ɑ/, /i/, /ʃ/, and /s/ at a distance the child can usually hear them. The child is asked to clap his hands or to repeat each sound when he hears it. Amplification systems in the therapy room must be in good operating condition for the child to benefit from voice work. If group or individual auditory trainers are used, the speech pathologist must check the equipment before each use (Baldwin, 1975). This includes listening to each receiver and making sure the controls are operable.

GOALS OF THERAPY

The goals of therapy for children with a voice problem in the presence of a hearing loss are: (1) balanced resonance, without excessive hypernasality, hyponasality, or the cul-de-sac effect; (2) proper modal pitch level with appropriate expressive pitch variations; (3) control of loudness; (4) a clear laryngeal tone free from hypertension and hypotension; and (5) correct rate and rhythm of speaking.

Each goal is approached through the use of the 10 step voice therapy outline (Fig. 25). Included in this outline are the three basic procedures of voice therapy: listening training, teaching correct voice use, and habituation of correct voice use. The aspect of voice found to be most amenable to change is selected to begin concentrated listening training. However, with most children we work on several aspects of defective voice simultaneously. For example, because of the close interrelationship of loudness and pitch, these are often given simultaneous attention. Inappropriate use of rate may also be included in a simultaneous approach.

Carryover and habituation may prove to be especially slow in the presence of a hearing impairment (Miller, 1948). The habituation procedures described in Chapter 12 should be followed. Habituation, especially in children with hearing impairments, requires much time, patience, and perseverance on the part of the speech pathologist, the child, his family, and his teachers.

Voice Guide Lines

As we start voice therapy with a hearing-impaired child we have him follow guide lines for effective speaking based on Ewing and Ewing (1954, p. 214):

1. Speak at a suitable pitch level and rely mainly on lower-pitched tones rather than very high-pitched tones.

2. Study the speaking situation—see how many people are present and how big the room is; then decide whether to speak at ordinary conversational loudness, more loudly, or more quietly than usual.

3. Throw your voice well forward so everyone can understand you and remember, crisp consonants help intelligibility.

4. Never speak too quickly or too slowly; speak with a proper rate.

5. Speak rhythmically and with good intonation; use full sentences.

6. When you read aloud, recite in class, or act in plays think of the meaning of the words and how to phrase them so their meaning will be clear to others.

Our basic approach to voice therapy with the hearing impaired is illustrated by the following example:

Ellen was 11 years of age when we first knew her. She had a bilateral high frequency hearing loss sensorineural in nature, which had been diagnosed when she was 3 years old. Our audiological evaluation of her revealed an air and bone steep configuration with normal hearing sensitivity at 250 Hz dropping to 80 dB at 4000 Hz and 8000 Hz. Her air conduction hearing loss for the average 500–1000–2000 Hz was 43 dB right ear and 67 dB left ear. Her speech reception threshold was 40 dB right ear, 55 dB left

ear, and 40 dB sound field. Speech discrimination scores were 56% right ear, 60% left ear, and 58% sound field. Ellen wore a hearing aid in her right ear; her aided speech reception threshold was 25 dB and speech discrimination 62%. Prior to seeing us Ellen had had several years of therapy designed chiefly to improve her overall language ability and articulation.

The main features of our voice evaluation were: (1) Voice profile rating of 6, low modal pitch level, and 6 for monotone inflections. Her modal fundamental frequency was 195 Hz with a range of 185 to 205 Hz (2 semitones); normal is 265 Hz, range 220 to 310 (6 semitones). (2) Profile rating of 7 for slow rate. She spoke with three to four words per breath group with excessive duration time on syllables. Her reading rate on our "Zoo" passage was 41 words per minute, considered about 75 to 100 words too slow. (3) Profile rating of 6 for breathy laryngeal tone, with the notation of continuous phonation. Ellen's maximum phonation time was 5 sec, less than half the average for her age.

Our therapy plan for Ellen was a generalized approach where we would work on several parameters simultaneously. We wanted her to raise her modal pitch level 5 semitones to about middle C. During this process we planned to use pitch and loudness variation exercises to modify her monotone. We wanted to increase her rate of speaking; this had to be coordinated closely with work on her continuous phonation. For this dual task we had her practice reading sentences one word at a time; at the same time we increased her rate by having her say each word quickly to shorten syllable duration. Excessive breathiness was approached through a combined auditory, tactile, and visual program. We followed our 10 step therapy outline paying careful attention to the auditory aspects of breathiness. We had her feel with her hand the high air flow of a breathy vowel compared to the low air flow of a fully phonated vowel which can hardly be felt; for visual reinforcement we demonstrated the difference in air flow by showing her how a breathy vowel made a candle flame flicker while a loud clear vowel had little effect on the flame. We used breathing exercises and pushing exercises to increase her maximum phonation time and to eliminate the short breath groups.

A typical therapy session looked something like this: (1) breathing and pushing exercises; (2) raising voice pitch level as she phonated during these exercises; (3) skits in which she assumed characters using varying pitch inflections; (4) during these impersonations she would use varying rates, slow, average, and fast; (5) sentence practice to break up continuous phonation and speeding up rate by saying each word more quickly; (6) production of a clear voice free from breathiness; (7) regular carryover assignments written in her notebook so she had very specific and enjoyable voice projects to do at home and school.

Ellen was seen for 70 one hour sessions over a period of 1 year. At the end of this time she had a clearer laryngeal tone with the breathiness almost eliminated (rated *3*). Her modal pitch level was near middle C and she had increased her range so her voice sounded quite suitable for a 12 year old (rated *2*). Continous phonation, while still present at times, was not distracting because her rate of talking was getting close to 125 words per minute (rated *2*). Increased rate and widened pitch range had resulted in practically eliminating the monotone effect (rated *1*). Ellen now had better voice control and a more pleasant voice. She had therapy with us for an additional 6 months with continuing improvement and she was quite satisfied with her newly learned communication abilities.

RESONANCE

The resonance problem in a child with a hearing loss may be hypernasality, hyponasality, or the hollow muffled quality typical of cul-de-sac resonance. Sometimes there is a combination of two or more resonance parameters; often cul-de-sac resonance is a prominent feature.

The reduction of hypernasality is usually rated high on the list of voice parameters to be approached in the hearing impaired. Fletcher and Daly (1976) used TONAR II on a group of subjects with mean hearing loss

for the better ear of 83 dB HTL (ISO 1964). The subjects ranged in age from 7 to 21 years, with a mean age of 15.9. Compared to a group of normally hearing subjects, the impaired hearing group allowed a much greater proportion of the sound to escape through the nose than did those with normal hearing. Colton and Cooker (1968) compared perceived hypernasality in the oral reading of two groups: one consisted of 13 males and 15 females (mean age 18.74 years) with a mean hearing loss in the better ear of 90 dB; the other group was a matched group with normal hearing. A group of listeners judged the deaf speakers as more hypernasal than the normally hearing subjects.

For establishing oral-nasal resonance balance in hearing-impaired children we suggest following the program described in Chapter 10. Our program emphasizes the auditory approach supplemented by visual, kinesthetic, and tactile aspects of establishing oral-nasal resonance balance. Ling (1975, p. 75) reminded us that hypernasality in a hearing-impaired child is due to auditory inability to monitor resonance. Ling stated the /m/, /n/, and /ŋ/ are poorly produced and the adjacent vowels and other consonants are distorted. Amplification in the 300 Hz range is essential for hearing these nasal sounds. Therefore, Ling (1975, p. 75) stated listening training for correction of hypernasality may be more successful if a high quality group aid is used. A high quality group or speech training aid may cover the range from 70 to 7000 Hz; this is in contrast to wearable hearing aids which do not always give amplification of the low frequencies (Ling, 1975, p. 68).

A typical resonance problem found in many hearing-impaired children is a combination of cul-de-sac resonance and hyponasality. This is often described as hollow muffled resonance. Cul-de-sac resonance is sometimes prevented by early hearing aid use and early attention to voice. Since it is usually associated with hyponasal or hypernasal speech, attention to proper nasal resonance may result in a modification of the cul-de-sac resonance. However, in some children it requires direct attention through a program based on listening training and supplemented by special techniques.

We will use this type of problem to illustrate methods for improving resonance following the therapy steps of the Resonance Balance Chart (Fig. 43). The program is begun with (Step 1) the speech pathologist explaining the rule about the use of proper resonance. Simple drawings help to show how the consonants /m/, /n/, and /ŋ/ are nasalized and that the velopharyngeal port is essentially closed for all other sounds. The child learns that one cause of cul-de-sac resonance is retracting the tongue "into a ball" in the back of the mouth. Then the basic listening training program is started following the procedures described in Chapters 7 and 10. This includes (Steps 2 and 3) (a) making the child aware of resonance differences in others, (b) gross discrimination of resonance differences in others, and (c) fine discrimination of differences in others. These three points are applied as follows: First, the speech pathologist produces vowels, words, and phrases with undesirable resonance on some productions and normal resonance on others. The child indicates when he hears the undesirable resonance. Initially amplification with an auditory trainer is useful to make sure the child receives a strong signal. Soon, however, the child should use his own hearing aid. Second, the speech pathologist produces undesirable resonance and normal resonance samples requiring the child to discriminate between the two by indicating which is which. Third, the speech pathologist randomly produces sounds with varying degrees of resonance imbalance from severe imbalance through moderate and mild imbalance to normal resonance for the child to discriminate. Then (Steps 4 and 5) the listening training program is applied to the child's own voice. He is made aware of resonance defects in himself, followed by gross and fine discrimination of differences of resonance in his own voice. The speech pathologist prepares recordings of the child's voice. The child listens to these recordings of his own productions following the pattern used in discriminating resonance imbalance in the speech pathologist's voice. Now he must become aware of excessive resonance imbalance in his recordings, identifying only the very worst ones. Next he listens to his recordings, identifying the productions with excessive resonance imbalance and those with normal resonance. Then he discriminates very fine differences in his own productions ranging from excessive resonance imbalance to normal.

When the child can identify and discriminate resonance imbalance of varying degrees and normal resonance in both others and

himself, he is ready to begin control of resonance in himself (Steps 6 and 7). The recordings of the child are used as models of production. The child listens to these recordings and does negative practice of varying degrees of resonance imbalance contrasted with his productions of normal resonance. In this way the child obtains voluntary control of resonance and is able to reduce or eliminate undesirable resonance.

Boone (1966) felt cul-de-sac quality is due to a focus of resonance in the pharyngeal area related to retraction of the tongue toward the pharyngeal wall. He recommended the following exercise designed to keep the tongue low in the mouth with the tongue tip forward and to increase oral resonance. Have the child start with a whispered repetitive /tɑ/, /tɑ/, /tɑ/, /tɑ/ and then whisper /dɑ/, /sɑ/, and /zɑ/ in the same way. The exercise is repeated using voice. These alveolar tongue-tip sounds should be practiced in rapid drill for about 5 min four or five times daily. Boone also used the consonants /w/, /p/, /b/, /f/, /v/, /θ/, /ð/, and /l/ combined with vowels having a high oral focus, such as /i/, /ɪ/, /e/, /ɛ/, and /æ/. Carryover (Steps 8, 9, and 10) is now systematically approached following procedures described in the next chapter. The speech pathologist should realize that carryover of new resonance patterns may be difficult for some hearing-impaired children (Ling, 1975, p. 68).

Many additional techniques should be used with the hearing-impaired child to help him learn better use of resonance. Often a hearing-impaired child has poor resonance on the nasals /m/, /n/, /ŋ/. Therefore, the speech pathologist should concentrate on improving both oral and nasal resonance, maintaining a careful distinction between the two. The use of the instruments listed on p. 157 helps the child discriminate between hypernasal, hyponasal, and normal resonance and can be an aid in the production of improved resonance. The child should be taught the kinesthetic and tactile sensations that signal to him the adequate use of resonance. The child can learn tactile sensations by placing his fingers lightly on the speech pathologist's nose, comparing the presence of vibrations during hypernasal speech with the absence of vibrations during non-nasal speech. The child then does the same on himself. A series of vowels with /m/, /n/, and /ŋ/ can be used, for example /u–n/, /ɑ–n/, /o–n/, /i–n/.

Magner (1971, pp. 253–254) stated resonance methods developed for work with hearing children should be used with the hearing impaired. Sometimes special exercises to control breathing, tongue movements, and the muscles of the soft palate are useful. Improvement of articulation of /m/, /n/, and /ŋ/ will often help improve resonance balance. Sometimes lowering the pitch of the voice helps reduce hypernasality. Shifting pitch downward results in a lowering of the tongue carriage. This allows for more orality of sound production and reduces cul-de-sac resonance. Magner recommended giving children help toward increasing the kinesthesia of oral speech contrasted to nasal speech. Syllable drills with voiceless consonants preceding and following vowels aid in developing this type of kinesthesia. For example, have the child practice /ta, ta, ta/ then /tat, tat, tat/. Magner further stated that reducing hypernasality often results from the use of /h/ in vowel drill: for example, /ɑ–hɑ/, /o-ho/, /u-hu/.

Calvert and Silverman (1975, pp. 184–185) suggested that the speech pathologist imitate the child's hypernasal voice even exaggerating it so the child can recognize his undesirable resonance. Exercises concentrating on directing breath through the oral cavity should be used. Having the child inhale and exhale through a wide open mouth and then holding the position helps to develop the kinesthesia of velar movement. Combining nasal consonants with a vowel spoken with force also helps develop this kinesthesia. For example, we have the child practice syllable groups of the following type, being sure he explosively says each of the vowels. An abrupt glottal attack must be avoided.

/ŋɑ, ŋɑ, ŋɑ/, /ŋo, ŋo, ŋo/
/mi, mi, mi/, /mu, mu, mu/
/næ, næ, næ/, /nɔ, nɔ, nɔ/

The following exercises were recommended by Haycock (1933, pp. 100–102), and are to be performed with the child observing himself in a mirror.

1. Instruct the child to open his mouth, lower the back of the tongue and place the tongue tip firmly behind the lower incisors. Holding this tongue position, have the child breathe in and out strongly several times.

2. Have the child close his lips, inhale through the nose, then open the mouth for the exhalation. While he does this the tongue should be low in the mouth and the throat relaxed.

3. With his mouth wide open, have the child inhale through the nose and exhale through his mouth.

4. Have the child phonate /ŋ-ɑ/ several times, noting the visual, auditory, kinesthetic, and tactile differences between them.

5. Have the child say a series of vowel sounds followed by /ŋ/, for example /u-o-ɑ-i-ŋ/, prolonging the /ŋ/. Have the child do the same exercise followed by /m/ and then by /n/.

Vorce (1974, pp. 60–61) suggested exercises for resonance designed for children 7 to 9 years of age. The following are for improving oral resonance: (1) Tell the child to say rapidly the syllables /bʌ/, /dʌ/, /gʌ/. Repeating them several times promotes rapid movement of the lips, tongue, and velum. Next have the child combine these consonants with vowels in rhythmic groups, for example, /bo, do, go/, /bi, di, gi/. (3) Now have the child say vowels such as /i/, /ɑ/, /u/ accompanied by rhythmic movements. Using a specific rhythm have him pat his hands on the table as he says the vowels. The following exercises are to develop improved nasal resonance: (1) Have the child prolong /m/ and /n/ having him note the "tickle" in the lips for /m/ and in the nose and tongue for /n/. (2) Ask him to prolong the series /m-n-ŋ/ on one continuous breath. Have him note the vibrations in the face and head. (3) Tell him to keep the tongue relaxed as he prolongs the nasals in a syllable, for example, /hɑm-hɑm-hɑm-/, /hɑn-hɑn-hɑn-/, /hɑŋ-hɑŋ-hɑŋ-/.

Vorce (1974, p. 72) suggested for children 10 to 12 years of age these exercises to help in developing oral-nasal resonance balance. (1) For oral resonance ask the child to practice plosives with vowels in breath groups. Each group should be said on one breath. Have the child concentrate on orality of the sounds, avoiding hypernasality. /bi/; /bi/ /be/; /bi/ /be/ /bɑ/; /bi/ /be/ /bɑ/ /bu/; /bi/ /be/ /bɑ/ /bu/ /bɔ/. A good exercise to improve nasal resonance using /h/ is suggested. Have the child repeat the following three times prolonging the nasal sounds and being sure to keep the speech musculature relaxed: /hʌm/, /hʌn/, /hʌŋ/. For oral-nasal resonance balance have the child practice /hʌŋ-gʌ/ with the /g/ exploded into the following vowel. Vorce stated this exercise is especially good for lazy velums and muffled voices. Other examples are /hʌŋ-gɑ/, /hʌŋ-gi/, /hʌŋ-gu/.

Additional resonance practice exercises are (after Van Dusen, 1953, p. 142).

1. Say the first sound being sure it vibrates your nose; pause, and then say the second sound without hypernasality.

/m/——/ɑ/
/n/——/o/
/ŋ/——/ɔ/

Next turn them around:

/ɑ/——/m/
/o/——/n/
/ɔ/——/ŋ/

2. Do the same with syllables:

/mɑ/——/bɑ/
/no/——/do/
/ŋɔ/——/gɔ/

Turn them around:

/bɑ/——/mɑ/
/do/——/no/
/gɔ/——/ŋɔ/

3. Now use words.

mop——top
not——dot
/ŋɔk/——gawk

Turn them around.

top——mop
dot——not
gawk——/ŋɔk/

4. Use also phrases and sentences.

We have given sample exercises to improve resonance in the hearing-impaired child These can be used by the speech pathologist as a basis for developing additional exercises.

PITCH

The modal pitch level of a child with a hearing loss should be checked periodically and compared with norms for his age to make sure the high pitch of childhood does not persist as he matures. Although individuals vary, young hearing-impaired children generally use a fundamental frequency within the normal range. For example, Meckfessel (1965) found deaf boys 7 and 8 years of age had a mean fundamental frequency of 292 Hz and normally hearing boys 289 Hz. Also, Ermovick (1965) found the mean fundamental frequency of deaf girls the same age was 235 Hz and of normally hearing girls 245 Hz. All these figures fall within the normal limits of our pitch tables (Tables 1 and 2). However, a group of deaf males 17 and 18 years of age had a mean fundamental frequency of 184 Hz and the normally hearing group 130 Hz (Meckfessel, 1965), a difference of one-half octave which is significant. The normally hearing group is comparable to our norms (Table 1) while the mean of the deaf boys is definitely higher than our acceptable limits. The situation is a little different for girls of this age. No statistical difference was found between the mean fundamental frequencies of 256 Hz for the deaf girls and 230 Hz for normally hearing girls (Ermovick, 1965). However, while the figure for hearing girls is within our acceptable limits (Table 2) the mean for deaf girls is slightly above our upper limit. Boone (1966), commenting on this study, stated there was wide variation among the older deaf girls with some of them having very high pitch; these girls should be taught to use a lower modal pitch level.

Differences have been found, however, at a young age. Jones (1971) reported on the fundamental frequency of cry samples of 40 young children with severe to profound hearing loss and a control group of 24 normally hearing children all 4 years of age or younger. The results indicated the hearing-impaired youngsters consistently demonstrated a higher fundamental frequency than the normally hearing children.

According to Nickerson (1975) pitch problems of the deaf are of two general types, inappropriate modal pitch and improper intonation. Intonation problems consist of two major types, monotone voice and excessive or erratic pitch variations. Modal fundamental frequency is higher than normal and is less stable. Jones (1967) in reviewing research on 'deaf voice' reported the deaf have patterns of vowel sound production that are imprecise. Also, they have nontypical glottic and velopharyngeal adjustments in connected speech resulting in different quality and resonance. There are distortions of transitions between consonants and vowels, and durational differences. Nickerson (1975) stated improper use of muscles or the use of inappropriate muscles or muscle groups may account for some of the pitch variations from vowel to vowel. Also excessive variations in pitch may be the result of inappropriate muscle contractions causing a tensing or slackening of the vocal cords.

The basic procedures for improvement of pitch can be built around the 10 steps on the pitch chart (Fig. 38). If any of these steps proves to be especially difficult for a child with a hearing loss, the speech pathologist can take emphasis off the chart temporarily until the child has mastered the difficult steps.

Pitch Listening Training

Hearing-impaired children can benefit from concentrated listening training to improve pitch discrimination. Gengel (1969) stated the capacity of hearing-impaired children to make fine discriminations of pitch is not as poor as many people feel and that with practice they can improve their performance. Gengel compared two groups of hearing-impaired children, one classified as deaf and the other as hard of hearing, with a group of normally hearing children on their ability to discriminate differences between paired pure tones. Various pure tones were compared with two standard frequencies, 250 Hz and 500 Hz. It was found that about half of the hearing-impaired children were able to discriminate differences in frequencies when the difference was 4% at the two standard frequencies. (A semitone change in vocal music is approximately 6%.) This level of performance compared favorably with the performance of children with normal hearing sensitivity.

The speech pathologist should apply the basic listening training program described in Chapters 7 and 9 to pitch. The child learns to identify undesirable pitch in others, and then proceeds to gross discrimination and fine discrimination of pitch differences in others. A tape recorder can be used to establish better pitch discrimination. The speech pathologist first records his own voice using a high pitch and then a very low pitch and asks the child to make gross discriminations. Ling (1976, p. 208) suggested initially varying the pitch of the voice by at least 8 semitones for discrimination training. If a frequency indicator is used the two tones should differ about 100 to 120 Hz for a woman's voice and 60 to 70 Hz for a man's voice. The speech pathologist proceeds to three different levels—high, middle, and low—with the middle tone at the

child's optimum modal level. The child makes fine discrimination between these three levels. Later the pitch differences between the tones can be reduced for discriminating even smaller differences. If the child initially is unable to distinguish pitch differences in the speech pathologist's voice, a piano, musical instrument, toy horn, or toy xylophone may be used to present widely different tones for discrimination. The speech pathologist later returns to discrimination of voice.

Some hearing-impaired children may be able to proceed through the stages of listening training with only slightly more practice than children with normal hearing. For others special methods of developing pitch discrimination may be needed. Visual aids are helpful in developing pitch discrimination. Ling (1976, p. 208) suggested giving visual cues to the child by accompanying high tones with a hand stretched high above the head and then indicating low tones with a hand below the waist. Later the hand signals are eliminated and the child must discriminate pitch by voice alone. Vorce (1974, p. 51) suggested the child can imitate the teacher in physical movements to reinforce "high" or "low." Lines can be drawn at various levels on the blackboard and a car or airplane moved up and down the lines to indicate pitch changes. Lights of different colors can be flashed when different pitches are presented (Streng et al. 1958, p. 322). When working with young children appropriate mechanical toys can be activated when various pitch levels are presented, for example, a bird for high pitch, a clown for medium pitch, and a dancing bear for low pitch. An older child can view an oscilloscope or the VU meter of a pitch indicator to aid him in identifying various pitches produced by the speech pathologist. Flash cards can be used or stimuli can be written on the chalkboard with placement of the words indicating pitch level:

Gross Discrimination (two levels):

Fine Discrimination (three levels):

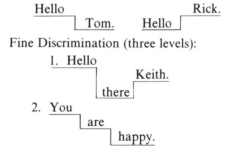

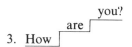

3. How _are_ _you?_

The training can be made more interesting by varying the child's responses as well as the stimuli. Grammatico (1975) showed pictures to a child of two different objects, for example, a birthday cake and an airplane. The teacher sings a song about one, with the child indicating the appropriate item. At first the child can watch the teacher's face, but later he should be able to discriminate songs, sentences, phrases, and individual sounds, adequate and inadequate vocal parameters, without watching the source of the sounds. The child can be asked to lift his hands above his head for a high tone, touch his shoulders for a medium tone, and stoop toward the floor for a low tone (Streng et al. 1958, p. 214). The head, waist, or knees could be touched for other intermediate tones. Magner (1971, p. 253) stated the use of musical instruments with the child going up and down stair steps according to the pitch level heard helps him understand pitch differences. Streng et al. (1958, p. 214) used stairs or steps for responding. The child can climb to the top step when he hears a high tone and return to lower steps and the floor for intermediate and low tones.

As the child improves in pitch discrimination the teacher can read or tell stories using a variety of pitch for different characters (Streng et al. 1958, p. 214). Magner (1971, p. 253) suggested using stories in which pitch can be dramatized, for example, *The Three Bears* and *Billy Goat Gruff*. The child can be asked to indicate which character is being impersonated.

Teaching Correct Pitch Use

Before a child is ready to be taught correct use of pitch he should listen discriminatingly to his own use of pitch. The first step is to make the child aware of undesirable pitch use in his own voice. The child listens to recordings of his voice made in various situations to identify undesirable pitch use. Examples of desirable pitch use are also identified. Gross discrimination practice of these two widely different levels of pitch is done. The training proceeds to the final step, fine discrimination of three levels of pitch: high, normal, and low. Examples of these are isolated in his recordings and the child is shown the differences. Discrimination practice of the

three levels continues until the child becomes proficient in judging his own pitch use. The singing voice can be used in a similar manner (Presto, 1943). The speech pathologist should check with the classroom and music teachers to coordinate training in pitch discrimination with other discrimination training the child is receiving.

Now the child is ready for the two major aspects of learning correct pitch use: (1) using a suitable modal pitch level within an appropriate pitch range, and (2) using appropriate pitch intonation and inflection patterns. The program for teaching correct pitch described in Chapters 7 and 9 should be followed. Additional techniques may be necessary for the hearing-impaired child. The following procedures for developing control of pitch are based on Streng et al. (1958, p. 230): (1) the child imitates the teacher as he hums gliding up and down the scale; (2) the teacher hums middle C, B, or B flat below middle C. The child feels the vibrations in the teacher's face and throat and then imitates these notes; (3) the child imitates specific notes produced by the teacher using tactile and kinesthetic cues; (4) the teacher hums /m/ at the child's optimum pitch while the child says the following syllables at this pitch: /m/-/ɑ/, /m/-/ɑ/, /mɑ/; /m/-/ɔ/, /m/-/ɔ/, /mɔ/; /m/-/o/, /m/-/o/, /mo/; the child then hums one octave higher and produces these syllables at this pitch; the child does the same thing one-half octave higher than his optimum pitch; (5) the child speaks short sentences in a monotone at the correct pitch level; (6) the child then uses normal variations of pitch while saying the same sentences; (7) the child uses variations of pitch while telling stories and participating in dramatic sketches. Synchronous reading may be helpful (Berry and Eisenson, 1956, p. 467; Greene, 1964, pp. 221–222; Van Riper, 1959). The speech pathologist reads in unison with the child on a binaural trainer. The intensity of the speech pathologist's voice is gradually increased until the child hears only the speech pathologist's voice. He then may follow the pitch variations he hears. This can be done to help obtain correct pitch level, inflections, and rhythm. This should be done carefully to be sure the child is actually following the pitch variations he hears. There are children's records available with accompanying pictures and stories. Carefully chosen records may be useful for synchronous reading. Children with hearing impairments should be taught to sing at a very early age. Singing enables hearing-impaired children to maintain or to develop more suitable pitch and inflections in their speech.

Direct methods for teaching pitch control are often useful. Ling (1976, p. 210) suggested the teacher vocalize at three levels on separate breaths at high, middle, and low points in the child's vocal range with the middle one the desired level for the child. Then the child can duplicate these levels to get the feeling of the new desired level. Ling (1976, p. 208) suggested that to obtain a lower pitch have the child prolong vowels as he lowers his chin towards his chest keeping the arms and shoulders relaxed. Then to obtain high pitch have the child raise his head and stretch his neck as he prolongs vowels. Attention should be focused on the auditory aspects of pitch with head movements eliminated as soon as possible. Another way to get lower pitch suggested by Ling is to have the child press on his own thyroid cartilage. Pitch can be oscillated by alternating pressure on the cartilage—producing a quavering production which can be fun. Pitch levels can be scanned in this way with correct levels identified and isolated.

As the child begins to be able to control pitch many direct exercises can be used. We have found a set of exercises based on Van Dusen (1953, pp. 107–109) useful with many hearing-impaired children. These exercises can be used for scanning to search for the desirable modal level, to isolate and control pitch breaks, and for improvement of expression. These involve practicing vowels, syllables, words, and sentences at three levels: high, modal, and low. Instruments can be used with these exercises to help the child control pitch. Examples are given below. Vary the vowels, consonants, and sentences.

1. Vowel drill

High	/ɑ/		/ɑ/	
Modal		/o/	/o/	/o/
Low		/u/	/u/		/u/

2. Syllable drill

High	/bɑ/		/bɑ/	
Modal		/bo/	/bo/	/bo/
Low		/bu/	/bu/		/bu/

3. Word drill

High	boy		bat	
Modal		box	book	box
Low		boat		boat

4. Sentence drill

High	saw		Cupcakes		
Modal	I	the		are	good.
Low		dog.		very	

Pronovost (1977, p. 207) stressed the importance of teaching intonational features of language to the deaf. For intonation training Grammatico (1975) suggested the teacher should use frequent changes in intonation, asking the child to indicate the level of intonation; for example, a child's name can be said at three different pitch levels, high, middle, and low, asking the child to respond indicating which one he heard. Then have him say his own name at the three levels. Vorce (1974, pp. 61–62) suggested using a system of markings for developing intonation, such as using arrows to indicate pitch changes. Vorce also suggested practice associating intonation with emotional tones. This can be done using pictures showing anger, fear, love. The child can be asked to say a sentence with the intonation pattern expressing the emotion depicted. For older children and teenagers Vorce (1974, p. 80) suggested continuing work with intonation and pitch variations and use of voice for expression of emotion through dramatics and short skits. Videotaping also provides motivation and opportunity for practice of the newly learned intonation patterns.

Disturbed mutation can be a problem in a hearing-impaired adolescent. The methods described in Chapters 7 and 9 can be used for these young people. Engleberg (1962) described the following program he used in working on a falsetto voice in a deaf female 20 years of age. Phonate while the head is extended backward. Phonate on request at a lower pitch. Phonate at the highest pitch, dropping suddenly to the lowest pitch. The sounds to be used with this technique are /ɑ/, /o/, and /i/, /mɑ/, and the word *mama*. Counting from 1 through 10 is used, paying particular attention to pitch control and avoiding forced respiration. Sessions are also devoted to improving vocal inflection, progressing from reading to general conversation.

The deflection of the needle on the meter of the pitch indicator is particularly useful in indicating to the hard of hearing adolescent when his pitch level is appropriate and when he is making adequate use of pitch inflections. This aids the adolescent in exploring vocal ranges and gives him a visual indication of the appropriate pitch level (Boone, 1966). The youth can be taught to produce the desired pitch level by checking his pitch on the pitch indicator and then asking him to note the kinesthetic and tactile sensations when he produces the desired pitch. The speech pathologist should immediately compare this with the person's old inappropriate pitch by comparing the tactile and kinesthetic sensations of the two.

Voice therapy for improving pitch control and intonation patterns continues until a child or teenager has acquired optimal use of these parameters. All sensory channels should be used for teaching, with the child eventually depending on the auditory channel as much as he and his hearing aid allow.

LOUDNESS

The modification of loudness follows the general pattern of listening training, learning to produce the desired level, and habituation. The 10 step loudness chart (Fig. 36) is appropriate for use with a hearing-impaired child. To introduce loudness concepts the following special techniques were recommended by Streng et al. (1958, pp. 212–213): (1) compare loud stomping with tiptoeing, loud clapping with soft clapping, and loud music with soft music; (2) play a hide and seek game as the child searches for a hidden toy; play music with the loudness regulated according to the nearness of the child to the toy; (3) the child sings or hums softly and then loudly to relate the concept of loudness or softness to his own voice; (4) teach the child to increase speech intensity in noisy surroundings and decrease it in quiet places; take him into both types of situations. We recommend calling attention to auditory, kinesthetic, and tactile cues to show him correct loudness in the presence of varying levels of background noise.

Ewing and Ewing (1954, p. 214) stated appropriate loudness levels for hearing-impaired children have to be determined by a person with normal hearing. This can be done by using the VU meter of a group auditory trainer. Children can compare their VU meter readings with the teacher's and in this way learn when they are speaking at ordinary conversational loudness and at quieter and louder levels. The intensity indicator of a recorder, an oscilloscope, or sound level meter can also be used in teaching the child to use a desired loudness. The child watches the visual indicator as he uses different loudness levels with the speech pathologist telling him when the loudness level is adequate. In this way the child can coordinate the visual indication with what he hears and feels as he is speaking and can adjust his loudness level accordingly. He can be given supervised practice on different levels in different situations until he has a feeling for the level most suitable for each. Work on appropriate loudness can be incorporated into the general auditory training program and combined with procedures to improve other parameters of voice. Repeated verbal comments on appropriate loudness in various situations will be effective in helping the child correct any deficiency in the use of appropriate loudness.

Ewing and Ewing (1954, pp. 151–152) suggested the words *loud* and *quiet* can be demonstrated to the hearing-impaired child in terms of the amount of effort he uses as he beats a drum. A game "The Old Man" can be played where a whispered voice is used when he is asleep, and then a loud voice is used to waken him, and an even louder voice to make him angry. Ling (1976, pp. 203–205) suggested having the child do brief, loud vocalizations while playing a similar game—"Wake up the Teacher." Vowels, words, and short phrases can be used. The teacher keeps his eyes closed until a specific loudness level is reached. Work on speaking louder as the distance from the teacher is increased can be part of the game. Mechanical toys and voice-operated or hand-switched instruments can also be used; they can be activated only when the voice is as loud as desired. We described some of these instruments in Chapter 9.

Ling (1976, pp. 203–205) suggested methods of practicing soft utterances. For this the teacher stays asleep while the child vocalizes quietly, but wakens when he is too loud. Next the child practices whispered speech. Feeling the force of the breath stream on the hand during a whisper helps monitor loudness. This can also be done by showing the child the effect of an adequate whisper on a candle flame. Ling stated speech during loudness practice of loud, quiet, and whispered speech should be of at least 3 sec duration.

A child can learn varying degrees of loudness such as *very loud, loud, rather loud, quiet, very quiet* through modifying his own muscular efforts as he beats a drum. His ability to monitor loudness while playing a drum is transferred to his use of voice at different distances and in situations that require variations in voice loudness (Ewing and Ewing, 1954, pp. 151–152). We use four loudness levels—*very loud, loud, just right,* and *too soft.* Pictures can be placed in the child's notebook illustrating the levels. These can be pictures of people speaking at different loudness levels (Fig. 35); they can also be pictures of vehicles, machines, or animals which make different levels of noise, or they can be pictures of children engaging in activities ranging from quiet to noisy. The child can be asked to point to the appropriate picture as he and the speech pathologist use each different level of voice.

Van Dusen's (1953, pp. 107–109) format, which we used for pitch control can be adapted to loudness control for the hearing-impaired child. Using a sound level indicator of some type helps the child monitor his loudness during the exercises. Now instead of three pitch levels, the instructions include four levels of loudness, very loud, loud, just right, and too soft.

Carefully planned loudness modification programs help the hearing impaired to communicate effectively. Attention should center on maintaining an adequately loud voice while avoiding one that is overly loud.

LARYNGEAL TONE

Voice therapy designed to improve resonance, pitch, and loudness in the hearing impaired adds flexibility to the voice and often has the added effect of eliminating or modifying problems of laryngeal tone such as harshness, breathiness, and hoarseness. Programs for persistent harshness or hoarseness following procedures for laryngeal dysfunction described in Chapters 8 and 9 should be used when indicated. If the laryngeal tone is hoarse and if the analysis of vocal abuse reveals any abuses being used excessively and to a severe degree, the speech pathologist should develop a program of elimination or modification. Positive laryngeal findings such as vocal nodules definitely indicate the necessity for such a program. In the absence of pathology a program of elimination or modification of vocal abuse serves as a preventive measure for developing pathology. The program for vocal abuse in Chapters 8 and 9 adapted to the needs of the hearing-impaired child should be followed.

Vocal Abuse

Many hearing-impaired children use various forms of vocal abuse. Some of these abuses occur during play and sports activity as part of the pattern of usual exuberance and enthusiasm exhibited by all participants. Other vocal abuses may occur as a child forces phonation in an attempt to be understood.

Ling (1976, p. 213) stated the most common cause of vocal abuse in hearing-impaired children is undue laryngeal tension. The tension may be the result of hard glottal attacks and overusing exertion exercises to obtain voicing. Generalized body tension and the habitual use of inappropriate pitch also contribute to excessive laryngeal tension. Remedial work should include establishing new habits of voicing by vocalizing while holding all but essential muscles relaxed. The teacher should approach voice and speech work with the child in a relaxed easy manner; as a result the child will have a relaxed easy voice. Vorce (1974, p. 49) also stated care should be taken to avoid tension in teaching situations; this will insure that the child will have a natural pleasant voice. Calvert and Silverman (1975, pp. 185–186) stated a strident voice in a hearing-impaired child may be the result of a deaf speaker talking with much generalized constriction and tension in the glottal and supraglottal areas. To demonstrate this the teacher can have the child place his fingers just above her (the teacher's) larynx and have him compare the muscular tension he feels as the teacher uses exaggerated muscle tension and normal muscle action. Then the child can be shown how to modify muscular tension in his own neck. If stridency is associated with bunching the tongue in the back of the mouth, the child can be shown how to keep his tongue forward. Mirror work on tongue positioning is useful.

Breathiness

Special attention should be given to breathiness because it is a frequently encountered laryngeal dysfunction in children with hearing impairments. Breathy voice occurs when there is not enough tension in the vocal cords and they fail to approximate firmly (Ling, 1976, p. 211). Breathiness may be related to a deaf person's use of very short phrases separated by unnecessarily frequent inhalations; also excessive force on plosives preceding vowels may result in breathiness on the vowels (Calvert and Silverman, 1975, p. 185). For this problem we suggest applying our complete program of listening training to breathiness. The procedures described in Chapter 8 for hypofunction are useful in eliminating breathiness. We have found Froeschels' pushing exercises especially valuable in reducing breathiness.

Hudgins (1937) felt elimination of breathiness depends upon the ability to adjust the laryngeal muscles in proper relationship to breath pressure in forming speech sounds. Hudgins found the following series of exercises useful in reducing breathiness in a group of profoundly deaf children with breathy voices; they can be used for all hearing-impaired children.

1. Have the child hold his breath for a reasonable period with the chest slightly inflated and the mouth open. Ask the child to pant in this position, exhaling and inhaling small puffs of air at the rate of about 2 or 3 a sec. This is designed to teach control of the breath supply by use of chest and abdominal muscles.

2. Have the child assume the inflated chest position with the mouth open and exhale a series of puffs of air between inhalations. He is to stop the breath flow between each puff of air. The child does not inhale until he has completed the series of puffs. The number of puffs must be specified, using four or six at first. Each series is followed by a rapid inhalation through the mouth. Do not allow the child to use his entire breath supply in any one series, and do not allow him to revert to the panting exercise. The speed of the pulses should approximate the rate of syllables in normal speech.

3. The next step is designed to develop normal vocal attack. At first have the child produce a tone briefly to make sure he is using the proper amount of tension in the larynx. Proper tension is present when breathiness is absent. Then have him phonate a prolonged /ɑ/. If the tone does not retain a natural quality throughout its duration, the child should be stopped and asked to start over. When he can use a good voice on /ɑ/, he is then asked to produce /u/ and /i/ in the same way.

4. Have the child phonate repetitive vowels on puffs of air, first using /ɑ/ and later proceeding to the /u/ and /i/. The child should start with a series of four or six syllables on a single breath and gradually increase the number. He should maintain good posture and proper laryngeal adjustment, avoiding breathiness on the tone. At first each series consists of a single vowel. Then he is asked to change from one vowel to another in a series, for example, /ɑ/, /u/, /i/, /u/, /i/, /ɑ/. The rate of the vowel production should correspond to normal speaking rate.

5. The basic procedure of the preceding exercise is used, but this time ask the child to alternate a loud and soft vowel within each series. This requires a slight adjustment of the vocal cords to the rate of air flow. This exercise can be varied by having him accent every third vowel as well as having him use other patterns of accent. It can be done on a series containing a single vowel and proceed to varying the vowel within a series.

6. Have the child alternate a whisper and vocalization in a series of vowels. This is done on a single exhalation. The sounds are produced rapidly and intensity is held constant. The air flow is stopped between sounds with the child inhaling only between series. He should begin with only four syllables in a series.

7. The child is asked to produce /hɑ/ and /ɑ/ alternately. He should not prolong or emphasize the /h/. He can proceed to /u/ and /i/ in the same manner, and then go on to alternating the vowels in a single series. As the exercises are perfected and breathiness diminishes, more complex combinations of vowels and consonants can be used. The child should use phrases at a normal speech rate and be able to maintain desirable voice quality.

To correct breathiness Ling (1976, p. 212) suggested exercises involving exertion, for example, games where the child holds his breath in anticipation of speaking. The child can be selected as the one to signal the beginning of a race. He is told to hold his breath with his mouth open ready to say "Go." Then the teacher signals the start of the race and the child phonates. This results in good vocal cord closure and the cords are tense enough for a strong voice production. Repetition of this and other anticipatory games helps improve tonicity of the laryngeal muscles.

To reduce breathiness Calvert and Silverman (1975, p. 185) suggested holding a strip of paper in front of the mouth to check its flutter; noting the clouding of moisture on a mirror held in front of the mouth also calls attention to breathiness. To help economize air use have a child count on one breath and then keep increasing the length of the counting. For more fluency each number can be connected by *and* such as *one-and-two-and-three.* Calvert and Silverman also suggested attaining proper glottal action by having the child hold a weight such as a stack of books, or having him push against a table, as he says vowels, words, and sentences.

The laryngeal tone of the hearing-impaired child should be clear and vocal abuse eliminated to insure clarity. Special attention should be centered on voice production free from breathiness.

RATE AND RHYTHM

A hearing-impaired child usually has difficulty maintaining suitable rate and rhythm of speaking. Some speak with an excessively slow rate and inappropriate rhythm patterns. The amount of phonation time on syllables is a frequent problem among the hearing impaired; some children should increase their time and others shorten it for improved rate, rhythm, and speech intelligibility. Other children may have the problem of continuous phonation, voicing unvoiced sounds as well as voiced sounds.

Improving voice and speech of the hearing-impaired child should include teaching the rhythm, intonation, and sound patterns characteristic of the language. Language rhythm is a distinctive stress pattern involving variations in loudness, time, and pitch; time involves both duration and rate (Ervin, 1971). Correct use of stress on syllables helps the hearing-impaired child improve rhythm and intonation. This involves raising the pitch of the voice, lengthening the vowel in the syllable, and extending the length of the whole syllable (Magner, 1971, p. 262).

Fletcher and Daly (1976) reported on reading rates for two groups, the first, aged 7 through 21 years, with a mean loss in the better ear of 83 dB HTL (ISO 1964) and the second a comparable group with normal hearing. The results were 95 words per min

for the hearing impaired and 173 words per min for the other group. These rates can be compared to Franke's (1939) acceptable limits of 140 to 185 words per min.

A child's slow rate of speaking may be related to lack of breath control. For example, he may need to take a breath every few words and not have enough breath to finish a phrase. The speech pathologist should plan a program of improvement stressing methods of proper breathing for speech and handling imbalance of muscular tension. Our method of modifying rate using the rate chart (Fig. 39) is useful for most children with hearing losses. With some children it is sufficient to make a simple, direct request for more rapid rate and to urge the child to maintain a rhythmic flow of speech if he lags. However, it appears only selected hearing-impaired children can improve intelligibility by increasing the rate of speaking. Thus before increasing rate in a hearing-impaired child, the speech pathologist should check the effect of increased rate on intelligibility. Only those children who have improved intelligibility as a result of increased rate should be instructed to maintain the increased rate habitually. This recommendation is based on a study by Tato and Arcella (1962). They studied the relationship of speech rate to intelligibility in a group of deaf subjects. They measured habitual speech rates on familiar written passages. The average rate was 0.47 sec a syllable and the range was from 0.30 to 0.76. A comparable group of hearing children averaged 0.20 sec and ranged from 0.17 to 0.27 sec. After a month's training the deaf subjects' rate was reduced to 0.28 sec a syllable and ranged from 0.20 to 0.42, which was close to the rate for normal children. The intelligibility of the deaf group was judged by a group of listeners to improve markedly in 27% of the cases, to show no significant change in 36%, and to deteriorate markedly in the other 37%.

Colton and Cooker (1968) demonstrated that hearing-impaired persons speak significantly slower than normally hearing speakers. The total time for the hearing-impaired speakers averaged 8 to 10 sec/sentence and normally hearing speakers averaged 3 to 4 sec/sentence. It is suggested the slower speaking rate of deaf speakers results in perceived hypernasality and that the hypernasality is not caused by velopharyngeal dysfunction. Thus an increase in the speaking rate of the deaf may reduce perceived hypernasality. We therefore suggest that the severely hearing-impaired or deaf child who speaks at a slow tempo with perceived hypernasality be given instruction to increase his rate of talking.

The results of a study by Hood and Dixon (1969) suggest that in some persons improvement of speech rhythm might result from a reduction of phonation time of syllables and an increase in the rate of talking. Intelligibility may be improved as a result. In this way a hearing-impaired person's speech rhythm improves and his speech is easier to understand and more pleasant.

Whitehead and Jones (1976) studied vowel duration in three groups of male adults: a hearing-impaired group with pure tone averages in the better ear from 73 to 81 dB HL (ANSI 1969), a deaf group with losses from 92 to 103+ dB HL, and a normally hearing group. They found longer vowel durations in the hearing-impaired and deaf groups when compared to the vowel durations found in the normally hearing group. Durational measures on the three groups led the authors to conclude that a hearing-impaired population who receives some auditory input can learn the timing system in the same way a normally hearing population does, but a deaf population does not appear to learn these durational differences to the same extent. The authors therefore suggested it would seem that the hearing impaired who have some residual hearing would be capable of developing normal vowel duration patterns. This study shows that those with impaired hearing have longer mean durations for vowels than do normal subjects, thus lending support to the fact that the hearing impaired and deaf are apt to sound as if they have more continuous phonation than the normally hearing person. The authors maintain there are indications that those classified as hearing impaired in their study could benefit in instruction to shorten vowel duration.

Some deaf children have not learned to phonate when voicing is required. Ling (1976, p. 201-203) suggested exercises teaching a young child to vocalize at least 3 sec. Once he has learned this, correct length of vocalization can be transferred to speech. Ling suggested the following techniques to increase phonation time:

1. The teacher moves a desired toy toward the child as long as there is vocalization.

2. The teacher pours sand or liquid into a container having the child vocalize until it overflows.

3. The child or the teacher draws a line on the chalkboard as the child vocalizes. See how long the line can be made, but set limits to begin to teach limited vocalization.

4. An electric train or windmill can be switched on as the child vocalizes and off when he should quit.

5. Musical chairs can be played with the child vocalizing while the music is on. Adapt the exercises to get the child to imitate up to four separate vocalizations differing in length and on one breath. Try to obtain vocalizations through the auditory channel, but visual and tactile stimuli may be necessary. Signal lights work nicely here. Be sure the child uses an easy vocal attack and that the vocalizations are free from tension.

Pronovost (1977, pp. 203-204) stated many deaf individuals are likely to produce separate phonemes and words with many pauses as a result of having been taught to articulate speech sounds as precisely as possible. One goal of therapy, therefore, is producing properly sustained phonation on voiced sounds in words. Pronovost suggested that full phonation be taught older children and adults who demonstrate difficulty with spoken sentences by seeming to concentrate on articulation rather than durational features. Practice can start with nonsense expressions. Varying word durations enables the hearing-impaired person to become conscious of the role of duration in word and sentence stress. The concepts of speaking words with *long* duration contrasted with *short* duration and *slow* contrasted with *fast* can be used to illustrate phonation durations and stress patterns.

Millin (1971) stated continuous phonation is sometimes present in persons with congenital or profound hearing losses of long duration. Continuous phonation consists of voicing unvoiced speech sounds. This distorts the transitions between phonemes and reduces speech intelligibility. Continuous phonation is not always easily perceived; it is more easily perceived in a slow talker than in a fast talker. The cause of continuous phonation is obscure, but Millin pointed out is may be due to the emphasis placed on voicing in the training of the hearing impaired. A child with continuous phonation should be taught to cease voicing unvoiced sounds. Millin (1971) suggested the following procedures to break up continuous phonation. Have the child practice abruptly ceasing speech production after each word. To do this, sentences can be written on the chalkboard. The child reads the sentences word-by-word as the teacher points to each word. This allows the child to hesitate and cease phonation between words. Sometimes it is helpful if the teacher signals silence by a gesture. When a child understands what is required of him the teacher simply draws a vertical line after each word as it is read as a cue to cease phonation between words. Millin stated the distinct separation between words may be somewhat unnatural but it produces an immediate and marked improvement in speech intelligibility. Then with practice children are able to produce relatively fluent spontaneous speech with brief but distinct pauses between words. After this, individual phonemes are approached so the child can learn how to voice and unvoice sounds correctly, for example /k-g/, /t-d/, /p-b/. Finally smooth rhythmic speech can be taught through using pauses only when appropriate for meaning and between breath groups. With some children it may be best to reverse the plan of attack, that is starting with phoneme voicing and unvoicing and proceeding to sentence practice.

Programs of coordinating gross bodily movements with music (van Uden, 1960, pp. 19/3–12) can be used to improve the rate and rhythm of speaking. All children with impaired hearing should do a great deal of carefully supervised group singing, with emphasis on using correct rate, rhythm, and pitch. Harris (1971, pp. 186–192) felt the use of music and rhythm is an excellent way of developing natural speech. She observed that some hearing-impaired children use better inflections in their speech following exercises with music; since the child breathes more freely when he is active this may promote improved coordination of speech and breathing. Gilmore (1966) recommended the use of percussion instruments and rhythmic activities involving the whole body for the development of basic rhythmic patterns of speech. Magner (1971, p. 260) suggested playing a recording of a story and having the child follow it in print as he listens. Then the child can begin to read orally along with the recording and attempt to imitate the speech rhythm.

Teaching correct rate of speaking, seeing that proper phonation time is spent on syllables and improving the rhythm of speaking generally makes speech more intelligible and more pleasant for the listener.

The therapy objectives for hearing-impaired children presented in this chapter are exemplified by the procedures we used with a 7-year-old boy.

Jim had an unaided speech reception threshold of 80 dB and aided speech reception of 45 dB (ISO 1964). His habitual pitch was too high and uncontrolled and his laryngeal tone was breathy. He habitually talked too loud and did much uncontrolled shouting. He used abrupt glottal attacks and his rate of speaking was too slow.

Therapy was initiated with work on pitch, and other problems were approached after the first session. Listening training for pitch began with awareness of differences in others. The speech pathologist read a story using a very high pitch intermittently on words. Jim signalled by pressing a button which activated a red light each time he heard the high pitch. When he learned accurately and reliably to recognize the occurrence of high pitch in the speech pathologist's voice, he was ready to do gross discrimination of differences. He was given the task of recognizing the extremes of very high pitch and very low pitch in the speech pathologist's voice. He pushed the appropriate button on a switch panel—red for too high and yellow for too low. When he could accurately discriminate gross pitch differences he then went on to fine discrimination of differences. He was taught to recognize each level of pitch as the speech pathologist used three levels ranging through very low, correct, and very high. He used the switch panel to activate appropriate lights. A green light was added to indicate correct pitch level.

After Jim had completed the program of listening to others he was ready to apply these procedures to the pitch of his own voice. His own recordings were used to develop awareness of the high pitch and to develop gross and fine discrimination of pitch levels in his voice. He was then ready to be taught conscious control of pitch. Jim was first asked to speak words on two pitch levels: too high and correct. When he had gained voluntary control over these two levels he then produced at will a very high pitch and a very low pitch. Next he produced three levels of pitch, high, middle, and low, selecting the middle one as the correct pitch level for his own use. After practicing the correct pitch level Jim began transfer of his new pitch into habitual use. This was done in a limited way at first with the speech pathologist. Then outside assignments were added until he used adequate voice pitch in all situations.

The elimination of the abrupt glottal attack was incorporated into the ongoing program. Jim was taught the kinesthetic cues of abrupt, explosive vocalization contrasting these to the sensations felt during an easy initiation. Jim was taught to shout in an easier, effortless way following the program suggested by Uris (1962) (Chapter 8). We worked on increasing rate and decreasing breathiness while we worked on pitch. As a result of the therapy program, Jim gained control over his use of loudness and pitch and eliminated the vocal abuses. He had a more pleasant voice with improved quality. His rate of speaking was normal and his speech intelligibility had improved.

SUMMARY

Each child with a hearing loss may need to work toward a different combination of goals. He may need to be shown how to use balanced resonance without excessive hypernasality or hyponasality free from the cul-de-sac effect. A correct modal pitch level with appropriate inflections is necessary. The loudness of voice may need adjustment to an appropriate level. A clear laryngeal tone free from harshness, hoarseness, or breathiness is desirable. Eliminating or modifying vocal abuse assures better voice hygiene. Teaching correct rate and rhythm of speaking may make speech more intelligible. Often several parameters are simultaneously approached for a unified program of voice improvement. This program must be adapted to each child's needs and his hearing ability and coordinated with the total auditory and speech program.

TWELVE

Habituation, Family Role, Dismissal, Reports

Throughout voice therapy children are encouraged to use newly learned voice behavior at school, in the home, and during play. Additional carryover programs are presented in this chapter to assure consistent use of new voice parameters. The role of the family in voice therapy including carryover is discussed. Criteria are presented for evaluating progress and determining when children have benefited maximally from therapy. Finally, writing progress and dismissal reports are outlined.

HABITUATION OF NEW VOICE PATTERNS

The habitual use of new voice patterns is essential for the completion of successful voice therapy. The habituation program must be planned carefully following definite procedures. Planned supervision is necessary. Permanent habituation must not be left to chance. The speech pathologist should carefully explain the goal of each habituation assignment and have the child help plan the assignment (Engel, Brandriet, Erickson, Gronhovd, and Gunderson, 1966). Some children find habituation relatively easy while others find it difficult. A few children have trouble using new voice patterns because the old way sounds natural to them. Any change in voice will alter this auditory monitoring sometimes with an uncomfortable feeling. A child with a soft voice may have difficulty in talking more loudly; the louder voice feels unnatural so practice is necessary for the child to get used to a new level of loudness (Pronovost and Kingman, 1959, p. 113).

The child must be strongly motivated to use his new vocal patterns habitually. Several aspects of a child's voice may have been changed during the period of voice therapy. Changes may have taken place in pitch, loudness, and quality in addition to modifications of vocal abuse habits. All aspects add up to

a multidimensional habituation project that requires much patience from the child, parents, and speech pathologist (Wilson, 1961). The amount of responsibility for carryover placed on a child depends upon his age. Carryover responsibility in a 4 year old is different from that of a 17 year old. The activities and instructions vary according to age, too. The younger the child the more the speech pathologist depends upon other people in the environment, such as the parents and teachers, in carrying out programs to help a child habituate new voice patterns.

Habituation must be structured to enable the child to use his new voice *some* (Step 8), *most* (Step 9) and *all* the time (Step 10). At first the child uses his new vocal pattern only a few minutes at a time. Assignments may include situations with the speech pathologist, certain school situations, and special times at home and at play. Later the periods of carryover are extended to whole sessions with the speech pathologist, class hours, mealtimes, and play periods, then to half days or evenings, and finally to the use of the new vocal pattern consistently and permanently. Each voice therapy session should provide a child with some type of carryover activity. In fact, carryover may begin with the first therapy session. As each new voice habit is taught the child immediately begins carryover. Thus at any one point he may be working on different carryover stages of several new habits. When a child is introduced to a new vocal pattern, he is asked to use this pattern only with the speech pathologist. Soon he can use it outside the clinic in certain school situations and during special times at home and at play. A special audiotape technique described by Haley (1972) for use with articulation can be used for habituation of newly learned vocal behavior. "Beep" signals from a bell or buzzer are audiotaped at set intervals from 3 to 1 sec for a total time of 30 to 60 sec.

When a child hears a beep he responds in a predetermined manner. For example, a child who has just learned *easy* glottal attack can be given a list of words and asked to say a word with easy attack each time he hears a beep. Beeps are first spaced 3 seconds apart, then 2 seconds and finally 1 second. Brief prearranged situations between the child and his parents or teachers should be constructed to exercise control over the new patterns (Wilson, 1961). In some instances a new voice should be used first with strangers, then be brought into use with friends and family (Van Riper, 1972, p. 166). We feel this is especially true in cases of falsetto voices and in problems where there is quite a decided change in the voice. Later the speech pathologist might ask the child to use a lower pitch when he talks to five different people at home.

Children should not be allowed to practice on their own until the speech pathologist is sure they know how to do their exercises correctly (Van Thal, 1961). The speech pathologist should practice each assignment with the child so it can be done easily and accurately; he may accompany the child on some outside situations especially those designed to practice voice control under emotional conditions or in distracting situations such as exciting games and conversations (Engel et al. 1966).

We have found the use of a notebook with the child, parents, and teachers aids in habituating new patterns. Pictures of activities with the child's family and friends can be placed in the notebook with labels "I now use my new voice with my family and friends" (Fig. 44). The notebook can be used to have a child report assignments in writing (Engel et al. 1966). When a child has learned to control certain types of vocal behavior in his daily life he should be appropriately rewarded. For young children a program of rewards can be developed with parents; older children and teenagers can develop their own system of rewards. In this way correct vocal responses can become habitual. Creative dramatics under the direction of the speech pathologist aids in habituation. Creative dramatics can be used as an adjunct to speech therapy especially to bridge the gap between clinic sessions and everyday speaking. No scripts or technical aids are needed; the speech pathologist guides the children in planning and producing the dramatization of a story or situation. Throughout the session emphasis is placed on good voice use (McIntyre and McWilliams, 1959).

As therapy progresses the habituation time is extended to whole sessions with the speech pathologist, class hours, mealtimes, play periods, then half days or evenings, and finally to overall habituation. When a child and others report the consistent use of newly learned vocal patterns carryover is complete.

To assure long-term habituation of new vocal habits periodic check-ups for the child should be scheduled after the concentrated voice therapy program has been completed. Appointments should be made with the speech pathologist and various members of the voice team. Periodic visits to the speech pathologist serve as reminders of good voice use to both the parent and child and tend to perpetuate the use of the new voice (Wilson, 1961). Extended follow-up programs make it possible to evaluate the effectiveness of voice therapy procedures and to make sure the voice habits have become permanent.

ROLE OF THE FAMILY IN VOICE THERAPY

When working with children with voice problems it is necessary to enlist the cooperation of the family as supportive personnel. The parents' cooperation is essential in obtaining necessary medical, dental, and psychological examinations and treatment. The parents should be actively engaged in the voice program including evaluation, therapy, and habituation. The role of the parents during active voice therapy depends a great deal

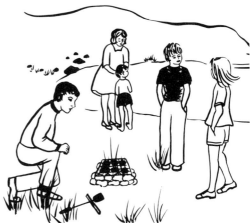

"I now use my new voice with my family and friends."

Fig. 44. Habituation. Illustration by Geraldine Balsam.

upon the type of voice problem and the type of therapy.

The family's role is particularly important when a child has vocal nodules or any other voice problem related to vocal abuse. The successful management of vocal nodules in children requires great patience in securing family comprehension, cooperation, and motivation (Arnold, 1963). Both the child and his parents should cooperate in eliminating vocal abuse (Murphy, 1967). Parents should understand the unfavorable vocal effects of excessive screaming (Luchsinger, 1965, p. 184). The reduction of vocal abuse requires the concentrated effort of those involved in the child's life, including his family, teachers, and friends; the child should not be nagged but it is advisable to have an organized home program for eliminating vocal abuse (Baynes, 1967). Consideration of the psychosomatic aspects of vocal nodules necessitates not only checking the child but also his family, and in some cases therapy includes counseling for the family (Withers and Dawson, 1960).

A child's voice problem which is the result of imitation of others in his environment presents a real problem for the speech pathologist. Counseling the child and involving the family in voice reeducation are indicated to give the child insight into the situation. If at all possible the child should be kept away from the person or other child he is imitating (Klinger, 1962).

In order to gain family support and cooperation for voice therapy with a child, the speech pathologist must take into consideration the feelings and attitudes of the family toward the child and his problem. There may be specific problems in the home. Wilson (1972) reported on the family structure of 1000 voice-disordered children. Factors investigated were divorce, separation, abnormal living conditions, numerous adults in the home environment, abnormal parent-child relationships, and unusual sibling relationships, including children from different marriages. Incidence of these factors in the families was 42%. This is in contrast to the estimate of social workers and sociologists indicating 21% of the families in St. Louis County had some degree of "family pathology." Webster (1966) stated no matter what the cause of the child's communication problem it can be assumed the child and his parents have some anxiety in their communication with each other and with their interpersonal relationships. Many parents express guilt to some degree and are concerned about what has caused their child's problem. Parents may appear overly aggressive to cover their fears about the situation. It is natural for parents to have defenses against feelings of guilt with the defenses taking the form of hostility toward the child or the speech pathologist. The speech pathologist can do much to relieve the guilt feelings of parents by careful counseling regarding the child's voice problem and its cause.

The active participation of parents is especially necessary in cases of laryngeal dysfunction when vocal abuse and vocal misuse are felt to contribute not only to the original cause of the problem but also to the continuation of the problem. Moore (1971b, pp. 135–136) stated interviews with parents and other members of a child's family have two purposes: (1) to seek methods to reduce the amount of talking and vocal abuse in a child with vocal pathology and (2) to help guide the parents toward the creation and maintenance of a quieter environment at home and during play. Ask parents to monitor vocal abuse periods and to help the child reduce shouting and loud singing by a program of rewards. To dramatize the amount of talking done Moore suggested having the family observe 5 to 15 min of silence during a usually talkative time such as mealtime, setting up a system of rewards for not talking and punishments for talking.

In most instances when vocal behavior is being altered parents can be given specific instructions and a program can be worked out for their help with assignments at home. Fudala (1973) stated that parents should be given home assignments after observing the actual techniques being used by the speech pathologist. Fudala added that children whose parents willingly assist them in speech assignments achieve better results than those whose parents are reluctant to help them. Parents of young hearing-impaired children should become teachers. Bennett (1974) suggested a series of home programs to provide information on speech and language and to outline speech training procedures. Parents first observe the speech pathologist and then are observed by the speech pathologist as they work with their child. Records of home training procedures should be kept so parents can chart both their own effectiveness and their child's progress. Individual conferences either in person or by phone are essential at first. When written assignments are given to a child instructions to the parents can be included.

Daily logs should be kept by the parent and the child. Phillips and Mordock (1974, p. 352) suggested asking parents to put a chart on the kitchen wall to record positive behavior. Also the child can be given stars, plastic tokens, pennies, and praise when target behavior is attained. Rewards such as a movie or horseback riding are given when specific numbers of points have been entered on the chart. Immediate reinforcers, if needed, can be given at close intervals. To increase a child's ability to delay gratification reinforcement is gradually spaced out. Children should be told they are being rewarded because they are asked to do things that are hard for them such as keeping quiet when they would like to shout. Very small gradual positive changes in behavior should be carefully observed and rewarded.

The target behavior and the criteria for acceptability should be set for parents. Carpenter and Augustine (1973) suggested giving mothers the speech pathologist's telephone number with instructions to call if any problems are encountered or if the child's performance is below criterion level (e.g. 50%) for two consecutive days. Or when the child gets 80% correct performance of the desired behavior for 2 consecutive days, mothers are asked to call to receive instructions for the next step. At the end of a week mothers are asked to send the speech pathologist the results of the home assignments. The suggestions of Carpenter and Augustine can be used in training parents to assist in eliminating vocal misuse and vocal abuse. Also these methods can be used to conduct programs for carryover of improved voice and speech.

Wing and Heimgartner (1973) presented a sequence of carryover for practice at home. They recommended logs be kept of the work and progress. We have applied their basic program to the problem of reducing throat clearing:

First Day. Establish baselines of throat clearing. Have the child read for 5 min. No attention should be called to throat clearings or to the parent's tallying. Next for 5 min have the child tell a story in spontaneous connected speech. Enter the results on a chart. Again no mention is made of throat clearing and tallying is done out of sight of the child.

Second Day. Reduce throat clearing. Five minutes of oral reading is followed by 5 min of spontaneous talking with the child attempting to limit throat clearing during both activities. The parent tallies the clearings during each activity in sight of the child. Enter the results on the chart. Reward the child if he reduces the number of throat clearings to 50% of the 1st day baseline.

Third Day. Reduce throat clearing. Plan a 10 min conversation between child and parent. Both the child and parent now tally throat clearings independently. Enter the results on a chart. Give a reward at 80% reduction of the 1st day baseline.

Fourth Day. Reduce throat clearing. This is an unstructured unplanned conversation between child and parent. Each one tallies the clearings. Enter results on a chart after 10 min. Keep on talking for another 5 min. Tally and enter the results on the chart. Reward for 80% reduction of the 1st day baseline.

Bush and Bonachea (1973) described a program of weekly meetings for parents. Their program was for children with language problems, but the basic program can be adapted to voice problems. They brought small groups of parents together weekly in a social setting at school to exchange experiences about their children. Soon parents began advising each other about how to solve problems. For example, in dealing with a screamer the advice might be not to say "Shut up," but rather to give him a quiet activity to do and a reward for being quiet. Meetings can feature videotapes of voice therapy sessions, such as controlling vocal abuse during games, simple plays, and puppet shows. These can be used to show the parents techniques they can use at home. Each week instructions are given the parents for specific home projects. These are usually family activities where better voice hygiene is practiced and they should be presented as recreational or fun activities not as homework. This results in the child receiving positive attention from his family and he progresses more rapidly toward the goal of good voice use. Group meetings also result in warmer relationships among family members and between the school and the family.

PROGRESS AND DISMISSAL CRITERIA

At specific points in a therapy program the speech pathologist should review and rate the child's progress in therapy. This is necessary for periodic reports during a program of voice therapy and when a child is dismissed from therapy. We will present four systems that can be used to describe progress and also as dismissal criteria.

Brodnitz's (1963) categories for determining outcome of vocal rehabilitation are: *Successful*—children who are able to produce a satisfactory voice which reflects good physiological use, is esthetically pleasing, and will continue to be satisfactory under varying conditions of use; *Improved*—children who have a much improved and useable voice, but whose voice still has some traces of the undesirable quality, pitch, or resonance; *Poor*—children who have not obtained a better voice as a result of adequate medical and voice therapy attention; *Discontinued Treatment*—this category is for children who terminated therapy so early in the program an opinion on progress is not indicated. Brodnitz (1963) in defining criteria of success in voice therapy stated both the speech pathologist and the person himself should consider whether or not the voice therapy was a success.

Boone (1974) listed five dismissal criteria for voice patients: (1) Improved status of laryngeal lesions, such as reduced thickening or reddening, or the reduction or elimination of additive lesions such as nodules. (2) The voice sounds normal or near normal. (3) The person is satisfied with the voice changes and he experiences no vocal fatigue, throat dryness or tightness, or loss of voice. (4) No improvement in laryngeal pathology or in the clarity of the laryngeal tone. (5) This category is reserved for persons who themselves terminate therapy without any improvement in voice or laryngeal condition.

Toohill (1975) reported on the classification of results of treatment of 77 prepubertal children with vocal nodules. Vocal rehabilitation was considered *complete* if there was a clear laryngeal tone with no hoarseness, normal pitch, and a normal laryngoscopic examination. Voice *improvement* was designated if there was a decrease in the degree of hoarseness, progress in the elimination of vocal abuse, and a diminution in nodule size. Voice was considered *unimproved* if the laryngeal tone remained hoarse, if there was no decrease in vocal abuse, and the vocal nodule size remained unchanged.

Cooper (1971a, p. 611; 1973, p. 277; 1977, p. 40) suggested the following criteria, based on visual, auditory, and sensory impressions, for completing voice therapy. The laryngologist reports on the visual, the patient and speech pathologist evaluate the auditory, and the patient himself makes the sensory judgment. (1) *Excellent.* The larynx including the vocal cords is normal, the modal pitch is the optimal, and the laryngeal tone is clear 90 to 100% of the time. The person reports no feeling of irritation or discomfort in the laryngeal or pharyngeal areas. (2) *Good.* The larynx and vocal cords are basically normal, but slight inflammation may be present. The person correctly uses pitch and has a clear tone 80 to 90% of the time. The patient reports only occasional throat discomfort or irritation. (3) *Fair.* There is some laryngeal inflammation and lesions are reduced. The person has 70 to 80% correct pitch use and clear tone. He experiences some irritation or discomfort during or after speaking.

These four systems of criteria for progress and dismissal are similar in their basic approaches for determining degree of success in vocal rehabilitation. The speech pathologist can select one system or combine them as desired. In essence, ratings of improvement must be made based upon the results of physical appearance seen by the laryngologist, the auditory and physical parameters observed by the speech pathologist, and the report by the child himself as he perceives the auditory effects of his voice and his positive or negative physical feelings as he speaks. Many factors should be reviewed including the use a child demands of his voice. In some instances the child and his parents may be well satisfied to have an improved voice even though some undesirable aspects are still present. On the other hand, parents of a child who does a great deal of singing at school or in a choir may have higher standards regarding the results of vocal rehabilitation.

PROGRESS AND DISMISSAL REPORTS

Progress and dismissal reports should be prepared by the speech pathologist. These require careful evaluation by the speech pathologist. Reports become part of the child's permanent record in the speech pathologist's files and copies are sent to other members of the voice team. When appropriate, copies also become part of the child's school health and academic records.

Periodic reports should be written approximately every 3 months. Sometimes it is ap-

Name of Child _____ Date of Report _____
Address _____
Voice Problem _____
Number of Sessions _____ Average Length of Session _____
Date Began _____ Date Ended _____

1. Voice Status at Beginning of Report Period:

2. Outline of Treatment:

3. Voice Status at End of Report Period:

4. Recommendations:

Speech Pathologist _____ Title _____
Agency _____
Address _____ Telephone _____

Fig. 45. Voice rehabilitation report.

propriate and convenient to have the reports coincide with other periodic reports such as school grading periods or end of semester reports. Voice therapy reports should be brief and concise usually not more than one typewritten page. Longer reports are necessary when the child is transferred from one agency to another.

Figure 45 is the report form we use. This was modified from one developed at The Child Guidance and Speech Correction Clinic, Jacksonville, Florida. It can be used for both periodic reports and final reports. The form contains four divisions: voice status at beginning of report period, outline of voice therapy, voice status at end of report period, and recommendations.

1. Voice status at beginning of report period. This should contain a basic description of the child's voice problem and ratings on the general voice profile and special profiles at the beginning of the report period.

2. Outline of treatment. Basic and special remediation procedures are outlined. Limitations on voice use and any advice or instructions are included.

3. Voice status at end of report period. The speech pathologist reevaluates the child's voice by administering current voice profiles. These profiles are reported along with the speech pathologist's overall impression of progress. Brodnitz (1963) suggested comparing the new use of voice with previous inadequate use by listening to tape recordings taken prior to therapy and during therapy. Brodnitz pointed out the individual speech pathologist may be somewhat prejudiced in his judgment; thus it is advisable to have the child's voice evaluated by other speech pathologists also. Dismissal criteria are assigned and the child's status on each one explained.

4. Recommendations. Progress reports include recommendations for continued voice therapy with considerations for change in frequency or length of sessions or for a change in the individual-group ratio, reevaluation by the voice team or any of its members, or additional examinations or tests. Final report recommendations should specify frequency of rechecks indicating the specialists to be consulted.

SUMMARY

New and improved voice patterns must be used habitually in all situations. Successful carryover is the result of carefully planned activities following specific methods. Picture notebooks for younger children and tallying charts for teenagers provide means of recording data showing success in using new vocal parameters. A reward system aids motivation for carryover. Families play an important role in helping children at all stages of vocal rehabilitation. Of particular importance is the help they can actively give a younger child and the support they can give a teenager. Improvement in voice is based on the positive physical changes seen by the laryngologist, improved laryngeal tone and oral-nasal resonance observed by the speech pathologist and the child himself, and improvement in the sensory feelings reported by the child. Progress and dismissal reports are prepared by the speech pathologist to inform other professionals of children's progress in voice improvement and dismissal from active voice therapy.

REFERENCES

Adler, S. (1960). Some techniques for treating the hypernasal voice. *J. Speech Hear. Disord. 25:* 300–302.

Alfaro, V. R. (1960). Psychogenic influences in otolaryngology. *Arch. Otolaryngol. 71:* 11–17.

Allen, B., and Peterson, G. E. (1942). Laryngeal inflammation in a case of falsetto. *J. Speech Disord. 7:* 175–178.

Anderson, V. A. (1977). *Training the Speaking Voice*, Ed. 3. Oxford University Press, New York.

Anderson, V. A., and Newby, H. A. (1973). *Improving the Child's Speech*, Ed. 2. Oxford University Press, New York.

Andrews, A. H., Jr., and Moss, H. W. (1974). Experiences with the carbon dioxide laser in the larynx. *Ann. Otol. Rhinol. Laryngol. 83:* 462–470.

Andrews, J. R. (1973). Applying principles of instructional technology in evaluating speech and language services. *Lang. Speech Hear. Serv. Schs. 4:* 66–71.

Andrews, M. L. (1975). Some communication problems encountered in voice therapy with children. *Lang. Speech Hear. Serv. Schs. 6:* 183–187.

Andrews, M. L., and Madeira, S. S. (1977). The assessment of pitch discrimination ability in young children. *J. Speech Hear. Disord. 42:* 279–286.

Anonymous (1964a). Clinical suggestions. *W. Mich. Univ. J. Speech Ther. 1:* 6.

Anonymous (1964b). Helpful hints. *W. Mich. Univ. J. Speech Ther. 1:* 6–7.

Anonymous (1966). Clinical helps. *W. Mich. Univ. J. Speech Ther. 3:* 11.

Arnold, G. E. (1962). Vocal nodules and polyps: Laryngeal tissue reaction to habitual hyperkinetic dysphonia. *J. Speech Hear. Disord. 27:* 205–216.

Arnold, G. E. (1963). Vocal nodules. In Voice problems and laryngeal pathology, by J. F. Daly (Moderator). *N. Y. State J. Med. 63:* 3096–3110.

Arnold, G. E. (1964). Clinical application of recent advances in laryngeal physiology. *Ann. Otol. Rhinol. Laryngol. 73:* 426–442.

Arnold, G. E. (1965). Physiology and pathology of speech and language. In *Voice-Speech-Language. Clinical Communicology: Its Physiology and Pathology*, edited by R. Luchsinger and G. E. Arnold, pp 337–791. Wadsworth Publishing Company, Belmont.

Arnold, G. E. (1966). Advances in laryngeal physiology and their clinical application. *Eye Ear Nose Throat Mon. 45:* 78–84.

Aronson, A. E. (1971). Early motor unit disease masquerading as psychogenic breathy dysphonia: A clinical case presentation. *J. Speech Hear. Disord. 36:* 115–124.

Aronson, A. E. (1973). *Psychogenic Voice Disorders: An Interdisciplinary Approach to Detection, Diagnosis and Therapy: Audio Seminars in Speech Pathology.* W. B. Saunders Co., Philadelphia.

Aronson, A. E., Brown, J. R., Litin, E. M., and Pearson, J. S. (1968a). Spastic dysphonia. I. Voice, neurologic and psychiatric aspects. *J. Speech Hear. Disord. 33:* 203–218.

Aronson, A. E., Brown, J. R., Litin, E. M., and Pearson, J. S. (1968b). Spastic dysphonia. II. Comparison with essential (voice) tremor and other neurologic and psychogenic dysphonias. *J. Speech Hear. Disord. 33:* 219–231.

Aronson, A. E., Peterson, H. W., Jr., and Litin, E. M. (1964). Voice symptomatology in functional dysphonia and aphonia. *J. Speech Hear. Disord. 29:* 367–380.

ASHA Executive Council (1964). The speech clinician's role in the public school. A statement by the American Speech and Hearing Association. *Asha. 6:* 189–191.

Aston, W. (1973). Bo the blinking dog helps children learn to speak. *Volta Rev. 75:* 214–215.

Atkinson, C. J. (1952). Vocal responses during controlled aural stimulation. *J. Speech Hear. Disord. 17:* 419–426.

Austin, M. D., and Leeper, H. A., Jr. (1975). Basal pitch and frequency level variation in male and female children: A preliminary investigation. *J. Commun. Dis. 8:* 307–315.

Baker, D. C., Jr. (1954). Congenital disorders of the larynx. *N. Y. State J. Med. 54:* 2458–2462.

Baker, D. C., Jr. (1962). Laryngeal problems in singers. *Laryngoscope 72:* 902–908.

Baker, D. C., Jr. (1963). Polypoid vocal cord. In Voice problems and laryngeal pathology, by J. F. Daly (Moderator). *N. Y. State J. Med. 63:* 3096–3110.

Baldwin, R. L. (1975). Characteristics of quality programs for hearing impaired children. *Volta Rev. 77:* 436–439.

Balick, S., Spiegel, D., and Greene, G. (1976). Mime in language therapy and clinician training. *Arch. Phys. Med. Rehabil. 57:* 35–38.

Bangs, J. L., and Freidinger, A. (1949). Diagnosis and treatment of a case of hysterical aphonia in a thirteen-year-old girl. *J. Speech Hear. Disord. 14:* 312–317.

Barnes, I. J., and Morris, H. L. (1967). Interrelationships among oral breath pressure ratios and articulation skills for individuals with cleft palate. *J. Speech Hear. Res. 10:* 506–514.

Barr, T. (1938). Hoarseness. *Tex. State J. Med. 34:* 553–555.

Barton, R. T. (1960). The whispering syndrome of hysterical dysphonia. *Ann. Otol. Rhinol. Laryngol. 69:* 156–164.

Batza, E. M. (1971). Vocal abuse in rock-and-roll singers. Report of five representative cases. *Cleve. Clin. Q. 38:* 35–38.

Batza, E. M., and Parker, W. (1971). Hyponasality associated with patulous eustachian tubes: Report of a case. *J. Speech Hear. Disord. 36:* 410–413.

Bawden, P. D. (1968). Allergies and their possible effect on speech. Unpublished essay for master's degree, Wayne State University, Detroit, Michigan.

Baynes, R. A. (1965). Clinical observations of children with voice disorders. *J. Mich. Speech Hear. Assoc. 1:* 10–12.

Baynes, R. A. (1966). An incident study of chronic hoarseness among children. *J. Speech Hear. Disord. 31:* 172–176.

Baynes, R. A. (1967). Voice therapy with children: A global approach. *J. Mich. Speech Hear. Assoc. 3:* 11–14.

Baynes, R. A., and Wendling, D. (1965). Clinical observations of children with voice disorders. *Asha. 7:* 393.

Beebe, H. H. (1951). Teaching the congenitally deaf to speak. In *The Chewing Approach in Speech and Voice Therapy*, edited by D. A. Weiss and H. H. Beebe, pp 52–69. S. Karger Pub., Basel-New York.

Beebe, H. H. (1976). Pioneer in auditory/oral training. *Newsounds 1:* 2.

Beebe, H. H. (1977). Deaf children can learn to hear. *Hear. Aid J. 30:* 6, 34–36.

Beeden, A. G. (1972). The bifid uvula. *J. Laryngol. Otol. 86:* 815–819.

Bennett, C. (1974). Speech pathology and the hearing impaired child. *Volta Rev. 76:* 550–557.

Beranek, L. L. (1947). Airplane quieting. II. Specification of acceptable noise levels. *Trans. Am. Soc. Mech. Engin. 69:* 97–100.

Beranek, L. L., and Rudmose, H. W. (1947). Sound control in airplanes. *J. Acoust. Soc. Am. 19:* 357–364.

Berg, F. S. (1970). Educational audiology. In *The Hard of Hearing Child. Clinical and Educational Management*, edited by F. S. Berg and S. G. Fletcher, pp 275–318. Grune and Stratton, New York.

Berg, F. S. (1976). *Educational Audiology: Hearing and Speech Management.* Grune & Stratton, New York.

Berner, R. E. (1962). Hazards of adenotonsillectomy in the child with cleft palate. *J. Am. Med. Assoc. 181:* 558–559.

Bernstein, L. (1967). Treatment of velopharyngeal incompetence. *Arch. Otolaryngol. 85:* 67–74.

Bernthal, J. E., and Beukelman, D. R. (1977). The effect of changes in velopharyngeal orifice area on vowel intensity. *Cleft Palate J. 14:* 63–77.

Berry, M. F., and Eisenson, J. (1956). *Speech Disorders. Principles and Practices of Therapy.* Appleton-Century-Crofts, Inc., New York.

Bess, F. H., Gale, D. W., Aarni, J. D., and Redfield, N. P. (1974). Attenuation characteristics of recreational helmets. *Ann. Otol. Rhinol. Laryngol. 83:* 119–124.

Bess, F. H., and Poyner, R. E. (1972). Snowmobile engine noise and hearing. *Arch. Otolaryngol. 95:* 164–168.

Bess, F. H., and Poyner, R. E. (1974). Noise-induced hearing loss and snowmobiles. *Arch. Otolaryngol. 99:* 45–51.

Beving, B., and Eblen, R. E. (1973). "Same" and "different" concepts and children's performance on speech sound discrimination. *J. Speech Hear. Res. 16:* 513–517.

Bicknell, P. G. (1973). Mild hypothyroidism and its effects on the larynx. *J. Laryngol. Otol. 87:* 123–127.

Billeaud, F. P. (1971). Vocal rest as a technique in dysphonia. *J. Commun. Disord. 4:* 263–265.

Bindra, D., Williams, J. A., and Wise, J. S. (1965). Judgments of sameness and difference: Experiments on decision time. *Science 150:* 1625–1627.

Bingham, D. S., Van Hattum, R. J., Faulk, M. E., and Taussig, E. (1961). Program organization and management. In Research Committee of the American Speech and Hearing Association, public school speech and hearing services. *J. Speech Hear. Disord.,* Monogr. Suppl. 8.

Black, J. W. (1949). The intensity of oral responses to stimulus words. *J. Speech Hear. Disord. 14:* 16–22.

Black, J. W. (1950). Some effects upon voices of hearing tones of varying intensity and frequency while reading. *Speech Monogr. 17:* 95–98.

Black, J. W. (1961). Relationships among fundamental frequency, vocal sound pressure, and rate of speaking. *Lang. Speech 4:* 196–199.

Black, M. E. (1964). *Speech Correction in the Schools.* Prentice-Hall, Inc., Englewood Cliffs.

Black, M. E. (1970). *School Speech Therapy: A Source Book.* Stanwix House, Inc., Pittsburgh.

Bless, D. M., and Saxman, J. H. (1970). Maximum phonation time, flow rate, and volume change during phonation: normative information on third-grade children. Paper presented ASHA Convention.

Bloch, P. (1960). New limits of vocal analysis. *Folia Phoniatr. 12:* 291–297.

Blood, G. W., and Hyman, M. (1977). Children's preception of nasal resonance. *J. Speech Hear. Disord. 42:* 446–448.

Bloomer, H. H., and Wolski, W. (1968). Office examination of palatopharyngeal function. *Clin. Pediatr. (Phila.) 7:* 611–618.

Boland, J. L., Jr. (1953). Voice therapy for hoarse voice. *J. Okla. State Med. Assoc. 46:* 109–113.

Boles, R. (1968). Laryngeal lesions in the young. *Postgrad. Med. 43:* 177–182.

Bolt, Beranek, and Newman, Inc. (1965). Noise in automobiles: Report on a second set of tests conducted by Bolt, Beranek, and Newman, Inc., for J. Walter Thompson Company and the Ford Motor Company on 29 April 1965.

Report No. 1249, Job No. 181176, 14 May 1965.

Boone, D. R. (1966). Modification of the voices of deaf children. *Volta Rev. 68:* 686–692.

Boone, D. R. (1973). Voice therapy for children. *Human Commun. 1:* 30–43.

Boone, D. R. (1974). Dismissal criteria in voice therapy. *J. Speech Hear. Disord. 39:* 133–139.

Boone, D. R. (1977). *The Voice and Voice Therapy*, Ed. 2. Prentice-Hall, Inc., Englewood Cliffs.

Boone, D. R., and Prescott, T. E. (1972). Content and sequence analyses of speech and hearing therapy. *Asha 14:* 58–62.

Borlak, J., and Moller, K. T. (1976). Phonetic context and hypernasality in two groups of cleft palate speakers. *Human Commun. 1:* 23–33.

Bowler, N. W. (1964). A fundamental frequency analysis of harsh vocal quality. *Speech Monogr. 31:* 128–134.

Bowman, S. A., Shanks, J. C., and Manion, M. W. (1972). Effect of prolonged nasotracheal intubation on communication. *J. Speech Hear. Disord. 37:* 403–406.

Bown, J. C. (1971). The expanding responsibilities of the speech and hearing clinician in the public schools. *J. Speech Hear. Disord. 36:* 538–542.

Bown, J. C. (1972). A communication model for evaluation and remediation. *Except. Child. 38:* 385–394.

Bown, J. C. (1973). The communication disorders specialist as a support team member of a resource program. *Lang. Speech Hear. Serv. Schs. 4:* 77–78.

Brackett, I. P. (1946). Intelligibility related to pitch. *Speech Monogr. 13:* 24–31.

Bradford, L. J., Brooks, A. R., and Shelton, R. L., Jr. (1964). Clinical judgment of hypernasality in cleft palate children. *Cleft Palate J. 1:* 329–335.

Brennan, D. G., and Leeper, H. A., Jr. (1974). The clinical efficiency of four oral breath pressure measures. *J. Commun. Disord. 7:* 247–255.

Brodnitz, F. S. (1954). Voice problems of the actor and singer. *J. Speech Hear. Disord. 19:* 322–326.

Brodnitz, F. S. (1955). Post-operative vocal rehabilitation in benign lesions of the vocal cord. *Folia Phoniatr. 7:* 193–200.

Brodnitz, F. S. (1958a). The pressure test in mutational voice disturbances. *Ann. Otol. Rhinol. Laryngol. 67:* 235–240.

Brodnitz, F. S. (1958b). Vocal rehabilitation in benign lesions of the vocal cords. *J. Speech Hear. Disord. 23:* 112–117.

Brodnitz, F. S. (1961). Contact ulcer of the larynx. *Arch. Otolaryngol. 74:* 70–80.

Brodnitz, F. S. (1962). The holistic study of the voice. *Q. J. Speech 48:* 280–284.

Brodnitz, F. S. (1963). Goals, results and limita-

tions of vocal rehabilitation. *Arch. Otolaryngol. 77:* 148–156.

Brodnitz, F. S. (1966). Rehabilitation of the human voice. *Bull. N. Y. Acad. Med. 42:* 231–240.

Brodnitz, F. S. (1967a). Review of A. T. Murphy, *Functional Voice Disorders, J. Commun. Disord. 1:* 100–101.

Brodnitz, F. S. (1967b). Semantics of the voice. *J. Speech Hear. Disord. 32:* 325–330.

Brodnitz, F. S. (1969). Functional aphonia. *Ann. Otol. Rhinol. Laryngol. 78:* 1244–1258.

Brodnitz, F. S. (1971a). *Vocal Rehabilitation.* Ed. 4. American Academy of Ophthalmology and Otolaryngology, Rochester, Minnesota.

Brodnitz, F. S. (1971b). Hormones and the human voice. *Bull. N. Y. Acad. Med. 47:* 183–191.

Brodnitz, F. S. (1976). Spastic dysphonia. *Ann. Otol. Rhinol. Laryngol. 85:* 210–214.

Brodnitz, F. S., and Froeschels, E. (1954). Treatment of vocal nodules by chewing method. *Arch. Otolaryngol. 59:* 560–565.

Brooks, A. R., and Shelton, R. L., Jr. (1963). Incidence of voice disorders other than nasality in cleft palate children. *Cleft Palate Bull. 13:* 63–64.

Brookshire, R. H. (1967). Speech pathology and the experimental analysis of behavior. *J. Speech Hear. Disord. 32:* 215–227.

Brookshire, R. H. (1973). The use of consequences in speech pathology: Incentive and feedback functions. *J. Commun. Disord. 6:* 88–92.

Brown, J. F. (1975). *Dictionary of Speech and Hearing—Anatomy and Physiology.* Speech and Hearing Service, Sacramento, California.

Brown, W. S., Jr., Murry, T., and Hughes, D. (1976). Comfortable effort level: An experimental variable. *J. Acoust. Soc. Am. 60:* 696–699.

Bryce, D. P. (1974). *Differential Diagnosis and Treatment of Hoarseness.* C. C Thomas, Springfield.

Bryngelson, B. (1954). The functional falsetto voice. *Speech Teacher 3:* 127–128.

Buck, L. A., Gallant, R. V., and Freshley, N. (1973). A communication therapy program in a hearing and speech center. *J. Commun. Disord. 6:* 53–65.

Buck, M. (1954). Post-operative velo-pharyngeal movements in cleft palate cases. *J. Speech Hear. Disord. 19:* 288–294.

Buck, M., and Harrington, R. (1949). Organized speech therapy for cleft palate rehabilitation. *J. Speech Hear. Disord. 14:* 43–52.

Burke, H. A., Jr. (1968). Endocrine aspects of otolaryngology. *Laryngoscope 78:* 857–862.

Bush, C., and Bonachea, M. (1973). Parental involvement in language development: The PAL program. *Lang. Speech Hear. Serv. Schs. 4:* 82–85.

Bzoch, K. R. (1964). The effects of a specific

pharyngeal flap operation upon the speech of forty cleft-palate persons. *J. Speech Hear. Disord.* 29: 111–120.

Callahan, N. (1958). Vocal cord strain. *South. Med. J.* 51: 1578–1584.

Calnan, J. (1954). Submucous cleft palate. *Br. J. Plast. Surg.* 6: 264–282.

Calnan, J., and Renfrew, C. E. (1961). Blowing tests and speech. *Br. J. Plast. Surg.* 13: 340–346.

Calnan, J. S. (1971a). Permanent nasal escape in speech after adenoidectomy. *Br. J. Plast. Surg.* 24: 197–204.

Calnan, J. S. (1971b). Congenital large pharynx. *Br. J. Plast. Surg.* 24: 263–271.

Calvert, D. R., and Silverman, S. R. (1975). *Speech and Deafness.* Alexander Graham Bell Assoc. for the Deaf, Inc., Washington, D.C.

Canfield, W. H. (1964). A phonetic approach to voice and speech improvement. *Speech Teacher* 8: 42–46.

Cardoso, A., and Gomes, S. (1972). A bullet in the vocal cord. *J. Laryngol. Otol.* 86: 1073–1074.

Carney, P., and Sherman, D. (1971). Severity of nasality in three selected speech tasks. *J. Speech Hear. Res.* 14: 396–407.

Carpenter, R. L., and Augustine, L. E. (1973). A pilot training program for parent-clinicians. *J. Speech Hear. Disord.* 38: 48–58.

Carter, A. L., Ricker, K. S., and Corsini, D. A. (1972). Relational judgment of sound intensity by young children. *Percept. Psychophys.* 11: 1–4.

Casper, J. (1972). Hypernasality: Functional or organic. *Public School News*, Winter, 1972, 1, 2, 4.

Cavanagh, F. (1955). Vocal palsies in children. *J. Laryngol. Otol.* 69: 399–418.

Chandler, J. R. (1972). Avulsion of the larynx and pharynx as the result of a water ski rope injury. *Arch. Otolaryngol.* 96: 365–367.

Chaplin, J. P. (1968). *Dictionary of Psychology.* Dell, New York.

Cherry, J., and Bordley, J. E. (1966). Surgical correction of choanal atresia. *Ann. Otol. Rhinol. Laryngol.* 75: 911–919.

Clauson, G. M., and Kopatic, N. J. (1975). Teacher attitudes and knowledge of remedial speech programs. *Lang. Speech Hear. Serv. Schs.* 6: 206–210.

Clemis, J. D. (1976). Allergic factors in management of middle ear effusions. *Ann. Otol. Rhinol. Laryngol.* 85: 259–262.

Clerf, L. H. (1952). Laryngeal disease and voice therapy. In *Proceedings of the First Institute on Voice Pathology, and the First International Meeting of Laryngectomized Persons.* Cleveland Hearing and Speech Center, Cleveland.

Coleman, R. O. (1976). A comparison of the contributions of two voice quality characteristics to the perception of maleness and femaleness in the voice. *J. Speech Hear. Res.* 19: 168–180.

Collins, E. G. (1964). *A Guide to Diseases of the Nose, Throat and Ear for General Practitioners and Students.* Williams & Wilkins Company, Baltimore.

Colton, R. H., and Cooker, H. S. (1968). Perceived nasality in the speech of the deaf. *J. Speech Hear. Res.* 11: 553–559.

Connelly, M. K., Wilson, F. B., and Leeper, H. A., Jr. (1970). A group voice therapy technique for decreasing vocal abuse in children with vocal nodules. *J. Mo. Speech Hear. Assoc.* 3: 7–18.

Cook, T. A., Cohn, A. M., Brunschwig, J. P., Goepfert, H., Butel, J. S., and Rawls, W. E. (1973). Laryngeal papilloma: Etiologic and therapeutic considerations. *Ann. Otol. Rhinol. Laryngol.* 82: 649–655.

Cooper, M. (1971a). Modern techniques of vocal rehabilitation for functional and organic dysphonias. In *Handbook of Speech Pathology and Audiology*, edited by L. E. Travis, pp 585–616. Prentice-Hall, Inc., Englewood Cliffs.

Cooper, M. (1971b). Papillomata of the vocal folds: A review. *J. Speech Hear. Disord.* 36: 51–60.

Cooper, M. (1973). *Modern Techniques of Vocal Rehabilitation.* C. C Thomas, Springfield.

Cooper, M. (1974). Spectrographic analysis of fundamental frequency and hoarseness before and after vocal rehabilitation. *J. Speech Hear. Disord.* 39: 286–297.

Cooper, M. (1975). A response to Mueller. *J. Speech Hear. Disord.* 40: 278–279.

Cooper, M. (1977). Direct vocal rehabilitation. In *Approaches to Vocal Rehabilitation*, edited by M. Cooper and M. H. Cooper, pp 22–42. C. C Thomas, Springfield.

Cooper, M., and Nahum, A. M. (1967). Vocal rehabilitation for contact ulcer of the larynx. *Arch. Otolaryngol.* 85: 41–46.

Cooper, M., and Yanagihara, N. (1971). A study of the basal pitch level variations found in the normal speaking voices of males and females. *J. Commun. Disord.* 3: 261–266.

Costello, J. M. (1977). Programmed instruction. *J. Speech Hear. Disord.* 42: 3–28.

Cracovaner, A. J. (1959). Hyperkeratosis of the larynx. *Arch. Otolaryngol.* 70: 287–291.

Cullinan, W. L., and Counihan, D. T. (1968). Some factors affecting the size of Q values for speech ratings. *Percept. Mot. Skills* 27: 531–536.

Cunningham-Grant, J. D. S. (1972). Maximum phonation time in children 6 through 8 years of age. Unpublished master's thesis, State University of New York at Buffalo.

Curry, E. T. (1940). The pitch characteristics of the adolescent male voice. *Speech Monogr.* 7: 48–62.

Curtis, J. F. (1967). Disorders of voice. In *Speech Handicapped School Children*, Ed. 3. By W. Johnson, S. F. Brown, J. F. Curtis, C. W. Edney, and J. Keaster, pp 175–228. Harper and Row, New York.

Daly, D. A. (1974). Quantitative measurement of nasality in EMR children. *J. Commun. Disord. 7:* 287–293.

Daly, D. A. (1977). Bioelectronic measurement of nasality in trainable mentally retarded children. *J. Speech Hear. Disord. 42:* 436–439.

Damitz, J. C., and Dill, J. L. (1940). Chronic hoarseness: Report of three hundred consecutive cases. *Ann. Otol. Rhinol. Laryngol. 49:* 996–1007.

Damsté, P. H. (1973). Vocal disorders. A guide to their diagnosis. *ORL (Basel) 35:* 149–153.

Darley, F. L., Aronson, A. E., and Brown, J. R. (1975). *Motor Speech Disorders.* W. B. Saunders Co., Philadelphia.

Darley, F. L., Brown, J. R., and Goldstein, N. P. (1972). Dysarthria in multiple sclerosis. *J. Speech Hear. Res. 15:* 229–245.

Deal, R. E., McClain, B., and Sudderth, J. F. (1976). Identification, evaluation, therapy, and follow-up for children with vocal nodules in a public school setting. *J. Speech Hear. Disord. 41:* 390–397.

Dedo, H. H. (1976). Recurrent laryngeal nerve section for spastic dysphonia. *Ann. Otol. Rhinol. Laryngol. 85:* 451–459.

Des Roches, C. P. (1976). Speech therapy services in a large school system: A six-year overview. *Lang. Speech Hear. Serv. Schs. 7:* 207–219.

DeWeese, D. D., and Saunders, W. H. (1973). *Textbook of Otolaryngology*, Ed. 4. C. V. Mosby Company, St. Louis.

DeWeese, D. D., and Saunders, W. H. (1977). *Textbook of Otolaryngology*, Ed. 5. C. V. Mosby Company, St. Louis.

Dickson, S., and Jann, G. R. (1974). Diagnostic principles and procedures. In *Communication Disorders, Remedial Principles and Practices*, edited by S. Dickson, pp. 2–49. Scott, Foresman and Company, Glenview, Ill.

Diedrich, W. M. (1971). Procedures for counting and charting a target phoneme. *Lang. Speech Hear. Serv. Schs.* No. 5.

Diedrich, W. M. (1973). *Charting Speech Behavior.* University of Kansas Bureau of Child Research, Lawrence, Kansas.

Diehl, C. F., and Stinnett, C. D. (1959). Efficiency of teacher referrals in a school speech testing program. *J. Speech Hear. Disord. 24:* 34–36.

Domenec, O. (1973). Laryngoscopy with the "Storz" cold light nasopharyngoscope. *Acta Otorhinolaryngol. Iber. Am. 24:* 201–205.

Draper, M. H., Ladefoged, P., and Whitteridge, D. (1960). Expiratory pressures and air flow during speech. *Br. Med. J. 18:* 1837–1843.

Drudge, M. K. M., and Philips, B. J. (1976).

Shaping behavior in voice therapy. *J. Speech Hear. Disord. 41:* 398–411.

Duffy, R. J. (1970). Fundamental frequency characteristics of adolescent females. *Lang. Speech 13:* 14–24.

Dunlap, K. (1932). *Habits: Their Making and Unmaking.* Liveright, New York. (Reissued 1972 by Liveright).

Dweck, R. (1975). A study of elementary school children with hoarse voices. Unpublished master's project, State University of New York at Buffalo.

Eisenson, J., and Eisenson, A. M. (1974). *Voice and Diction*, Ed. 3. Macmillan Publishing Company, New York.

Eisenson, J., and Ogilvie, M. (1977). *Speech Correction in the Schools*, Ed. 4. Macmillan Publishing Company, New York.

Ellis, M. (1959). Remarks on dysphonia. *J. Laryngol. Otol. 73:* 99–103.

Emanuel, F. W., Lively, M. A., and McCoy, J. F. (1973). Spectral noise levels and roughness ratings for vowels produced by males and females. *Folia. Phoniatr. 25:* 110–120.

Encyclopedia Americana—International Edition. (1976). Americana Corp., New York.

Engel, D. C., Brandriet, S. E., Erickson, K. M., Gronhovd, K. D., and Gunderson, G. D. (1966). Carryover. *J. Speech Hear. Disord. 31:* 227–233.

Engleberg, M. (1962). Correction of falsetto voice in a deaf adult. *J. Speech Hear. Disord. 27:* 162–164.

Erickson, R. (1974). Assessing voice. *W. Mich. Univ. J. Speech Ther. 11:* 7–9.

Ermovick, D. A. (1965). A spectrographic analysis comparing connected speech of deaf subjects and hearing subjects. Unpublished master's thesis, University of Kansas.

Ervin, J. C. (1971). Implications of an understanding of English rhythm for teaching speech to children with impaired hearing. *J. Speech Hear. Assoc. Va. 12:* 7–11.

Ewing, I. R., and Ewing, A. W. G. (1954). *Speech and the Deaf Child.* Volta Bureau. Washington, D. C.

Fabricant, N. D. (1962). Some facts about dysphonia. *Eye Ear Nose Throat Mon. 41:* 729–738.

Fairbanks, G. (1960). *Voice and Articulation Drillbook*, Ed. 2. Harper and Brothers, New York.

Fairbanks, G., Herbert, E. L., and Hammond, J. M. (1949). An acoustical study of vocal pitch in seven- and eight-year-old girls. *Child Dev. 20:* 71–78.

Fairbanks, G., Wiley, J. H., and Lassman, F. M. (1949). An acoustical study of vocal pitch in seven- and eight-year-old boys. *Child Dev. 20:* 63–69.

Fairman, H. D. (1972). Papillomatosis of the larynx. *Proc. R. Soc. Med. 65:* 619–624.

Ferguson, G. B. (1955). Organic lesions of the larynx produced by misuse of the voice. *Laryngoscope 65:* 327–336.

Filter, M. D. (1974). Proprioceptive-tactile-kinesthetic feedback in voice therapy. *Lang. Speech Hear. Serv. Schs. 5:* 149–151.

Fisher, H. B. (1975). *Improving Voice and Articulation,* Ed. 2. Houghton Mifflin Co., Boston.

Fisher, H. B., and Logemann, J. (1970). Objective evaluation of therapy for vocal nodules: A case report. *J. Speech Hear. Disord. 35:* 277–285.

Fletcher, H. (1953). *Speech and Hearing in Communication.* D. Van Nostrand Co., Princeton.

Fletcher, S. G. (1972). Contingencies for bioelectronic modification of nasality. *J. Speech Hear. Disord. 37:* 329–346.

Fletcher, S. G., and Daly, D. A. (1976). Nasalance in utterances of hearing impaired speakers. *J. Commun. Disord. 9:* 63–73.

Flower, R. M. (1959). Voice training in the management of dysphonia. *Laryngoscope 69:* 940–946.

Flowers, C. R., and Morris, H. L. (1973). Oral-pharyngeal movements during swallowing and speech. *Cleft Palate J. 10:* 180–190.

Flugrath, J. M. (1969). Modern-day rock-and-roll music and damage-risk criteria. *J. Acoust. Soc. Am. 45:* 704–711.

Flugrath, J. M., Irwin, J. A., Wolfe, B. N., Jr., Krone, B., and Parnell, M. (1971). Temporary threshold shift and rock-and-roll music. *J. Aud. Res. 11:* 291–293.

Fomon, S., Bell, J. W., Lubart, J., Schattner, A., and Syracuse, V. R. (1966). Otolaryngology and speech therapy. *Eye Ear Nose Throat Mon. 45:* 71–76.

Fox, D. R., and Blechman, M. (1975). *Clinical Management of Voice Disorders.* Cliffs Notes, Lincoln, Nebraska.

Fox, D. R., and Johns, D. (1970). Predicting velopharyngeal closure with a modified tongue-anchor technique. *J. Speech Hear. Disord. 35:* 248–251.

Frable, M. A. S. (1962). Hoarseness, a symptom of premenstrual tension. *Arch. Otolaryngol. 75:* 66–68.

Frank, D. I. (1940). Hoarseness: New classification and brief report of four interesting cases. *Laryngoscope 50:* 472–478.

Franke, P. (1939). A preliminary study validating the measurement of oral reading rate in words per minute. Unpublished master's thesis, University of Iowa. Cited in T. D. Hanley and W. L. Thurman (1970). *Developing Vocal Skills,* Ed. 2., p. 148. Holt, Rinehart and Winston, Inc., New York.

Fred, H. L. (1962). Hoarseness due to phonation by the false vocal cords: Dysphonia plicae ventricularis. *Arch. Intern. Med. 110:* 472–475.

Freedman, S. R., and Garstecki, D. C. (1973). Child-directed therapy for a nonorganic voice disorder: A case study. *Lang. Speech Hear. Serv. Schs. 4:* 8–12.

Freeman, G. G. (1961). County speech services: A clinical program in the public schools. *Asha 3:* 46–47.

Freeman, G. G. (1969). Innovative school programs: The Oakland schools plan. *J. Speech Hear. Disord. 34:* 220–225.

French, N. R., Carter, C. W., Jr., and Koenig, W., Jr. (1930). The words and sounds of telephone conversations. *Bell System Tech. J. 9:* 290–324.

Freud, E. D. (1962). Functions and dysfunctions of the ventricular folds. *J. Speech Hear. Disord. 27:* 334–340.

Frick, J. V. (1960). The incidence of voice defects among school-age speech defective children. *Penn. Speech Ann. 17:* 61–62.

Froeschels, E. (1940). Laws in the appearance and the development of voice hyperfunctions. *J. Speech Disord. 5:* 1–4.

Froeschels, E. (1943). Hygiene of the voice. *Arch. Otolaryngol. 38:* 122–130.

Froeschels, E. (1952). Chewing method as therapy. *Arch. Otolaryngol. 56:* 427–434.

Froeschels, E., and Jellinek, A. (1941). *Practice of Voice and Speech Therapy. New Contributions to Voice and Speech Pathology.* Expression Company, Boston.

Froeschels, E., Kastein, S., and Weiss, D. A. (1955). A method of therapy for paralytic conditions of the mechanisms of phonation, respiration and glutination. *J. Speech Hear. Disord. 20:* 365–370.

Fudala, J. B. (1973). Using parents in public school speech therapy. *Lang. Speech Hear. Serv. Schs. 4:* 91–94.

Fuller, C. W. (1970). Differential diagnosis. In *The Hard of Hearing Child. Clinical and Educational Management,* edited by F. S. Berg, and S. G. Fletcher, pp 203–215. Grune and Stratton, New York.

Gacek, R. R. (1976). Hereditary abductor vocal cord paralysis. *Ann. Otol. Rhinol. Laryngol. 85:* 90–93.

Gengel, R. W. (1969). Practice effects in frequency discrimination by hearing impaired children. *J. Speech Hear. Res. 12:* 847–856.

Gillespie, S. K., and Cooper, E. B. (1973). Prevalence of speech problems in junior and senior high schools. *J. Speech Hear. Res. 16:* 739–743.

Gilmore, M. E. (1966). Rhythm, language, and the deaf child. *Volta Rev. 68:* 160–165.

Glenn, J. W., and Kleiner, N. (1968). Speaker identification based on nasal phonation. *J. Acoust. Soc. Am. 43:* 368–371.

Goda, S. (1966). Speech therapy with selected patients with congenital velopharyngeal inadequacy. *Cleft Palate J. 3:* 268–274.

Gonzales, J. B., and Aronson, A. E. (1970). Palatal lift prosthesis for treatment of anatomic and neurologic palatopharyngeal insufficiency. *Cleft Palate J. 7:* 91–104.

Goode, R. L., and Ross, J. (1972). Velopharyngeal insufficiency after adenoidectomy. *Arch. Otolaryngol. 96:* 223–226.

Gould, W. J. (1973). The Gould laryngoscope. *Trans. Am. Acad. Ophthalmol. Otolaryngol. 77:* ORL 139–141.

Gould, W. J. (1975). Quantitative assessment of voice function in microlaryngology. *Folia Phoniatr. 27:* 190–200.

Goumaz, C.-F. (1973). Laryngotracheal sequelae of prolonged intubation in newborn infants. *ORL (Basel) 35:* 1–14.

Grammatico, L. F. (1975). The development of listening skills. *Volta Rev. 77:* 303–308.

Gray, B. B., England, G., and Mohoney, J. L. (1965). Treatment of benign vocal nodules by reciprocal inhibition. *Behav. Res. Ther. 3:* 187–193.

Greene, M. C. L. (1964). *The Voice and Its Disorders*, Ed. 2. J. B. Lippincott, Philadelphia.

Greene, M. C. L. (1972). *The Voice and Its Disorders*, Ed. 3. Pitman Publishing Corp., New York.

Grey, P. (1973). Microlaryngostroboscopy and "singers' nodes". *J. Otolaryngol. Soc. Aust. 3:* 525–527.

Gupta, V. (1977). *Tractor Performance Pocket Book, 1977 Summary of Tractor Test Reports on Current Models as Tested by Nebraska Tractor Testing Cab.* Continental Publishing Co., Inc., Ralston, Nebraska.

Gutzmann, H. (1910). Diagnostik und Therapie der funktionellen Stimmstoerungen. *Med.-Paedagog. Monatsschr. f. d. ges. Sprachheilkunde 20:* 55. Cited by Brodnitz, F. S. (1958). The pressure test in mutational voice disturbances. *Ann. Otol. Rhinol. Laryngol. 67:* 235–240.

Gylling, U., and Soivio, A. I. (1965). Submucous cleft palates. Surgical treatment and results. *Acta Chir. Scand. 129:* 282–287.

Hagerty, R., and Hoffmeister, F. S. (1954). Velopharyngeal closure: An index of speech. *J. Plast. Reconstr. Surg. 13:* 290–298.

Hahn, E. (1955). Role-playing, creative dramatics and play therapy in speech correction. *Speech Teacher 4:* 233–238.

Haley, L. (1972). The use of beep tape to speed up articulatory responses. *Lang. Speech Hear. Serv. Schs. 3:* 35–36.

Hall, J. W., and Jerger, J. (1976). Acoustic reflex characteristics in spastic dysphonia. *Arch. Otolaryngol. 102:* 411–415.

Hamlet, S. L. (1973). Vocal compensation: An ultrasonic study of vocal fold vibration in normal and nasal vowels. *Cleft Palate J. 10:* 267–285.

Hanf, C., and Corso, J. (1966). Intensity of the voice and the theory of activation. *Am. J. Psychol. 79:* 226–233.

Hanley, T. D., and Peters, R. (1971). The speech and hearing laboratory. In *Handbook of Speech Pathology and Audiology*, edited by L. E. Travis, pp 75–140. Prentice-Hall, Inc., Englewood Cliffs.

Hanley, T. D., and Steer, M. D. (1949). Effect of level of distracting noise upon speaking rate, duration and intensity. *J. Speech Hear. Disord. 14:* 363–368.

Hanley, T. D., and Thurman, W. L. (1970). *Developing Vocal Skills*, Ed. 2. Holt, Rinehart and Winston, Inc., New York.

Hardingham, M., and Walsh-Waring, G. P. (1975). The treatment of a congenital laryngeal web. *J. Laryngol. Otol. 89:* 273–279.

Harper, P. (1970). A visible speech aid. *Volta Rev. 72:* 349–352.

Harrington, R. (1950). Children with voice disorders. In *Speech Problems of Children*, edited by W. Johnson, pp 190–203. Grune and Stratton, New York.

Harris, C. M., and Weiss, M. R. (1964). Effects of speaking condition on pitch. *J. Acoust. Soc. Am. 36:* 933–936.

Harris, G. M. (1971). *Language for the Preschool Deaf Child*, Ed. 3. Grune and Stratton, New York.

Harris, H. H. (1972). Management of injuries to the larynx and trachea. *Laryngoscope 82:* 1924–1929.

Hauth, L. (1961). Voice improvement. The speech teacher's responsibility. *Speech Teacher 10:* 48–52.

Haycock, G. S. (1933). *The Teaching of Speech*. Hill and Ainsworth, Ltd., Stoke-on-Trent, England. Reprintings by Volta Bureau, Washington, D. C.

Heaver, L. (1958). Psychiatric observations on the personality structure of patients with habitual dysphonia. *Logos 1:* 21–26.

Hengerer, A. S., Strome, M., and Jaffe, B. F. (1975). Injuries to the neonatal larynx from long-term endotracheal tube intubation and suggested tube modification for prevention. *Ann. Otol. Rhinol. Laryngol. 84:* 764–770.

Hess, D. A. (1976). A new experimental approach to assessment of velopharyngeal adequacy. Nasal manometric bleed testing. *J. Speech Hear. Disord. 41:* 427–443.

Hixon, T. J., Saxman, J. H., and McQueen, H. D. (1967). The respirometric technique for evaluating velopharyngeal competence during speech. *Folia Phoniatr. 19:* 203–219.

Hochberg, I. (1975). Most comfortable listening for the loudness and intelligibility of speech. *Audiology 14:* 27–33.

Holbrook, A. (1977). Instrumental analysis and

control of vocal behavior. In *Approaches to Vocal Rehabilitation*, edited by M. Cooper and M. H. Cooper, pp 65–75. C. C Thomas, Springfield.

Holbrook, A., and Crawford, G. H. (1970). Modifications of vocal frequency and intensity in the speech of the deaf. *Volta Rev. 72:* 492–497.

Holbrook, A., and Meador, M. N. (1969). A device for automatic modification of vocal frequency and intensity. *South. Speech J. 35:* 154–162.

Holbrook, A., Rolnick, M. I., and Bailey, C. W. (1974). Treatment of vocal abuse disorders using a vocal intensity controller. *J. Speech Hear. Disord. 39:* 298–303.

Holinger, L. D., Holinger, P. C., and Holinger, P. H. (1976). Etiology of bilateral abductor vocal cord paralysis. A review of 389 cases. *Ann. Otol. Rhinol. Laryngol. 85:* 428–436.

Holinger, P. H., and Brown, W. T. (1967). Congenital webs, cysts, laryngoceles and other anomalies of the larynx. *Ann. Otol. Rhinol. Laryngol. 76:* 744–752.

Holinger, P. H., Johnston, K. C., Conner, G. H., Conner, B. R., and Holper, J. (1962). Studies of papilloma of the larynx. *Ann. Otol. Rhinol. Laryngol. 71:* 443–447.

Holinger, P. H., Johnston, K. C., and McMahon, R. J. (1952). Hoarseness in infants and children. *Eye Ear Nose Throat Mon. 31:* 247–251.

Holinger, P. H., Johnston, K. C., and Schiller, F. (1954). Congenital anomalies of the larynx. *Ann. Otol. Rhinol. Laryngol. 63:* 581–606.

Holinger, P. H., Lutterbeck, E. F., and Bulger, R. (1972). Xeroradiography of the larynx. *Ann. Otol. Rhinol. Laryngol. 81:* 806–808.

Holinger, P. H., and Schild, J. A. (1972). Pharyngeal, laryngeal and tracheal injuries in the pediatric age group. *Ann. Otol. Rhinol. Laryngol. 81:* 538–545.

Holinger, P. H., Schild, J. A., and Maurizi, D. G. (1968). Internal and external trauma to the larynx. *Laryngoscope 78:* 944–954.

Holland, A. L. (1967). Some applications of behavioral principles to speech problems. *J. Speech Hear. Disord. 32:* 11–18.

Hollien, H., and Copeland, R. H. (1965). Speaking fundamental frequency (SFF) characteristics of mongoloid girls. *J. Speech Hear. Disord. 30:* 344–349.

Hollien, H., and Malcik, E. (1962). Adolescent voice change in southern Negro males. *Speech Monogr. 29:* 53–58.

Hollien, H., and Malcik, E. (1967). Evaluation of cross-sectional studies of adolescent voice change in males. *Speech Monogr. 34:* 80–84.

Hollien, H., Malcik, E., and Hollien, B. (1965). Adolescent voice change in southern white males. *Speech Monogr. 32:* 87–90.

Hollien, H., and Michel, J. F. (1968). Vocal fry as a phonational register. *J. Speech Hear. Res. 11:* 600–604.

Hollien, H., Moore, P., Wendahl, R., and Michel, J. (1966). On the nature of vocal fry. *J. Speech Hear. Res. 9:* 245–247.

Hollien, H., and Paul, P. (1969). A second evaluation of the speaking fundamental frequency characteristics of postadolescent girls. *Lang. Speech 12:* 119–124.

Hood, R. B., and Dixon, R. F. (1969). Physical characteristics of speech rhythm of deaf and normal-hearing speakers. *J. Commun. Disord. 2:* 20–28.

Hudgins, C. V. (1937). Voice production and breath control in the speech of the deaf. *Am. Ann. Deaf 82:* 338–363.

Huff, J. S. (1972). Laryngeal trauma. *Minn. Med. 55:* 348.

Huff, J. S., and Magielski, J. E. (1976). Surgical treatment of laryngeal injuries. *Otolaryngol. Clin. North Am. 9:* 393–401.

Huffman, L., and McReynolds, L. (1968). Auditory sequence learning in children. *J. Speech Hear. Res. 11:* 179–188.

Hunt, D., and Hunt, K. (1964). *Pantomime. The Silent Theater.* Atheneum, New York.

Irwin, R. B. (1965). *Speech and Hearing Therapy, Clinical and Educational Principles and Practices.* Stanwix House, Pittsburgh.

Isshiki, N., Honjow, I., and Morimoto, M. (1969). Cineradiographic analysis of movement of the lateral pharyngeal wall. *Plast. Reconstr. Surg. 44:* 357–363.

Isshiki, N., Okamura, H., and Morimoto, M. (1967). Maximum phonation time and air flow rate during phonation: Simple clinical tests for vocal function. *Ann. Otol. Rhinol. Laryngol. 76:* 998–1007.

Isshiki, N., Okamura, H., Tanabe, H., and Morimoto, M. (1969). Differential diagnosis of hoarseness. *Folia Phoniatr. 21:* 9–19.

Isshiki, N., and Takeuchi, Y. (1970). Factor analysis of hoarseness. *Stud. Phonol. 5:* 37–44.

Isshiki, N., and von Leden, H. (1964). Hoarseness: Aerodynamic studies. *Arch. Otolaryngol. 80:* 206–213.

Isshiki, N., Yanagihara, N., and Morimoto, M. (1966). Approach to the objective diagnosis of hoarseness. *Folia Phoniatr. 18:* 393–400.

Iwata, S., von Leden, H., and Williams, D. (1972). Air flow measurement during phonation. *J. Commun. Disord. 5:* 67–79.

Jackson, C. (1959). Hoarseness. In *Diseases of the Nose, Throat, and Ear*, Ed. 2, edited by C. Jackson and C. L. Jackson, p 576. W. B. Saunders Company, Philadelphia.

Jackson, C. (1967). Anomalies of the larynx. In *Otolaryngology*, edited by G. M. Coates and H. P. Schenck. Harper and Row, New York.

Jacobs, R. J., Philips, B. J., and Harrison, R. J. (1970). A stimulability test for cleft-palate children. *J. Speech Hear. Disord. 35:* 354–360.

Jacobson, E. (1938). *Progressive relaxation*, Ed. 2.

University of Chicago Press, Chicago. (Midway Reprint, 1974).

Jacobson, E. (1964). *Anxiety and Tension Control, A Physiologic Approach.* J. B. Lippincott Co., Philadelphia.

Jacobson, E. (1976). *You Must Relax,* Ed. 5. McGraw-Hill Book Co., Hightstown, New Jersey.

Jaffe, B. F. (1972). Postoperative hoarseness. *Am. J. Surg. 123:* 432–437.

James, H. P., and Cooper, E. B. (1966). Accuracy of teacher referrals of speech handicapped children. *Except. Child. 33:* 29–33.

Jensen, P. J. (1964). Hoarseness in cheerleaders. *Asha 6:* 406.

Jerger, J., and Jerger, S. (1970). Temporary threshold shift in rock-and-roll musicians. *J. Speech Hear. Res. 13:* 221–224.

Johnsen, S. (1973). What is prolonged intubation? *Acta Otolaryngol. (Stockh.) 75:* 377–378.

Johnson, P. E., and Ausband, J. R. (1972). Congenital myasthenia gravis with intermittent invagination of the posterior tracheal wall. *Ann. Otol. Rhinol. Laryngol. 81:* 772–777.

Johnson, T. H., Jr., and Feist, J. H. (1971). Laryngography: The procedure of choice for benign laryngeal lesions. *Am. J. Roentgenol. 111:* 109–114.

Johnson, T. S. (1976). *Vocal Abuse Reduction Program.* Department of Communicative Disorders, Utah State University.

Johnson, W., Darley, F. L., and Spriestersbach, D. C. (1963). *Diagnostic Methods in Speech Pathology,* Harper and Row, New York.

Jones, C. (1967). "Deaf voice"—A description derived from a survey of the literature. *Volta Rev. 69:* 507–508, 539–540.

Jones, H. H., and Oser, J. L. (1968). Farm equipment noise exposure levels. *Am. Ind. Hyg. Assoc. J. 29:* 146–151.

Jones, H. W., Hoerr, N. L., and Osol, A. (1949). *Blakiston's New Gould Medical Dictionary.* Blakiston Co., Philadelphia.

Jones, M. C. (1971). Diagnostic implications of acoustic cry features. *J. Commun. Disord. 4:* 310–316.

Kallen, L. A. (1959). What is "optimal" for the human voice? *Logos 2:* 40–48.

Kaplan, E. N., Jobe, R. P., and Chase, R. A. (1969). Flexibility in surgical planning for velopharyngeal incompetence. *Cleft Palate J. 6:* 166–174.

Kaplan, H. M. (1960). *Anatomy and Physiology of Speech.* McGraw-Hill Book Company, Inc., New York.

Kärjä, J., Jokinen, K., and Palva, A. (1975). Experiences with cryotherapy in otolaryngological practice. *J. Laryngol. Otol. 89:* 519–526.

Karlovich, R. S. (1968). Sensory interaction: Perception of loudness during visual stimulation. *J. Acoust. Soc. Am. 44:* 570–575.

Kasprzyk, P. L., and Gilbert, H. R. (1975). Vowel perturbation as a function of tongue height. *J. Acoust. Soc. Amer. 57:* 1545–1546.

Kelly, H. D. B., and Craik, J. E. (1952). Laryngeal nodes and the so-called amyloid tumour of the cords. *J. Laryngol. Otol. 66:* 339–358.

Kelly, J. C., and Steer, M. D. (1949). Revised concept of rate. *J. Speech Hear. Disord. 14:* 222–226.

Kelman, A. W., Gordon, M. T., Simpson, I. C., and Morton, F. M. (1975). Assessment of vocal function by air-flow measurements. *Folia Phoniatr. 27:* 250–262.

Kelsey, C. A., Ewanowski, S. J., Crummy, A. B., and Bless, D. M. (1972). Lateral pharyngeal-wall motion as a predictor of surgical success in velopharyngeal insufficiency. *N. Engl. J. Med. 287:* 64–68.

Kent, R. D. (1976). Anatomical and neuromuscular maturation of the speech mechanism: Evidence from acoustic studies. *J. Speech Hear. Res. 19:* 421–447.

Kenyon, E. L. (1928). Action and control of peripheral organs of speech: Psychologic principles, and scientific basis for methods of training. *J. A. M. A. 91:* 1341–1346.

Kerman, P. C., Singer, L. S., and Davidoff, A. (1973). Palatal lift and speech therapy for velopharyngeal incompetence. *Arch. Phys. Med. Rehabil. 54:* 271–276.

Kipfmueller, L. J., and Lang, B. R. (1972). Treating velopharyngeal inadequacies with a palatal lift prosthesis. *J. Prosthet. Dent. 27:* 63–72.

Kipnis, C. (1974). *The Mime Book.* Harper & Row, New York.

Kirchner, F. R. (1974). *Microcauterization in Otolaryngology.* American Academy of Ophthalmology and Otolaryngology, Rochester, Minn.

Kirchner, F. R. (1975). Microcauterization in pediatric patients. *Trans. Am. Acad. Ophthalmol. Otolaryngol. 80:* ORL 352–355.

Kirchner, F. R., and Duff, W. E. (1974). Treatment of laryngeal and ear strictures by microcauterization. *Laryngoscope 84:* 1326–1331.

Klinger, H. (1962). Imitated English cleft palate speech in a normal Spanish speaking child. *J. Speech Hear. Disord. 27:* 379–381.

Knight, H. S. (1973). Laryngological referrals: A serviceable procedure. *Lang. Speech Hear. Serv. Schs. 4:* 196–198.

Kodman, F., Jr. (1964). The team approach to hearing problems. *Maico Audiological Library Series,* Vol. 2, Report 10.

Koike, Y., and von Leden, H. (1969). Pathologic vocal initiation. *Ann. Otol. Rhinol. Laryngol. 78:* 138–147.

Kuras, J. E., and Findlay, R. C. (1974). Listening patterns of self-identified rock music listeners to rock music presented via earphones. *J.*

Aud. Res. 14: 51–56.

Laguaite, J. K. (1972). Adult voice screening. *J. Speech Hear. Disord. 37:* 147–151.

Laguaite, J. K. (1976). The use of hypnosis with children with deviant voices. *Int. J. Clin. Exp. Hypn. 24:* 98–104.

Laguaite, J., and Waldrop, W. F. (1964). Acoustic analysis of fundamental frequency of voices before and after therapy. *Folia Phoniatr. 16:* 183–192.

Landes, B. A. (1977). Management of hyperfunctional dysphonia and vocal tension. In *Approaches to Vocal Rehabilitation*, edited by M. Cooper and M. H. Cooper, pp 122–137. C. C Thomas, Springfield.

Lass, N. J., and Noll, J. D. (1970). A comparative study of rate characteristics in cleft palate and noncleft palate speakers. *Cleft Palate J. 7:* 275–283.

Launer, P. G. (1971). Maximum phonation time in children. Unpublished master's thesis, State University of New York at Buffalo.

Laupus, W. E., and Pastore, P. N. (1967). The larynx. In *Disorders of the Respiratory Tract in Children*, edited by E. L. Kendig, Jr., pp 204–212. W. B. Saunders Co., Philadelphia.

Laver, J. D. M. (1968). Voice quality and indexical information. *Brit. J. Disord. Commun. 3:* 43–54.

Lawson, J. (1957). *Mime. The Theory and Practice of Expressive Gesture with a Description of its Historical Development.* Sir Isaac Pitman & Sons, Ltd., London.

Lawson, L. I., Chierici, G., Castro, A., Harvold, P., Miller, E. R., and Owsley, J. Q., Jr. (1972). Effects of adenoidectomy on the speech of children with potential velopharyngeal dysfunction. *J. Speech Hear. Disord. 37:* 390–402.

Lebo, C. P., and Oliphant, D. S. (1968). Music as a source of acoustic trauma. *Laryngoscope 78:* 1211–1218.

Lebo, C. P., Oliphant, D. S., and Garrett, J. (1967). Acoustic trauma from rock and roll music. *Calif. Med. 107:* 378–380.

Leeper, H. A., Jr. (1976). Voice initiation characteristics of normal children and children with vocal nodules: A preliminary investigation. *J. Commun. Disord. 9:* 83–94.

Lerman, J. W. (1972). Voice disorders. In *Communicative Disorders: An Appraisal*, edited by A. J. Weston, pp 101–127. C. C Thomas, Springfield.

LeSaz, R. (1973). Value of a "favorites" and "unfavorites" inventory. *Lang. Speech Hear. Serv. Schs. 4:* 47–48.

Levbarg, J. J. (1939). Vocal therapy versus surgery for the eradication of singers' and speakers' nodules. *Eye Ear Nose Throat Mon. 18:* 81–82, 91.

Levitt, H., and Nye, P. W. Eds. (1971). *Sensory Training Aids for Hearing Impaired.* National Academy of Engineering, Washington, D. C.

Lewin, M. A., Heller, J. C., and Kojak, D. J. (1975). Speech results after Millard island flap repair in cleft palate and other velopharyngeal insufficiencies. *Cleft Palate J. 12:* 263–269.

Lewy, R. B. (1963). Practical aspects of psychiatry applied to otolaryngology. *Arch. Otolaryngol. 77:* 444–446.

Lichtenberg, F. S. (1966). A comparison of children's ability to make speech sound discriminations. *Volta Rev. 68:* 426–434.

Lierle, D., and Reger, S. (1958). The effect of tractor noise on auditory sensitivity of tractor operators. *Ann. Otol. Rhinol. Laryngol. 67:* 372–388.

Ling, D. (1975). Amplification for speech. In *Speech and Deafness*, by D. R. Calvert and S. R. Silverman, pp 64–88. Alexander Graham Bell Assoc. for Deaf, Inc., Washington, D. C.

Ling, D. (1976). *Speech and the Hearing-Impaired Child: Theory and Practice.* Alexander Graham Bell Assoc. for the Deaf, Inc., Washington, D. C.

Lintz, L. B., and Sherman, D. (1961). Phonetic elements and perception of nasality. *J. Speech Hear. Res. 4:* 381–396.

Lipscomb, D. M. (1969). High intensity sounds in the recreational environment: A hazzard to young ears. *Clin. Pediatr. (Phila.) 8:* 63–68.

Lively, M. A., and Emanuel, F. W. (1970). Spectral noise levels and roughness severity ratings for normal and simulated rough vowels produced by adult females. *J. Speech Hear. Res. 13:* 503–517.

Loré, J. M., Jr. (1950). Hoarseness in children. *Arch. Otolaryngol. 51:* 814–825.

Loré, J. M., Jr. (1973). *An Atlas of Head and Neck Surgery*, Vol. 2. Ed. 2. W. B. Saunders Co., Philadelphia.

Low, G., Crerar, M., and Lassers, L. (1959). Communication centered speech therapy. *J. Speech Hear. Disord. 24:* 361–368.

Lowry, L. D., Billings, B. L., and Leonard, J. E. (1974). Otolaryngic findings in a cleft palate population. *Cleft Palate J. 11:* 62–65.

Lubker, J. F., and Morris, H. L. (1968). Predicting cinefluorographic measures of velopharyngeal opening from lateral still x-ray films. *J. Speech Hear. Res. 11:* 747–753.

Lubker, J. F., Schweiger, J. W., and Morris, H. L. (1970). Nasal airflow characteristics during speech in prosthetically managed cleft palate speakers. *J. Speech Hear. Res. 13:* 326–338.

Luchsinger, R. (1965). Physiology and pathology of respiration and phonation. In *Voice-Speech-Language. Clinical Communicology: Its Physiology and Pathology,* edited by R. Luchsinger and G. E. Arnold, pp 3–334. Wadsworth Publishing Co., Belmont.

Lundquist, P.-G., Frithiof, L., and Wersäll, J.

(1975). Ultrastructural features of human juvenile laryngeal papillomas. *Acta Otolaryngol. (Stockh.) 80:* 137–149.

Luse, E., Heisse, J., and Foley, J. (1964). The vocal approach in the correction of cleft palate speech. *Folia Phoniatr. 16:* 123–129.

McCaskey, C. H. (1946). Aphonia. *Ann. Otol. Rhinol. Laryngol. 55:* 524–530.

McClosky, D. B. (1977). General techniques and specific procedures for certain voice problems. In *Approaches to Vocal Rehabilitation,* edited by M. Cooper and M. H. Cooper, pp 138–152. C. C Thomas, Springfield.

McDonald, E. T., and Baker, H. K. (1951). Cleft palate speech: An integration of research and clinical observation. *J. Speech Hear. Disord. 16:* 9–20.

McDonald, E. T., and Chance, B., Jr. (1964). *Cerebral Palsy.* Prentice-Hall, Inc., Englewood Cliffs.

McGlone, R. E. (1966). Vocal pitch characteristics of children aged one to two years. *Speech Monogr. 33:* 178–181.

McGlone, R. E. (1967). Air flow during vocal fry phonation. *J. Speech Hear. Res. 10:* 299–304.

McGlone, R. E., and Shipp, T. (1971). Some physiologic correlates of vocal-fry phonation. *J. Speech Hear. Res. 14:* 769–775.

McIntyre, B. M., and McWilliams, B. J. (1959). Creative dramatics in speech correction. *J. Speech Hear. Disord. 24:* 275–279.

McReynolds, L. V. (1970). Contingencies and consequences in speech therapy. *J. Speech Hear. Disord. 35:* 12–24.

McReynolds, L. V., and Huston, K. (1971). Token loss in speech imitation training. *J. Speech Hear. Disord. 36:* 486–495.

McWilliams, B. J. (1954). Some factors in the intelligibility of cleft palate speech. *J. Speech Hear. Disord. 19:* 524–527.

McWilliams, B. J., Bluestone, C. D., and Musgrave, R. D. (1969). Diagnostic implications of vocal cord nodules in children with cleft palate. *Laryngoscope 79:* 2072–2080.

McWilliams, B. J., and Bradley, D. P. (1965). Ratings of velopharyngeal closure during blowing and speech. *Cleft Palate J. 2:* 46–55.

McWilliams, B. J., Lavorato, A. S., and Bluestone, C. D. (1973). Vocal cord abnormalities in children with velopharyngeal valving problems. *Laryngoscope 83:* 1745–1753.

Mader, J. B. (1954). The relative frequency of occurrence of English consonant sounds in words in the speech of children in grades one, two, and three. *Speech Monogr. 21:* 294–300.

Magner, M. E. (1971). Techniques of teaching. In *Speech for the Deaf Child: Knowledge and Use,* edited by L. E. Connor, pp 245–264. Alexander Graham Bell Assoc. for the Deaf, Inc., Washington, D. C.

Manohar, P. D., and Jayaram, M., (1973). Prevalence of speech problems among school children of Mysore City. *J. All India Inst. Speech Hear. 4:* 126–130.

Marge, M. (1964). A factor analysis of oral communication skills in older children. *J. Speech Hear. Res. 7:* 31–46.

Martin, E. W. (1963). Client-centered therapy as a theoretical orientation for speech therapy. *Asha 5:* 576–578.

Martin, V. E. (1974). Consulting with teachers. *Lang. Speech Hear. Serv. Schs. 5:* 176–179.

Martin, V. E. (1975). Helping teachers decide when to refer. *Lang. Speech Hear. Serv. Schs. 6:* 154–155.

Mason, R. M., and Grandstaff, H. L. (1972). Evaluating the velopharyngeal mechanism in hypernasal speakers. *Lang. Speech Hear. Serv. Schs. No. 4,* 53–61.

Massengill, R., Jr. (1966). An objective technique for submucous cleft palate detection. *J. Plast. Reconstr. Surg. 37:* 355–359.

Massengill, R., Jr. (1972). *Hypernasality. Considerations in Causes and Treatment Procedures.* C. C Thomas, Springfield.

Massengill, R., Jr., and Brooks, R. (1973). A study of the velopharyngeal mechanism in 143 repaired cleft palate patients during production of the vowel /i/, the plosive /p/, and a /s/ sentence. *Folia Phoniatr. 25:* 312–322.

Massengill, R., Jr., and Phillips, P. P. (1975). *Cleft Palate and Associated Speech Characteristics.* Cliffs Notes, Inc., Lincoln, Nebraska.

Massengill, R., Jr., and Quinn, G. W. (1974). Adenoidal atrophy, velopharyngeal incompetence and sucking exercises: A two year follow-up case report. *Cleft Palate J. 11:* 196–199.

Massengill, R., Jr., Quinn, G. W., and Pickrell, K. L. (1971). The use of a palatal stimulator to decrease velopharyngeal gap. *Ann. Otol. Rhinol. Laryngol. 80:* 135–137.

Massengill, R., Jr., Quinn, G. W., Pickrell, K. L., and Levinson, C. (1968). Therapeutic exercise and velopharyngeal gap. *Cleft Palate J. 5:* 44–47.

Meckfessel, A. L. (1965). A comparison between vocal characteristics of deaf and normal hearing individuals. Unpublished master's thesis, University of Kansas.

Meskin, L. H., Gorlin, R. J., and Isaacson, R. J. (1964). Abnormal morphology of the soft palate: I. The prevalence of cleft uvula. *Cleft Palate J. 1:* 342–346.

Michel, J. F., Hollien, H., and Moore, P. (1965). Speaking fundamental frequency characteristics of 15-, 16-, and 17-year-old girls. *Lang. Speech 9:* 46–51.

Michelsson, K., and Sirvio, P. (1976). Cry analysis in congenital hypothyroidism. *Folia Phoniatr. 28:* 40–47.

Milisen, R. (1971). Methods of evaluation and

diagnosis of speech disorders. In *Handbook of Speech Pathology and Audiology*, edited by L. E. Travis, pp 635–672. Prentice-Hall, Inc., Englewood Cliffs.

Miller, D. (1973). Does cryosurgery have a place in the treatment of papillomata or carcinoma of the larynx? *Ann. Otol. Rhinol. Laryngol. 82:* 656–660.

Miller, E. (1948). A public school program for hard of hearing children. *J. Speech Hear. Disord. 13:* 256–259.

Miller, J. (1960). Speech and the preschool child. *Volta Rev. 62:* 315–317.

Miller, J. D. (1974). Effects of noise on people. *J. Acoust. Soc. Am. 56:* 729–764.

Millin, J. P. (1971). Therapy for reduction of continuous phonation in the hard-of-hearing population. *J. Speech Hear. Disord. 36:* 496–498.

Mills, J. H. (1975). Noise and children: A review of literature. *J. Acoust. Soc. Am. 58:* 767–779.

Missal, S. C. (1961). Food allergy in the ear, nose and throat practice of allergy. *Laryngoscope 51:* 512–523.

Moll, K. L. (1962). Velopharyngeal closure on vowels. *J. Speech Hear. Res. 5:* 30–37.

Moll, K. L. (1965). A cinefluorographic study of velopharyngeal function in normals during various activities. *Cleft Palate J. 2:* 112–122.

Moller, K. T., Starr, C. D., and Martin, R. R. (1969). The application of operant conditioning procedures to the facial grimace problem. *Cleft Palate J. 6:* 193–201.

Moncur, J. P., and Brackett, I. P. (1974). *Modifying Vocal Behavior.* Harper and Row, New York.

Montague, J. C., Jr. (1976). Perceived age and sex characteristics of voices of institutionalized children with Down's syndrome. *Percept. Mot. Skills. 42:* 215–219.

Montague, J. C., Jr., Brown, W. S., Jr., and Hollien, H. (1974). Vocal fundamental frequency characteristics of institutionalized Down's syndrome children. *Am. J. Ment. Defic. 78:* 414–418.

Montague, J. C., and Hollien, H. (1973). Perceived voice quality disorders in Down's syndrome children. *J. Commun. Disord. 6:* 76–87.

Montgomery, W. W., and Smith, S. A. (1976). Congenital laryngeal defects in the adult. *Ann. Otol. Rhinol. Laryngol. 85:* 491–497.

Moore, G. P. (1971a). Voice disorders organically based. In *Handbook of Speech Pathology and Audiology*, edited by L. E. Travis, pp 535–570. Prentice-Hall, Inc., Englewood Cliffs.

Moore, G. P. (1971b). *Organic Voice Disorders.* Prentice-Hall, Inc., Englewood Cliffs.

Moore, G. P., White, F. D., and von Leden, H. (1962). Ultra high speed photograpy in laryngeal physiology. *J. Speech Hear. Disord. 27:* 165–171.

Moore, M. V. (1967). Help for the child with a voice disorder. *Alabama School J. 84:* 30–31, 40, 42.

Moore, P. (1955). Treatment of voice defects following surgery. *Conn. Med. J. 19:* 180–183.

Moore, P., and Thompson, C. L. (1965). Comments on physiology of hoarseness. *Arch. Otolaryngol. 81:* 97–102.

Moore, P., and von Leden, H. (1958). Dynamic variations of the vibratory pattern in the normal larynx. *Folia Phoniatr. 10:* 205–238.

Moore, W. H., and Sommers, R. K. (1973). Phonetic contexts: Their effects on perceived nasality in cleft palate speakers. *Cleft Palate J. 10:* 72–83.

Morgan, D. B. (1948). A suggestive sign of allergy. *Arch. Dermatol. Syphilol. 57:* 1050.

Morris, H. L. (1966). The oral manometer as a diagnostic tool in clinical speech pathology. *J. Speech Hear. Disord. 31:* 362–369.

Morris, H. L. (1972). Cleft Palate. In *Communicative Disorders. An Appraisal*, edited by A. J. Weston, pp 128–160. C. C Thomas, Springfield.

Morris, H. L., and Smith, J. K. (1962). A multiple approach for evaluating velopharyngeal competency. *J. Speech Hear. Disord. 27:* 218–226.

Morris, H. L., Spriestersbach, D. C., and Darley, F. L. (1961). An articulation test for assessing competency of velopharyngeal closure. *J. Speech Hear. Res. 4:* 48–55.

Mosby, D. P. (1970). Psychotherapy versus voice therapy for a child with a deviant voice, a case study. *Percept. Mot. Skills 30:* 887–891.

Mosby, D. P. (1972). Appraising psychotherapeutic change in voice-deviant children with the Rorschach index of repressive style. *Percept. Mot. Skills 34:* 701–702.

Moses, P. J. (1959). Pathology and therapy of the singing voice. *Arch. Otolaryngol. 69:* 577–582.

Mueller, P. B. (1972). Vocal nodules in children. *J. Wisc. Speech Hear. Assoc. 9:* 5–15.

Mueller, P. B. (1975). Comment on "Spectrographic analysis of fundamental frequency and hoarseness before and after vocal rehabilitation" by Morton Cooper. *J. Speech Hear. Disord. 40:* 278.

Mulac, A., and Sherman, A. R. (1974). Behavioral assessment of speech anxiety. *Q. J. Speech 60:* 134–143.

Muma, J. R., Laeder, R. L., and Webb, C. E. (1968). Adolescent voice quality aberrations: Personality and social status. *J. Speech Hear. Res. 11:* 576–582.

Murphy, A. T. (1964). *Functional Voice Disorders.* Prentice-Hall, Inc., Englewood Cliffs.

Murphy, R. S. (1967). Hoarseness. *N. S. Med. Bull. 46:* 177–179.

Murry, T. (1971). Subglottal pressure and airflow measures during vocal fry phonation. *J. Speech Hear. Res. 14:* 544–551.

Mysak, E. D. (1966). Phonatory and resonatory

problems. In *Speech Pathology. An International Study of the Science*, edited by R. W. Rieber and R. S. Brubaker, pp 150–181. J. B. Lippincott Co., Philadelphia.

Mysak, E. D. (1971). Cerebral palsy speech syndromes. In *Handbook of Speech Pathology and Audiology*, edited by L. E. Travis, pp 673–695. Prentice-Hall, Inc., Englewood Cliffs.

Nation, J. E., and Aram, D. M. (1977). *Diagnosis of Speech and Language Disorders*. C. V. Mosby Co., St. Louis.

Neal, W. R., Jr. (1976). Speech pathology services in the secondary schools. *Lang. Speech Hear. Serv. Schs. 7:* 6–16.

Negus, V. E. (1939). The significance of hoarseness. *N. Y. State J. Med. 39:* 9–12.

Neiman, R. F., Mountjoy, J. R., and Allen, E. L. (1975). Myasthenia gravis focal to the larynx. *Arch. Otolaryngol. 101:* 569–570.

New, M. C. (1945). Speech suggestions for the hard of hearing. *Hearing News 13.*

Nichols, A. C. (1977). Motivations and manipulations in voice therapy. In *Approaches to Vocal Rehabilitation*, edited by M. Cooper and M. H. Cooper, pp 153–174. C. C Thomas, Springfield.

Nichols, A. C., Dembowski, P. J., and Dewey, A. L. (1971). The "soft-spoken" woman. I: "Comfortable" loudness and loudness adjustments. *J. Commun. Disord. 4:* 134–139.

Nickerson, R. S. (1975). Characteristics of the speech of deaf persons. *Volta Rev. 77:* 342–362.

Novak, A. (1972). The voice of children with Down's syndrome. *Folia Phoniatr. 24:* 182–194.

Novick, W. H. (1967). Traumatic stenosis of the trachea in children. *Laryngoscope 57:* 1351–1357.

Ogura, J. H. (1975). Voice rehabilitation following blunt trauma to the larynx. *Laryngoscope 85:* 181–185.

Oleske, J. M., and Kushnick, T. (1971). Juvenile papilloma of the larynx. *Am. J. Dis. Child. 121:* 417–419.

Olsen, B., Perez, D., Burk, K. W., and Platt, L. J. (1969). Respirometric-phonatory study of children with and without vocal nodules. Paper presented ASHA convention.

O'Neill, J. J., and McGee, J. A. (1962). Management of benign laryngeal tumors in children: Preoperative, operative and postoperative. *Ann. Otol. Rhinol. Laryngol. 71:* 480–488.

Orton, H. B. (1951). The significance of hoarseness. *New Orleans Med. Surg. J., 103:* 511–515.

Ouzts, J. W. (1969). Auditory temporary threshold shift following exposure to high-intensity and variable-peaked farm machinery noise. *J. Aud. Res. 9:* 64–70.

Owsley, J. Q., Jr., Chierici, G., Miller, E. R., Lawson, L. I., and Blackfield, H. M. (1967). Cephalometric evaluation of palatal dysfunction in patients without cleft palate. *J. Plast. Reconstr. Surg. 39:* 562–568.

Paisner, H. M., (1972). Nasal obstruction. *Postgrad. Med. 42:* 88–92.

Pannbacker, M. (1973). Speech therapy for cleft palate speakers. *Lang. Speech Hear. Serv. Schs. 4:* 157–173.

Pannbacker, M. (1975). Comment concerning "Incidence of chronic hoarseness among school-age children." *J. Speech Hear. Disord. 40:* 548–549.

Parisier, S. C., and Henneford, G. E. (1969). Surgical correction of acquired vocal cord webs. *Arch. Otolaryngol. 90:* 103–107.

Parker, B. L. (1972). The speech and language clinician on a learning center team. *Lang. Speech Hear. Serv. Schs. 3:* 18–23.

Peacher, G. (1952). Voice therapy for ulcers and nodules of the larynx. In *Proceedings of the First Institute on Voice Pathology, and the First International Meeting of Laryngectomized Persons.* Cleveland Hearing and Speech Center.

Peacher, G. M. (1963). Voice therapy. In *Voice problems and laryngeal pathology, symposium and panel discussion*, by J. F. Daly, Moderator. *N. Y. State J. Med. 63:* 3104–3107.

Pearsons, K. S., Bennett, R. L., and Fidell, S. (1976). *Speech Levels in Various Environments*. Bolt, Beranek and Newman Report No. 3281, prepared for Office of Resources and Development Environmental Protection Agency.

Perello, J. (1962). Dysphonies fonctionnelles: Phonoponose et phononevrose. *Folia Phoniatr. 14:* 150–205. Cited by A. E. Aronson, H. W. Peterson, Jr., and E. M. Litin (1964). Voice symptomatology in functional dysphonia and aphonia. *J. Speech Hear. Disord. 29:* 367–380.

Perello, J., and Tosi, O. (1974). Phonogram. *Folia Phoniatr. 26:* 289–290.

Perkins, W. H. (1957). The challenge of functional disorders of voice. In *Handbook of Speech Pathology*, edited by L. E. Travis, pp 832–877. Prentice-Hall, Inc., Englewood Cliffs.

Perkins, W. H. (1971). Vocal function: Assessment and therapy. In *Handbook of Speech Pathology and Audiology*, edited by L. E. Travis, pp 505–534. Prentice-Hall, Inc., Englewood Cliffs.

Perkins, W. H. (1977). *Speech Pathology. An Applied Behavioral Science*, Ed. 2. C. V. Mosby Co., St. Louis.

Philips, B. J. W. (1972). Stimulating language and speech development in cleft palate infants. In *Communicative Disorders Related to Cleft Lip and Palate*, edited by K. R. Bzoch, pp

231–238. Little, Brown and Co., Boston.

Phillips, D. (1976). Lecture. The practice of behavior therapy with children: A training seminar. Jan. 22–23, 1976, Philadelphia.

Phillips, D., and Mordock, J. B. (1974). Behavior therapy with children: Some general guidelines and specific suggestions. In *The Management of Childhood Behavior Problems in School and at Home*, edited by L. Daniels, pp 349–360. C. C Thomas, Springfield.

Phillips, P. P. (1975). *Speech and Hearing Problems in the Classroom.* Cliffs Notes, Inc., Lincoln, Nebraska.

Pitzner, J. C., and Morris, H. L. (1966). Articulation skills and adequacy of breath pressure ratios of children with cleft palate. *J. Speech Hear. Disord. 31:* 26–40.

Podol, J., and Salvia, J. (1976). Effects of visibility of a prepalatal cleft on the evaluation of speech. *Cleft Palate J. 13:* 361–366.

Pollack, D. (1970). *Educational Audiology for the Limited Hearing Infant.* C. C Thomas, Springfield.

Pont, C. (1965). Hoarseness in children. *W. Mich. Univ. J. Speech Ther. 2:* 6–8.

Porterfield, H. W., and Trabue, J. C. (1965). Submucous cleft palate. *Plast. Reconstr. Surg. 35:* 45–50.

Porterfield, H. W., Trabue, J. C., Terry, J. L., and Stimpert, R. D. (1966). Hypernasality in noncleft palate patients. *Plast. Reconstr. Surg. 37:* 216–220.

Powers, G. L., and Starr, C. D. (1974). The effects of muscle exercises on velopharyngeal gap and nasality. *Cleft Palate J. 11:* 28–35.

Presto, M. (1943). An experiment in voice control. *Volta Rev. 45:* 490–493.

Priest, R. E., Huff, J. S., and Banovetz, J. D. (1967). Laryngotracheal injuries. *Ann. Otol. Rhinol. Laryngol. 76:* 786–792.

Prins, D., and Bloomer, H. H. (1965). A word intelligibility approach to the study of speech change in oral cleft patients. *Cleft Palate J. 2:* 357–368.

Pronovost, W. (1977). Voice therapy for the hearing impaired. In *Approaches to Vocal Rehabilitation*, edited by M. Cooper and M. H. Cooper, pp 193–216. C. C Thomas, Springfield.

Pronovost, W., and Kingman, L. (1959). *The Teaching of Speaking and Listening in the Elementary School.* Longmans, Green and Co., New York.

Ptacek, P. H., and Sander, E. K. (1963). Maximum duration of phonation. *J. Speech Hear. Disord. 28:* 171–182.

Punt, N. A. (1974). Lubrication of the vocal mechanism. *Folia Phoniatr. 26:* 287–288.

Quigley, L. F., Jr. (1968). Pressure and cephalometric technics for evaluation of normal and cleft palate patients. II. Palatopharyngeal competency. *J. Dent. Res. 47:* 760–768.

Rabuzzi, D. D., and McCall, G. N. (1972). Spasmodic dysphonia: A clinical perspective. *Trans. Am. Acad. Ophthalmol. Otolaryngol. 76:* 724–728.

Rapp, D. J. (1972). *Allergies and Your Child.* Holt, Rinehart and Winston, New York.

Rapp, D. J., and Fahey, D. (1973). Review of chronic secretory otitis and allergy. *J. Asthma Res. 10:* 193–218.

Rees, M. (1958). Some variables affecting perceived harshness. *J. Speech Hear. Res. 1:* 155–168.

Rees, T. D., Wood-Smith, D., Swinyard, C. A., and Converse, J. M. (1967). Electromyographic evaluation of submucous cleft palate: A possible aid to operative planning. *Plast. Reconstr. Surg. 40:* 592–594.

Regnell, J. R., and Thomas, A. E. (1976). The voice chart: An objective approach to measurement of voice disorders. Paper presented at ASHA Convention. *Asha 18:* 683.

Rise, E. N. (1966). Velopharyngeal incompetence. *South. Med. J. 59:* 337–340.

Rochmis, L. N., and Doob, D. (1970). *Speech Therapy. A Group Approach for Schools and Clinics.* John Day Co., New York.

Roeser, R. J., Campbell, A., and Brown, B. (1976). The hearing health team—A one way street? *Audiol. Hear. Ed. 2:* 8–11.

Rogers, C. R. (1942). *Counseling and Psychotherapy.* Houghton-Mifflin Co., Boston.

Rogers, C. R. (1951). *Client-centered Therapy.* Houghton-Mifflin Co., Boston.

Rontal, E., Rontal, M., and Rolnick, M. I. (1975). Objective evaluation of vocal pathology using voice spectrography. *Ann. Otol. Rhinol. Laryngol. 84:* 662–671.

Rosedale, R. S., and Nowara, R. J. (1960). Etiology of hoarseness with an original classification. *Ohio Med. J. 56:* 334–338.

Rosenblith, W. A., Stevens, K. N., and the Staff of Bolt, Beranek, and Newman, Inc. (1953). *Handbook of Acoustic Noise Control. Vol. 2. Noise and Man.* Wright Air Development Center Technical Report 52–204.

Rubin, H. J. (1964). Role of the laryngologist in management of dysfunctions of the singing voice. *Trans. Pac. Coast Otoophthalmol. Soc. 45:* 57–77.

Rubin, H. J., and Lehroff, I. (1962). Pathogenesis and treatment of vocal nodules. *J. Speech Hear. Disord. 27:* 150–161.

Rupp, R. R., and Koch, L. J. (1969). Effects of too-loud music on human ears—But, Mother, rock'n roll HAS to be loud! *Clin. Pediatr. 8:* 60–62.

Salter, A. (1961). *Conditioned Reflex Therapy.* Capricorn, New York.

Salzinger, S., Salzinger, K., Portnoy, S., Eckman, J., Bacon, P. M., Deutsch, M., and Zubin, J.

(1962). Operant conditioning of continuous speech in young children. *Child Dev. 33:* 683–695.

Sanders, D. A. (1971). *Aural Rehabilitation.* Prentice-Hall, Inc., Englewood Cliffs.

Sanders, S. H. (1967). Infectious and allergenic conditions of the eye, nose and throat. *J. Miss. State Med. Assoc. 8:* 695–699.

Sansone, F. E., Jr., and Emanuel, F. W. (1970). Spectral noise levels and roughness severity ratings for normal and simulated rough vowels produced by adult males. *J. Speech Hear. Res. 13:* 489–502.

Saunders, E. A., and Miller, C. J. (1968). A study of verbal communication in mentally subnormal patients. *Br. J. Disord. Commun. 3:* 99–110.

Saunders, W. H. (1956). Dysphonia plicae ventricularis. *Ann. Otol. Rhinol. Laryngol. 65:* 665–672.

Saunders, W. H. (1964). The larynx. *Clinical Symposia 16:* 67–99.

Sawashima, M. (1966). Measurement of phonation time. *Jap. J. Logopedics Phoniatr. 7:* 23–28. Cited by Sawashima, M., Totsuka, G., Kobayashi, T., and Hirose, H. (1968). Surgery for hoarseness due to unilateral vocal cord paralysis. *Arch. Otolaryngol. 87:* 289–294.

Sawashima, M., Totsuka, G., Kobayashi, T., and Hirose, H. (1968). Surgery for hoarseness due to unilateral vocal cord paralysis. *Arch. Otolaryngol. 87:* 289–294.

Schendel, S. A., and Gorlin, R. J. (1974). Frequency of cleft uvula and submucous cleft palate in patients with Down's syndrome. *J. Dent. Res. 53:* 840–843.

Schiff, M. (1973). Nonauditory effects of noise. *Trans. Am. Acad. Ophthalmol. Otolaryngol. 77:* ORL 384–398.

Schlanger, B. B., and Gottsleben, R. H. (1957). Analysis of speech defects among the institutional mentally retarded. *Train. Sch. Bull. (Vinel.) 54:* 5–8.

Scholl, H. M. (1961). A holistic approach to the teaching of voice improvement. *Speech Teach. 10:* 200–205.

Schubert, K. (1963). Cough due to a large uvula. *Ger. Med. Mon. 8:* 413.

Schulz, R., Heller, J. C., Gens, G. W., and Lewin, M. (1973). Pharyngeal flap surgery and voice quality factors related to success and failure. *Cleft Palate J. 10:* 166–175.

Schweiger, J. W., Netsell, R., and Sommerfeld, R. M. (1970). Prosthetic management and speech improvement in individuals with dysarthria of the palate. *J. Am. Dent. Assoc. 80:* 1348–1353.

Senturia, B. H., and Wilson, F. B. (1968). Otorhinolaryngic findings in children with voice deviations. Preliminary report. *Ann. Otol. Rhinol. Laryngol. 77:* 1027–1042.

Shearer, W. H. (1972). Diagnosis and treatment of voice disorders in school children. *J. Speech Hear. Disord. 37:* 215–221.

Shelton, R. L., Jr. (1963). Therapeutic exercise and speech pathology. *Asha 5:* 855–859.

Shelton, R. L., Jr., Arndt, W. B., Jr., Knox, A. W., Elbert, M., Chisum, L., and Youngstrom, K. A. (1969). The relationship between nasal sound pressure level and palatopharyngeal closure. *J. Speech Hear. Res. 12:* 193–198.

Shelton, R. L., Jr., and Bosma, J. F. (1962). Maintenance of the pharyngeal airway. *J. Appl. Physiol. 17:* 209–214.

Shelton, R. L., Jr., Brooks, A. R., and Youngstrom, K. A. (1965). Clinical assessment of palatopharyngeal closure. *J. Speech Hear. Disord. 30:* 37–43.

Shelton, R. L., Jr., Hahn, E., and Morris, H. L. (1968). Diagnosis and Therapy. In *Cleft Palate and Communication,* edited by D. C. Spriestersbach and D. Sherman, pp 225–268. Academic Press, New York.

Sherman, D. (1970). Usefulness of the mean in psychological scaling of cleft palate speech. *Cleft Palate J. 7:* 622–625.

Sherman, D., and Linke, E. (1952). The influence of certain vowel types on degree of harsh voice quality. *J. Speech Hear. Disord. 17:* 401–408.

Sherman, D., and Moodie, C. E. (1957). Four psychological scaling methods applied to articulation defectiveness. *J. Speech Hear. Disord. 22:* 698–706.

Sherman, D., and Silverman, F. H. (1968). Three psychological scaling methods applied to language development. *J. Speech Hear. Res. 11:* 837–841.

Shipp, T. (1975). Vertical laryngeal position during continuous and discrete vocal frequency change. *J. Speech Hear. Res. 18:* 707–718.

Shipp, T., and Huntington, D. A. (1965). Some acoustic and perceptual factors in acute-laryngitic hoarseness. *J. Speech Hear. Disord. 30:* 350–359.

Shipp, T., and Izdebski, K. (1975). Vocal frequency and vertical larynx positioning by singers and nonsingers. *J. Acoust. Soc. Am. 58:* 1104–1106.

Shprintzen, R. J., Lencione, R. M., McCall, G. N., and Skolnick, M. L. (1974). A three dimensional cinefluoroscopic analysis of velopharyngeal closure during speech and nonspeech activities in normals. *Cleft Palate J. 11:* 412–428.

Shprintzen, R. J., McCall, G. N., and Skolnick, M. L. (1975). A new therapeutic technique for the treatment of velopharyngeal incompetence. *J. Speech Hear. Disord. 40:* 69–83.

Shupe, L. K. (1968). Speech intelligibility measures of cleft palate speakers before and after pharyngeal flap surgery. Unpublished Ph.D.

dissertation, State University of New York at Buffalo.

Siegel, A. W., and Allik, J. P. (1973). A developmental study of visual and auditory short-term memory. Learning Research and Development Center, U. of Pittsburgh.

Silverman, E. M., and Zimmer, C. H. (1975). Incidence of chronic hoarseness among school-age children. *J. Speech Hear. Disord. 40:* 211–215.

Silverman, S. R., and Davis, H. (1970). Hard-of-hearing children. In *Hearing and Deafness*, Ed. 3, edited by H. Davis and S. R. Silverman, pp 426–446. Holt, Rinehart, and Winston, New York.

Singleton, G. T., and Adkins, W. Y. (1972). Cryosurgical treatment of juvenile laryngeal papillomatosis. *Ann. Otol. Rhinol. Laryngol. 81:* 784–789.

Skelly, M., Donaldson, R. C., Scheer, G. E., and Guzzardo, M. R. (1971). Dysphonias associated with spinal bracing in scoliosis. *J. Speech Hear. Disord. 36:* 368–376.

Skinner, B. F. (1953). *Science and Human Behavior.* Free Press, New York.

Sloan, R. F., Brummett, S. W., Westover, J. L., Ricketts, R. M., and Ashley, F. L. (1964). Recent cinefluorographic advances in palatopharyngeal roentgenography. *Am. J. Roentgenol. 90:* 977–985.

Smith, R. O., Hemenway, W. G., English, G. M., Black, F. O., and Swan, H. (1969). Post-intubation subglottic granulation tissue: Review of the problem and evaluation of radiotherapy. *Laryngoscope. 79:* 1227–1251.

Sokoloff, M., and Rieber, R. W. (1966). Phonatory and resonatory problems. In *Speech Pathology. An International Study of the Science*, edited by R. W. Rieber and R. S. Brubaker, pp 321–336. North-Holland Publishing Co., Amsterdam.

Spriestersbach, D. C. (1958). Routine methods of examination and diagnosis of velopharyngeal incompetency—Speech aspects. *Cleft Palate Bull. 8:* 7–8.

Spriestersbach, D. C., Moll, K. L., and Morris, H. L. (1961). Subject classification and articulation of speakers with cleft palate. *J. Speech Hear. Res., 4:* 362–372.

Spriestersbach, D. C., and Powers, G. R. (1959). Articulation skills, velopharyngeal closure, and oral breath pressure of children with cleft palates. *J. Speech Hear. Res. 2:* 318–325.

Starr, C. D., and Wilson, F. B. (1976). Reliability considerations of a voice profiling system. *Human Commun. 1:* 47–56.

Stewart, J. M., Ott, J. E., and Lagace, R. (1972). Submucous cleft palate: Prevalence in a school population. *Cleft Palate J. 9:* 246–250.

Streng, A., Fitch, W. J., Hedgecock, L. D., Phillips, J. W., and Carrell, J. A. (1958). *Hearing Therapy for Children*, Ed. 2. Grune & Stratton, New York.

Strong, M. S., and Jako, G. J. (1972). Laser surgery in the larynx. *Ann. Otol. Rhinol. Laryngol. 81:* 791–798.

Strong, M. S., Jako, G. J., Polanyi, T., and Wallace, R. A. (1973). Laser surgery in the aerodigestive tract. *Am. J. Surg. 126:* 529–533.

Strother, C. R. (1942). Voice improvement. In *Foundations of Speech*, edited by J. M. O'Neill, pp 200–230. Prentice-Hall, Inc., New York.

Subtelny, D., and Koepp-Baker, H. (1956). The significance of adenoid tissue in velopharyngeal function. *J. Plast. Reconstr. Surg. 17:* 235–250.

Subtelny, J., Koepp-Baker, H., and Subtelny, D. (1961). Palatal function and cleft palate speech. *J. Speech Hear. Disord. 26:* 213–224.

Subtelny, J., Van Hattum, R. J., and Myers, B. B. (1972). Ratings and measures of cleft palate speech. *Cleft Palate J. 9:* 18–27.

Takagi, Y., McGlone, R. E., and Millard, R. T. (1965). A survey of the speech disorders of individuals with clefts. *Cleft Palate J. 2:* 28–31.

Tarlow, A. J., and Saxman, J. H. (1970). A comparative study of the speaking fundamental frequency characteristics in children with cleft palate. *Cleft Palate J. 7:* 696–705.

Tarneaud, J. (1958). The fundamental principles of vocal cultivation and therapeutics of the voice. *Logos 1:* 7–10.

Tato, J. M., and Arcella, A. I. (1962). La inteligibilidad en funcion della velocidad de la palabra hablada en los sordos desmutizados. *Acta Otorinolaringol. Iber. Am. 23:* 551–560. Cited by Quigley, S. P. (1966). Language research in countries other than the United States. *Volta Rev. 68:* 68–83.

Taylor, G. D. (1972). The bifid uvula. *Laryngoscope 82:* 771–778.

Templin, M. C., and Darley, F. L. (1969). *The Templin-Darley Tests—A Manual and Discussion of Articulation Testing*, Ed. 2. Bureau of Educational Research and Service, University of Iowa, Iowa City.

Thorn, K. (1947). 'Client-centered' therapy for voice and personality cases. *J. Speech Disord. 12:* 314–318.

Thurman, W. L. (1977). Restructuring voice concepts and production. In *Approaches to Vocal Rehabilitation*, edited by M. Cooper and M. H. Cooper, pp 230–255. C. C Thomas, Springfield.

Timcke, R., von Leden, H., and Moore, P. (1959). Laryngeal vibrations: Measurements of the glottic wave. Part II. Physiologic variations. *Arch. Otolaryngol. 69:* 438–444.

Tobias, J. V. (1959). Relative occurrence of phonemes in American English. *J. Acoust. Soc.*

Am. 31: 631.

Toohill, R. J. (1975). The psychosomatic aspects of children with vocal nodules. *Arch. Otolaryngol. 101:* 591–595.

Ulrich, R. F., and Pinheiro, M. L. (1974). Temporary hearing losses in teen-agers attending repeated rock-and-roll sessions. *Acta Otolaryngol. (Stockh.) 77:* 51–55.

Uris, D. (1962). Teen talk. *Todays Speech 10:* 15–16.

Van Demark, D. R. (1970). A comparison of the results of pressure articulation testing in various contexts for subjects with cleft palates. *J. Speech Hear. Res. 13:* 741–754.

Van Demark, D. R. (1971). Clinical research methodology in evaluating the therapeutic process. *Cleft Palate J. 8:* 26–35.

Van Demark, D. R. (1974a). Some results of speech therapy for children with cleft palate. *Cleft Palate J. 11:* 41–49.

Van Demark, D. R. (1974b). Assessment of velopharyngeal competency for children with cleft palate. *Cleft Palate J. 11:* 310–316.

Van Demark, D. R., Kuehn, D. R., and Tharp, R. F. (1975). Prediction of velopharyngeal competency. *Cleft Palate J. 12:* 5–11.

Van Demark, D. R., and Morris, H. L. (1977). A preliminary study of the predictive value of the IPAT. *Cleft Palate J. 14:* 124–130.

Van Dusen, C. R. (1953). *Training the Voice for Speech. A Guide to Voice and Articulation Improvement.* McGraw-Hill Book Co., Inc., New York.

Van Gelder, L. (1974a). Psychosomatic aspects of endocrine disorders of the voice. *J. Commun. Disord. 7:* 257–262.

Van Gelder, L. (1974b). Open nasal speech following adenoidectomy and tonsillectomy. *J. Commun. Disord. 7:* 263–267.

Van Hattum, R. J. (1974). Communication therapy for problems associated with cleft palate. In *Communication Disorders. Remedial Principles and Practices*, edited by S. Dickson, pp 297–355. Scott, Foresman and Co., Glenview, Ill.

Van Riper, C. (1959). Binaural speech therapy. *J. Speech Hear. Disord. 24:* 62–63.

Van Riper, C. (1963). *Speech Correction, Principles and Methods*, Ed. 4. Prentice-Hall, Inc., Englewood Cliffs.

Van Riper, C. (1972). *Speech Correction, Principles and Methods*, Ed. 5. Prentice-Hall, Inc., Englewood Cliffs.

Van Riper, C., and Dopheide, W. (1966). Diagnostic services in a training center. *Asha 8:* 37–39.

Van Riper, C., and Irwin, J. V. (1958). *Voice and Articulation.* Prentice-Hall, Inc., Englewood Cliffs.

Van Thal, J. H. (1961). Dysphonia. *Speech Pathol. Ther. 4:* 11–12.

van Uden, A. (1960). A sound perceptive method. In *The Modern Educational Treatment of Deafness*, edited by A. Ewing. Manchester University Press.

Villarreal, J. (1950). Consistency of judgments of voice quality. *South. Speech J. 15:* 10–20.

von Leden, H. (1958). The clinical significance of hoarseness and related voice disoders. *Lancet 78:* 50–53.

von Leden, H., and Isshiki, N. (1965). An analysis of cough at the level of the larynx. *Arch. Otolaryngol. 81:* 616–625.

Voorhees, I. W. (1934). The nonsurgical treatment of aphonia (hoarseness). *N. Y. State J. Med. 34:* 53–55.

Vorce, E. (1974). *Teaching Speech to Deaf Children.* Alexander Graham Bell Assoc. for the Deaf, Inc., Washington, D.C.

Walker, K. S. (1969). *Eyes on Mime. Language without Speech.* John Day Co., New York.

Ward, P. H., and Wepman, J. M. (1964). Pharyngeal implants for reduction of air space in velopharyngeal insufficiency. I. An experimental study. *Ann. Otol. Rhinol. Laryngol. 73:* 443–457.

Warren, D. W., Wood, M. T., and Bradley, D. P. (1969). Respiratory volumes in normal and cleft palate speech. *Cleft Palate J. 6:* 449–460.

Weatherley-White, R. C. A., Sakura, C. Y., Jr., Brenner, L. D., Stewart, J. M., and Ott, J. E. (1972). Submucous cleft palate. Its incidence, natural history and indications for treatment. *Plast. Reconstr. Surg. 49:* 297–304.

Webster, E. J. (1966). Parent counseling by speech pathologists and audiologists. *J. Speech Hear. Disord. 31:* 331–340.

Webster, E. J., Perkins, W. H., Bloomer, H. H., and Pronovost, W. (1966). Case selection in the schools. *J. Speech Hear. Disord. 31:* 352–358.

Webster's Seventh New Collegiate Dictionary (1963). G. C. Merriam, Springfield, Mass.

Weinberg, B., and Shanks, J. C. (1971). The relationship between three oral breath pressure ratios and ratings of severity of nasality for talkers with cleft palate. *Cleft Palate J. 8:* 251–256.

Weinberg, B., and Zlatin, M. (1970). Speaking fundamental frequency characteristics of five- and six-year-old children with mongolism. *J. Speech Hear. Res. 13:* 418–425.

Weiss, C. (1974). The speech pathologist's role in dealing with obturator-wearing school children. *J. Speech Hear. Disord. 39:* 153–162.

Weiss, D. A. (1948). Organic lesions leading to speech disorders. *Nerv. Child 7:* 29–37.

Weiss, D. A. (1950). The pubertal change of the human voice. *Folia Phoniatr. 2:* 127–158.

Weiss, D. A. (1971). *Introduction to Functional Voice Therapy.* S. Karger, Basel.

Wells, C. G. (1971). *Cleft Palate and its Associated*

Speech Disorders. McGraw-Hill Book Co., New York.

Werner-Kukuk, E., and von Leden, H. (1970). Vocal initiation. *Folia Phoniatr. 22:* 107–116.

Wertz, R. T., and Mead, M. D. (1975). Classroom teacher and speech clinician severity ratings of different speech disorders. *Lang. Speech Hear. Serv. Schs. 6:* 119–124.

West, R. W., and Ansberry, M. (1968). *The Rehabilitation of Speech*, Ed. 4. Harper and Row, New York.

Westlake, H., and Rutherford, D. (1966). *Cleft Palate*. Prentice-Hall, Inc., Englewood Cliffs.

Westphal, W. (1952). *Physikalisches Wörterbuch*. Springer, Vienna. Cited in R. Luchsinger and G. E. Arnold (1965). *Voice-Speech-Language. Clinical Communicology: Its Physiology and Pathology*. Wadsworth Publishing Co., Belmont.

White, F. W. (1946). Some causes of hoarseness in children. *Ann. Otol. Rhinol. Laryngol. 55:* 537–542.

Whitehead, R. L., and Jones, K. O. (1976). Influence of consonant environment on duration of vowels produced by normal-hearing, hearing-impaired, and deaf adult speakers. *J. Acoust. Soc. Am. 60:* 513–515.

Wiles, P., and Sweetnam, R. (1965). *Essentials of Orthopaedics*. Little, Brown, New York. Cited in Skelly, M., Donaldson, R. C., Scheer, G. E., and Guzzardo, M. R. (1971). Dysphonias associated with spinal bracing in scoliosis. *J. Speech Hear. Disord. 36:* 368–376.

Williams, G. C., and McReynolds, L. V. (1975). The relationship between discrimination and articulation training in children with misarticulations. *J. Speech Hear. Res. 18:* 401–412.

Williams, R. I. (1972). Allergic laryngitis. *Ann. Otol. Rhinol. Laryngol. 81:* 558–565.

Williamson, A. B. (1944). Diagnosis and treatment of 84 cases of nasality. *Q. J. Speech 31:* 471–479.

Wilson, D. K. (1961). Children with vocal nodules. *J. Speech Hear. Disord. 26:* 19–26.

Wilson, D. K. (1962a). The hearing team. *Volta Rev. 64:* 22–25.

Wilson, D. K. (1962b). Voice re-education of children with vocal nodules. *Laryngoscope 72:* 45–53.

Wilson, D. K. (1962c). Voice reeducation of adolescents with vocal nodules. *Arch. Otolaryngol. 76:* 68–73.

Wilson, D. K. (1966). Voice reeducation in benign laryngeal pathology. *Eye Ear Nose Throat Mon. 45:* 76–80.

Wilson, D. K. (1968). Voice therapy for children with laryngeal dysfunction. *South. Med. J. 61:* 956–958.

Wilson, D. K. (1972). Voice problems of hearing-impaired children. In *Proceedings of the International Congress on Education of the Deaf,* Stockholm 1970. Vol. 2, pp 497–501. Sveriges Lararforbund, Stockholm.

Wilson, D. K. (1977). Voice problems of children and teenagers. In *Approaches to Vocal Rehabilitation*, edited by M. Cooper and M. H. Cooper, pp 256–274. C. C Thomas, Springfield.

Wilson, F. B. (1971). Emotional stress may cause voice anomalies in kids. *J. A. M. A. 216:* 2085.

Wilson, F. B. (1972). The voice-disordered child: A descriptive approach. *Lang. Speech Hear. Serv. Schs. No. 4:* 14–22.

Wilson, F. B., and Rice, M. (1977). *A Programmed Approach to Voice Therapy*. Teaching Resources, Hingham, MA.

Wing, D. M., and Heimgartner, L. M. (1973). Articulation carryover procedure implemented by parents. *Lang. Speech Hear. Serv. Schs. 4:* 182–195.

Withers, B. T. (1961). Vocal nodules. *Eye Ear Nose Throat Mon. 40:* 35–38.

Withers, B. T., and Dawson, M. H. (1960). Psychological aspects. Treatment of vocal nodule cases. *Tex. State J. Med. 56:* 43–46.

Woesner, M. E., Braun, E. J., and Sanders, I. (1974). Xeroradiographic zonography of the larynx and hypopharynx. *Ann. Otol. Rhinol. Laryngol. 83:* 42–48.

Wolpe, J. (1973). *The Practice of Behavior Therapy*, Ed. 2. Pergamon Press, Inc., New York.

Wolski, W. (1967). Hypernasality as the presenting symptom of myasthenia gravis. *J. Speech Hear. Disord. 32:* 36–38.

Wolski, W., and Wiley, J. (1965). Functional aphonia in a fourteen-year-old boy: A case report. *J. Speech Hear. Disord. 30:* 71–75.

Wood, W., and Lipscomb, D. (1972). Maximum available sound-pressure levels from stereo components. *J. Acoust. Soc. Am. 52:* 484–487.

Wyatt, G. L. (1951). The application of Froeschels' chewing method in the treatment of disorders of the speaking voice. In *The Chewing Approach in Speech and Voice Therapy*, edited by D. A. Weiss and H. H. Beebe, pp 70–99. S. Karger, Basel.

Wyatt, G. L. (1977). The chewing method and the treatment of the speaking voice. In *Approaches to Vocal Rehabilitation*, edited by M. Cooper and M. H. Cooper, pp 274–299. C. C Thomas, Springfield.

Wynter, H. (1974). An investigation into the analysis and terminology of voice quality and its correlation with the assessment reliability of speech therapists. *Br. J. Disord. Commun. 9:* 102–109.

Yairi, E., Currin, L. H., Bulian, N., and Yairi, J. (1974). Incidence of hoarseness in school children over a 1-year period. *J. Commun. Disord. 7:* 321–328.

Yanagihara, N. (1967a). Hoarseness: Investigations of the physiological mechanisms. *Ann.*

Otol. Rhinol. Laryngol. 76: 472–488.

Yanagihara, N. (1967b). Significance of harmonic changes and noise components in hoarseness. *J. Speech Hear. Res. 10:* 531–541.

Yanagihara, N., and Koike, Y. (1967). The regulation of sustained phonation. *Folia Phoniatr. 19:* 1–18.

Yanagihara, N., Koike, Y., and von Leden, H. (1966). Phonation and respiration—Function study in normal subjects. *Folia Phoniatr. 18:* 323–340.

Yater, V. (1972). St. Louis County hearing clinician program. *Volta Rev. 74:* 247–255.

Yules, R. B., and Chase, R. A. (1968). Quantitative cine evaluation of palates and pharyngeal wall mobility in normal palates, in cleft palates, and in velopharyngeal incompetency. *Plast. Reconstr. Surg. 41:* 124–128.

Yules, R. B., and Chase, R. A. (1969). A training method for reduction of hypernasality in speech. *Plast. Reconstr. Surg. 43:* 180–185.

Zemlin, W. R. (1968). *Speech and Hearing Science. Anatomy and Physiology.* Prentice-Hall, Inc., Englewood Cliffs.

Zemmol, C. S. (1977). A priority system of caseload selection. *Lang. Speech Hear. Serv. Schs. 8:* 85–98.

Zerffi, W. A. C. (1939). Functional vocal disabilities. *Laryngoscope 49:* 1143–1147.

Zerffi, W. A. C. (1948). Voice reeducation. *Arch. Otolaryngol. 48:* 521–526.

Zerffi, W. A. C. (1952). Laryngology and voice production. *Ann. Otol. Rhinol. Laryngol. 61:* 642–647.

Zimmerman, J. D., and Canfield, W. H. (1968). Language, speech, and hearing therapy. In *Cleft Palate. A Multidiscipline Approach*, edited by R. B. Stark, pp 243–272. Harper and Row, New York.

Zwitman, D. H., and Calcaterra, T. C. (1973). The "silent cough" method for vocal hyperfunction. *J. Speech Hear. Disord. 38:* 119–125.

Zwitman, D. H., and Calcaterra, T. C. (1975). A case against teflon injection to lower vocal pitch. *J. Speech Hear. Disord. 40:* 499–501.

Zwitman, D. H., Gyepes, M. T., and Ward, P. H. (1976). Assessment of velar and lateral wall movement by oral telescope and radiographic examination in patients with velopharyngeal inadequacy and in normal subjects. *J. Speech Hear. Disord. 41:* 381–389.

Zwitman, D. H., Sonderman, J. C., and Ward, P. H. (1974). Variations in velopharyngeal closure assessed by endoscopy. *J. Speech Hear. Disord. 39:* 366–372.

Glossary

abduct. To move away from midline.

abrupt glottal attack (also coup de glotte, glottal stop). Buildup of air pressure beneath closed vocal cords with a sudden release of air or phonation.

acute. Abrupt onset with definite symptoms and of short duration.

adduct. To move toward midline.

adenoid (also pharyngeal tonsil). A mass of lymphoid tissue in posterior wall of nasopharynx.

adenoidectomy, lateral. Removal of the sides (external boundary) of the adenoid, leaving the midline bulk; also called lateral trim of the adenoid.

adventitious. Added, accidental, of sporadic occurrence (Webster, 1963, p. 13).

agenesis. Imperfect or incomplete development (Jones et al, 1949, p. 31).

allergen. An agent that produces a manifestation of allergy (Jones et al, 1949, p. 41).

amplitude. Extent of vibratory movement as in sound wave. Measured in decibels (dB) (Webster, 1963, p. 31).

amyloid. Protein with hyaline nature deposited in tissues as the result of tissue degeneration causing tumor-like structures (Jones, Hoerr, and Osol, 1949, p. 55).

angioma. Tumor composed of lymphatic vessels or blood (Jones et al, 1949, p. 66).

ANSI. American National Standards Institute.

anterior. Situated toward the front.

antigen. A substance which stimulates the production of antibodies or reacts to them (Jones et al, 1949, p. 77).

anxiety, speech. Apprehensiveness about speaking manifested by rigidity, inhibition, dysfluency, and agitation (Mulac and Sherman, 1974).

aperiodic. Irregular or random occurrence.

aphonia. Absence of all phonation.

appraisal, voice problem. Detailed description and evaluation of a voice problem.

apraxia. A motor articulatory disorder resulting from left cerebral hemisphere injury (Darley et al, 1975, p. 250).

asphyxiating thoracic dystrophy. Respiratory distress due to inherited disease where chest does not develop normally (Bowman et al, 1972).

aspirate. Voice: breathiness. Phoneme: /h/.

aspiration. The taking in of foreign bodies, food, or liquid into the respiratory system; also removal by suction (Webster, 1963, p. 52).

atrophy. Reduction in size.

autogenous. From within the organism, such as toxins, vaccines (Jones et al, 1949, p. 110).

aversive stimulus. Noxious stimulus, e.g. electric shock, which will be avoided if possible (Chaplin, 1968, p. 48).

avulsion. Forcible separation or detachment.

bifid. Divided into two parts.

bilateral. Two sides.

binaural. Both ears.

biofeedback. Instrumental information of body functions which can be used by a person to regulate his own behavior (Chaplin, 1968, p. 182).

bowed vocal cords. Vocal cords assume an elliptical or curved form resulting in imperfect approximation during phonation.

cauterization. Tissue destruction by heat: +800° C to +1120° C (Kirchner, 1974; 1975).

caudal. Away from the head.

cephalad. Toward the head.

cephalometric technique. Measurements of the head according to anatomical landmarks, e.g. using lateral x-ray films (Calnan, 1971b).

choanal atresia. Occluded posterior opening to nasal cavities, bilateral or unilateral.

chronic. Of extensive duration or recurring frequently.

cinefluorographic (also cinefluorography; cineradiographic). X-ray motion picture.

commissure. A place where two parts join or come together (Webster, 1963, p. 166).

condyloma acuminatum. Wart of the genital organs.

congenital. Present at birth.

continuous phonation. Voicing all phonemes, usually with increase in duration of vowels.

contralateral. Opposite; acting with a similar part on the other side of the body (Jones et al, 1949, p. 242).

corditis. Chronic inflammation of vocal cords.

coup de glotte. See *abrupt glottal attack*.

cricoarytenoid ankylosis. Injury, infection, or arthritic changes in the cricoarytenoid joint causing weak voice and hoarseness sometimes with pain (DeWeese and Saunders, 1977, p. 115).

criterion control (level). The number or per cent of responses during a specified time period.

cryosurgery. Destruction of tissue by freezing, −20° C to about −40° C (Kärjä et al, 1975; Miller, 1973; Singleton and Adkins, 1972).

cul-de-sac resonance. Hollow, muffled resonance focused in the pharyngeal area with posterior carriage of the tongue (Boone, 1966).

cyst. Sac with distinct wall filled with fluid, air, blood, or other material (Jones et al, 1949, p. 266).

denasal. See *hyponasal.*

dental prosthesis. See *speech aid, dental.*

dextral. Right side.

diagnosis. The identification or categorization of a disease from its signs and symptoms based on the appraisal.

diastasis. Simple separation or clefting of parts normally joined together (Jones et al, 1949, p. 292).

dicrotic dysphonia. See *vocal fry.*

dilatation. A state of being stretched or enlarged (Jones et al, 1949, p. 298).

dilation. The act of stretching or dilating; often used synonymously with dilatation (Jones et al, 1949, p. 298).

diplophonia. Double vibration in the vocal mechanism, e.g. one vocal cord vibrates at a perceivably different rate from the other cord (Perkins, 1977, p. 282).

distal. Far from point of attachment.

dysphagia. Difficulty in swallowing.

dysphonia. Partial loss of phonation.

dysphonia, hyperkinetic. Partial loss of phonation caused by overcontraction of laryngeal or respiratory muscles (Luchsinger, 1965, p. 303).

dysphonia plicae ventricularis (also ventricular phonation; hyperkinesia of false cords). Phonation with false vocal cords.

dysphonia, whispering. Speaking in a halting whisper without hoarseness; at times phonation is normal (Barton, 1960).

dyspnea. Difficult or labored breathing causing air hunger (Jones et al, 1949, p. 321).

dystonia. A disorder of, or reduced tonicity (Jones et al, 1949, p. 321).

edema. Excessive collection of fluid in tissue spaces causing swelling (Jones et al, 1949, p. 327).

effusion. A pouring out of fluid: serous, purulent, bloody; also the effused fluid (Jones et al, 1949, p. 327).

emphysema. Subcutaneous: air or gas accumulation in connective spaces under the skin due to trauma or infection. Pulmonary: increase in size of normal air spaces in the lungs and later with decreased elasticity of tissue (Jones et al, 1949, p. 336).

endoscopy. Visual examination of interior of body through natural outlets by instruments using lens systems or electric lights (Jones et al, 1949, p. 340).

falsetto (also light, loft). Highest voice register.

fibroma (also fibrotic tissue). Benign tumor consisting of whorls of white fibrous connective tissue (Jones et al, 1949, p. 380).

fibrotic tissue. See *fibroma.*

fistula. An opening that is abnormal—not natural.

flaccidity. Limp, soft, flabby, relaxed; exaggerated relaxation or overrelaxation of a muscle or muscles (Jones et al, 1949, p. 385; Webster, 1963, p. 316).

formants. Energy distribution in a complex sound by Hertz bands.

frequency. Number of complete vibrations or cycles per second as in sound wave; measured in Hertz.

glottal stop. See *abrupt glottal attack.*

glottal chink. Small opening in the glottis.

glottis. Space between the true vocal cords.

granulation tissue. Newly formed capillaries and fibroblasts become organized progressing to atrophy of blood vessels and maturation of connective tissue (Jones et al, 1949, p. 431).

habitual pitch level. See *modal frequency level.*

hematoma. Focus of blood clotting into solid mass becoming encapsulated by connective tissue (Jones et al, 1949, p. 450).

hemangioma. Tumor composed of blood vessels (Jones et al, 1949, p. 449).

HL. Hearing level.

HTL. Hearing threshold level.

hyalin. Glassy, clear, and structureless material—normal in cartilage matrix; abnormal in connective tissue degeneration (Jones et al, 1949, p. 475).

hyperemic. Reddened, excessive amount of blood.

hyperfunction. Excessive use of muscular force; overtense muscle tonus.

hyperkeratosis. A red, white, or pearly thickening or plaque.

hyperkinesia of false cords. See *dysphonia plicae ventricularis.*

hypernasal (also open nasality, nasal, or nasality). Excessive nasal resonance.

hypernasality, assimilation. Hypernasality on phonemes preceding or following /m/, /n/, and /ŋ/.

hypernasality, induced. Thin tense velum acts as a drumhead to increase nasality.

hyperplastic. Thickened; excessive formation of tissue (Jones et al, 1949, p. 484).

hypertrophy. Increase in size of an organ not due to natural growth (Jones et al, 1949, p. 485).

hypofunction. Lack of muscular force; overly lax muscle tonus.

hyponasality (also closed nasality and denasality). Inadequate nasal resonance.

inferior. Lower, underneath, or below.

ingest. To take into the body for digestion (Webster, 1963, p. 434).

injected. A blood vessel enlargement/distention.

in situ. Undisturbed; in a given position.

ISO. International Organization for Standardization.

intubation, endotracheal. Introduction of a tube into the larynx to assure air supply, for anesthesia or bronchoscopy (Jones et al, 1949, p. 516).

keel. Thin metal or Silastic temporary partition to separate surfaces of vocal cords (DeWeese and Saunders, 1977, p. 117).

laryngeal dysfunction. Abnormal or impaired functioning of the larynx.

laryngitis, nonspecific (also chronic laryngitis). Long-standing inflammatory changes in the laryngeal mucosa (DeWeese and Saunders, 1977, p. 107).

laryngitis, polypoid (also hypertrophic laryngitis, polypoid corditis, or polyposis of the vocal cords). Laryngitis resulting from small polypoid tumors on the vocal cords (Baker, 1963).

laryngocele. Air or fluid sac arising from the ventricle (Holinger and Brown, 1967).

laryngoesophageal cleft. Cleft of larynx and esophagus.

laryngomalacia (also congenital laryngeal stridor). Underdevelopment of cartilages of the larynx causing them to collapse into the airway upon inspiration (Saunders, 1964).

laryngopathia menstrualis. Voice changes just before and during menstruation.

laryngoscope. Instrument for direct examination of the larynx.

laser surgery, carbon dioxide (CO_2). Thermal tissue destruction by infrared light beam at a wave length of 10.6 μ (μ is symbol for micron unit equal to 1 millionth of a meter or 25,640th part of an inch) (*Encyclopedia Americana*, 1976, vol. 19, p. 32; Strong and Jako, 1972; Strong et al, 1973).

leukoplakia. Patchy white membrane.

lumen. The bore of a tube; cavity of a tubular organ (Webster, 1963, p. 503).

mesial. In or toward the middle or midline.

metastasis. Disease transfer to distant site from primary focus through lymph channels or blood vessels (Jones et al, 1949, p. 614).

modal frequency level (also modal pitch level, modal voice pitch level, habitual pitch level, fundamental frequency). Average pitch level of the voice used in speaking and reading, expressed in Hertz.

mucopus. A mucus and pus mixture.

mucosa. A mucous membrane.

mucous membrane. Membrane filled with mucous glands, lining body passages and cavities communicating outside the body (Webster, 1963, p. 555).

mucus. Liquid secreted by mucous glands.

multiple sclerosis. Chronic hardening of the various parts of the nervous system (Webster, 1963, p. 556).

mutation, bass. Precocious change of voice pitch in a boy to adult male level.

mutation, perverse. Girl's voice lowers an octave or more at puberty.

mutation, voice. Change in voice pitch due to growth of larynx.

myasthenia. Muscle weakness or debility.

myasthenia gravis. Neuromuscular transmission problem involving nerve impulses from motor nerve endings across the synapse to the motor end plate of skeletal muscles (Wolski, 1967).

nasal. See *hypernasal*.

nasal emission (also nasal snorting or fluttering). Audible air escape or production of phonemes through nasal cavity.

nasal flutter. Perceivable effect on nasal resonance when the nostrils are alternately occluded and unoccluded (Weiss, 1974).

negative practice. Conscious use of an involuntary habit to gain voluntary control.

neoplasm. New growth.

nodules, vocal (also singer's or screamer's nodules or nodes). Initially slight reddening, then localized swelling or thickening, in a mature nodule the thickening is replaced by fibrotic tissue, white or grayish in color (see Text, p. 33).

obturator. See *speech aid, dental*.

pachydermia, laryngis. Abnormal thickening of mucous membrane of larynx (Jones et al, 1949, p. 717).

palsy. See *paresis*.

papilloma. A wartlike neoplastic benign growth.

palpation. Use of hand to determine condition of body or underlying organs (Jones et al, 1949, p. 720).

paralysis. A complete loss of muscle sensation or function caused by nerve injury (Jones et al, 1949, p. 728).

paresis (also palsy). A partial or slight paralysis causing partial loss of sensation or function caused by nerve injury (Jones et al, 1949, pp. 728, 734).

patent. Open.

pedunculated. A narrow stalk to which is attached a tumor or polyp.

perturbation, frequency. Deranged or disturbed periodicity of sound vibration.

pharyngoplasty. Plastic surgery of the pharynx.

phonelegram. Print-out from a phonelescope for analyzing pitch (Hanley and Peters, 1971, p. 106).

plaque. A patch.

polyp. Tumor consisting of connective tissue, blood, or fluid.

posterior. Situated toward the back.

prognosis. The prediction of the outcome of a planned treatment procedure.

proprioceptive. Related to, of, or being, stimuli arising within the organism (Webster, 1963, p. 684).

prosthesis, dental. See *speech aid, dental.*

psychogenic. Originating in the mind or in emotional or mental conflict (Webster, 1963, p. 689).

psychosomatic. Pertaining to mind and body interaction and interdependence (Jones et al, 1949, p. 833).

purulent. Consisting of or forming pus (Jones et al, 1949, p. 839).

raphe. Ridge, furrow, or seam, indicating the line of junction of two symmetrical halves (Jones et al, 1949, p. 853).

retract. To draw back.

reverse phonation. Vocalizing on inhalation.

scoliosis. Lateral curvature of spine.

semitone. One-half of a whole musical tone.

sepsis. Toxic condition as a result of spread of bacteria or their products from a focus of infection (Webster, 1963, p. 790).

sessile. Attached by a broad base.

siccus. Dry.

sinister. Left side.

spastic dysphonia, incipient. Beginning spastic dysponia characterized by voice tremor and hoarseness.

spasticity. Exaggerated contraction or tension of muscle or muscles.

spectrographic analysis. Amplitude and frequency distribution of sound plotted as a function of time.

speculum. Ear: metal funnel-shaped instrument for straightening ear canal for examination. Nasal: metal pincher-like instrument for spreading the nares for examination of nasal passages (Jones et al, 1949, p. 954).

speech aid, dental (also obturator, dental prosthesis). An acrylic dental appliance used in treating palatal and velopharyngeal insufficiency.

stenosis. A narrowing or constriction.

stent. A compound or a mold to immobilize certain skin grafts.

stimulability test, voice. To determine improvement of voice after presentation of correct model.

stridor. Staccato, repetitive crowing or croaking noise during respiration, usually when inhaling.

stroboscope. Instrument with intermittent light source used to give the illusion of slowing, stopping, or reversing movement (Chaplin, 1968, p. 482).

superior. Upper, toward the top.

tonsils (also palatine or faucial tonsils). Masses of lymphoid tissue between anterior and posterior faucial pillars.

tracheostomy. Formation of an opening into the trachea and suturing the edges of this opening to an opening in the skin of the neck (Jones et al, 1949, p. 1072).

tracheotomy. The operation of cutting into the trachea (Jones et al, 1949, p. 1072).

tracheotomy tube. Metal or plastic tube for insertion into tracheal opening after tracheotomy.

transillumination. Outlining structures with a light.

tremor. Involuntary, usually rhythmic trembling of muscles (Jones et al, 1949, p. 1078).

tremor, essential. A coarse trembling of familial origin beginning in adolescence becoming progressively more pronounced in old age (Jones et al, 1949, p. 1078).

tumor. A new growth of cells or tissues independent of growth of the surrounding structures (Jones et al, 1949, p. 1094).

twang, regional. Hypernasality present on a dialectal basis.

ultrasound surgery. Thermal destruction of tissue by high frequency sounds. 9 MHz results in 20° C ± 2° C rise above body temperature (Fairman, 1972).

uniaural. One ear.

unilateral. One side.

valsalva maneuver. Testing patency of eustachian tubes by inflating middle ear with air by a forcible expiratory effort while holding nose and mouth closed (Jones et al, 1949, p. 1115).

vascular anomaly. Abnormal blood vessel.

vascular engorgement. Excessive amount of blood; hyperemia.

velopharyngeal insufficiency. Inadequate closure of velopharyngeal port due to cleft palate, submucous cleft palate, paralysis, structural deviations.

ventricular phonation. See *dysphonia plicae ventricularis.*

vocal fry (also dicrotic dysphonia, glottal fry). Lowest voice register; speaking in pulses at lowest possible pitch level.

web, laryngeal. Thin connective tissue attached to vocal cords or ventricular bands.

white noise. A sound containing all frequencies in a wide band of energy (Brown, 1975, p. 228).

Author Index

Subject Index